LIVE LONGEST

SUPER NEWTRITION

THE MICRO-NUTRIENT REVOLUTION

THE WORLD'S BEST DIET

Balanced, Expert, Sensible, Trusted

Medically Evidenced Best Beneficial Foods

PROTECT YOUR HEALTH

IMMUNE BOOSTING-ANTI-INFLAMMATORY

COVID-19 ADVICE

SUITABLE FOR BOTH VEGAN and MEAT EATERS

HAVE YOU GOT THE SMARTS?[1]

A 2020 study of 12 European countries is the first to show that the higher the educational status, the better the diet. As individual education level increased so did a healthier nutritional intake.

"Poor diet is linked to noncommunicable diseases, such as obesity, hypertension and cardiovascular disease and presents major health problems across Europe. In 2018, 59% of adults in the WHO European Region were overweight or obese and noncommunicable diseases are the leading cause of death, disease and disability in the region"

As you have bought this book this confirms you are smart.

Now get ready to top this up with the best advice, food and diet, you will ever get.

- Independent, unbiased
- Based on 50 years of international clinical experience
- Built on, but improves, the recognised World's Best Diet
- The food sources and benefits of the micronutrients
- No fads, no extremes, no crazy restrictions
- Simply the -

BEST

Balanced, Expert, Sensible, Trusted

---

[1] Inequalities in education and national income are associated with poorer diet: Pooled analysis of individual participant data across 12 European countries. *PLOS ONE*, 2020; 15 (5): e0232447 DOI: 10.1371/journal.pone.0232447

THE MEDITERRANEAN DIET

The term "Mediterranean diet" has been used to describe the eating habits of the Mediterranean inhabitants, particularly the inhabitants of Crete and Southern Italy, in the early 1960s.

Despite there being many Mediterranean Countries, they share a number of common ingredients that seem to donate more benefits than other diets.

The fact that the warmer Mediterranean coast had more olive trees to provide the oil for cooking or dressings, year-round fresh available fruit and vegetables, readily available fish and seafoods, established a fundamental difference from the diets of the colder or inland climates. They also had less cattle, so that butter, cream and meat were less available while dairy was provided mostly by preserved cheese and fermented products.

This warm, maritime geography established the fundamental common features of the Traditional Mediterranean Diets where human life prospered. There are also pockets of Mediterranean societies where the inhabitants live longer than the rest of the world.

The basis for Newtrition is the traditional Mediterranean Diet, voted by experts as the world's best, but now improved it in light of the latest evidence as well as identifying the micronutrients and the best micronutrient "super" foods.

The World's Best

In 2019 a panel of health experts examined and ranked 41 popular eating plans, concluding that the Mediterranean diet is the most universally beneficial for long-term health. Further down the list, U.S. News named vegetarian as 11th, vegan as 20th, Paleo as 33rd, and Whole30 and keto tied for 38th.

In 2020 they rated 35 diet plans and the Mediterranean Diet was again voted the best for long term health. But there is more, much more, that even improves on this Traditional Mediterranean Diet. Welcome to **Newtrition**

.

The Micronutrient Miracles

There are no essential foods — only essential nutrients

The Mediterranean Diet is voted the best of all diets.

But why and how?

And how can it be improved?

Research on over 56,000 Danes in 2019 reported that those consuming the most flavonoids had a 17% reduced risk for all-cause mortality, a 15% reduced risk for cardiovascular disease death and a 20% reduced risk for cancer mortality.[2]

Flavonoids are a big family of some 10,000 micronutrients about which we know very little – only some 200 have been studied in any detail.

But we are unlocking their secrets.

Micronutrients are not necessary for life, but it would seem they are increasingly being recognised as important for a long and healthy one.

And flavonoids are just one group of micronutrients.

There is no one super micronutrient. They contribute their health benefits by the amalgamation, the variety, the diversity, the array, the complete spectrum and *combination of all the ingredients from different foods* working in a symbiotic, blending and fusing partnership.

No one food supplies them all: We need a variety of foods.

Newtrition has researched the "super" foods which are highest in these beneficial micronutrients while *also* tweaking the Traditional Mediterranean Diet's amounts of fruit, vegetables, grains, seeds, nuts and protein in the light of the latest, best research.

Welcome to the world of Micronutrients and welcome to the Newtrition Micronutrient Revolution Diet.

---

[2] *Nature Communications* **volume 10**,
Article number: 3651 (2019) DOIhttps://doi.org/10.1038/s41467-019-11622-x

Dietary Flexibility:

The Hallmark of Humanity

The object of Newtrition is to provide you with the latest nutrition information based on the world's best research

It is a balanced approach based on human evolution – what we are meant to swallow, worked out after 2.8 million years of eating.

Humans prospered by being omnivores and flexible opportunists.

By necessity they had to eat whatever was available and this variety and flexibility resulted in them ingesting all the vitamins, minerals and micronutrients that made us the most successful survivor and animal on earth, and with the biggest brain.

Our ancestors also soon found what foods were poisonous.

Today, however, our food has altered. We are not really aware of this and we are now being poisoned – but very slowly and pleasantly. Hence the epidemics of obesity and heart disease. Newtrition, as well as providing the best diet, also identifies these damaging foods.

As well as the silly and the unqualified Bloggers and Gurus, there are some two to three million medical papers published every year. Many of these are funded by vested interests or rushed out as a 'publish or perish' necessity for academic researchers to keep their jobs or attract more money.

These vested interests have influenced research and results. But, in their greed, the micronutrients, progressively absent from the Western Diet, have mostly gone unnoticed, possibly because all they don't come in a package or obliged by religious ideology.

No one has all the answers but here is the best to current knowledge, free of vested, business or religious interests and providing new insights as to the beneficial micronutrients.

<u>The Mediterranean Diet</u> has been voted World's Best for past 3 years. BENEFITS: Newtrition updates and upgrades this

1. **Improved All-Cause Mortality**
2. **Less Heart Attacks and Strokes**
3. **Prevention of Cardiovascular Disease**
4. **Reduced Deaths in Patients with CVD**
5. **Improved Post Heart Attack Survival**
6. **Lower Inflammatory, Coag Markers, Triglycerides and BP, raised HDL**
7. **Lower Cholesterol & improved artery lining in men**
8. **Lipoprotein oxidation was reduced and lipid (LDL) fell**
9. **Metabolic Syndrome halved**
10. **Slower Aging**
11. **Long Lasting Benefits**
12. **Less Total Cancer**
13. **Less Uterine Cancer**
14. **Less Breast Cancer Risk**
15. **Less Colorectal Cancer**
16. **Less Prostate cancer**
17. **Less Diabetes**
18. **Less Age-Related Macular Degeneration (Blindness)**
19. **Brain Health and Protection**
20. **Less Alzheimer's**
21. **Less Depression**
22. **More Aged Physical Independence**
23. **Reduced Hip Fracture Risk in Women**
24. **Reduced Risk for Kidney Stones**
25. **Improved Survival of the elderly**
26. **Less Chronic Obstructive Pulmonary Disease**
27. **Reduced Apnoea-Hypopnoea Index**
28. **Improvement of erectile dysfunction.**
29. **Improved HDL**
30. **Further risk reduction in Cancer, CVD, Premature Death**
31. **Improved Memory**
32. **Bigger Brain**
33. **Less Gout**
34. **Less Asthma**
35. **Less Allergies**
36. **Improved Gut Microbiome**
37. **Promotes gut bacteria linked to 'healthy aging'**
38. **Improved bone density and less fractures in post-menopausal women**
39. **Improved IVF Results**
40. **More Long-Term Benefits than any other diet**

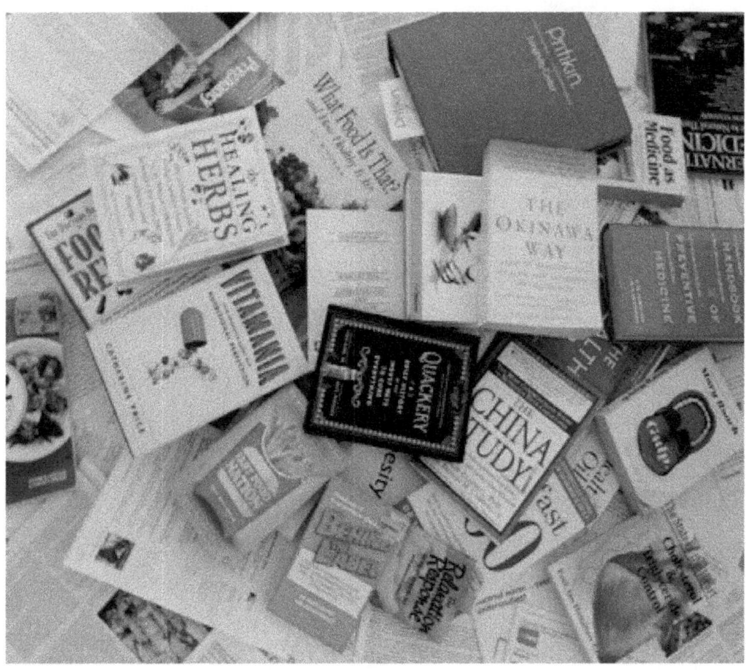

I have read thousands and thousands of medical journal nutrition articles and read (and thrown out) thousands of nutrition - diet books. Most are scams, fads and looney tunes.

But there are a few gems and, in this lot, tumbled at random from a bottom shelf of my bookcase, I can recommend:

- **The Okinawa Way**
- **Vitamania**
- **Gulp**
- **The Fast Food Nation**
- **Behind the Label**
- **What Food Is That**

and, nothing to do with nutrition, but in case you are wondering:

- **The Relaxation Response**
- **Quackery.**

There are, of course, many other good books on the subject but they would amount to one in 100, if that.
And now I even have reservations about some medical journal articles.

INTRODUCTION

This is a complete update and re-editing of my first Newtrition, a book written over 50 years of medical practice, for my patients, which, gratifyingly, sold out. It is much more than a diet book. It is a complete book of nutrition.

Confusion reigns as medical articles contradict medical articles and, in this era of 'Millennial Narcissism', the Internet has become the go-to source where Influencers and Celebs 'advise'. OMG! I have a chapter so you can read how frankly mad most are and also my 'History of Diets' which is a hoot of ridiculous and zany ideas.

My interest in nutrition was initiated by my Father and intensified when I was appointed to the World's First Coronary Care Unit. Cardiovascular Disease was our greatest killer, and still is. But it is preventable as are most illnesses.

But the main problem is that our food has changed more in the last 80 years than the previous 80,000 and Western society is now so structured that it is difficult to access the correct, unbiased medical information.

With the covid-19 social isolation I have now had time to check on some research authors, which has revealed some troubling concerns. And I am not alone.

I am not anti-vegetarian and not pro-meat, but many articles have progressively become so anti-meat that it raised my curiosity. They seem to be pushing an agenda based on religious zealotry and funding.

Newtrition is free of any such hidden agendas or bias.

Mileham Hayes Brisbane 2020.

Personal Disclaimer: *"I have no horse in this race"*

Today the different diets are ostensibly backed by science but, sadly, there seems no prophylactic against scientific and religious bias or business-vested interests. Incredibly, nutrition is not taught in medical schools and most clinicians are so busy that if we read how 200,000 people thrived on a diet of Gobi-Goobi Berries we kinda blindly accept it.

Doctors may resent Medical Reporters but there are some excellent investigative journalists with articles by Ian Leslie writing in the Guardian, Mary Tckovitz's in the British Medical Journal and Melinda Wenner Moyer in the Scientific American. I don't always agree with them (some have been stupidly wrong and inflammatory – they are, after all, journos) but I do think dogma should be challenged, but also then not replaced by their own dogma. Moyer wrote (10/02/17) *"Why Almost Everything Dean Ornish Says about Nutrition is Wrong"*. Dr Ornish is a low-fat advocate and gets the right of reply. But it is a most interesting article and what I liked most was her conclusion that, *"I have no horse in this race"*. We do need such independent analyses.

But again, this is a Journo's take on the truth – medical journalists depend for their jobs and livelihood on writing about medicine and, if that isn't a 'horse in the race' I don't know what is.

That said, I feel I 'have no horse in this race': I have no business, religious, cultist, faddist or food favorite bias (well some - mangoes) in this race. Just the world's best evidence and I very much doubt if any sales of this book will ever recoup the time, effort, thought and expense involved – I would have been financially much better off consulting and operating.

Numerous studies have found that when medical practitioners receive gifts from Drug Companies, Big Pharma, they are more disposed to prescribe their products. Some of these "gifts" include all-expenses paid luxury holidays overseas under the guise of a 'conference'. But further, University Departments are dependent on funding and donations and 'he who pays the piper, calls he tune'. In 50 years of clinical practice all I have ever received are cheap ball-point pens with the names of drugs I never used emblazoned on their sides, and I don't even get those now as the law has prohibited private practitioners from receiving such 'inducements'. But what about the Universities, Researchers and Hospitals? I am concerned that their articles are increasingly biased toward their Donors who, in effect, pay their salaries.

While I've stated how I have no vested interests, that, on reflection, is not quite accurate. I have a great vested interest in living longest-healthiest and to that end, I eat the Newtrition Diet as much as I can without becoming obsessive.

Live Longest is a Series covering all aspects of health. Newtrition is Book 1.

PREFACE

Newtrition provides the best diet for the longest, healthiest life. Above all it brings a sensible, balanced approach but based on authoritative research.

I say "sensible" because I have had to trawl through 4,600 years of faddists, loonies, zanies, crazies, dieticians, odd doctors and religious zealots ('the usual suspects'), all of whom thought they had the answer to what we should eat. Most were targeted at losing weight.

As it is human nature, the more difficult these diets were, the better they were thought to be but most fly in the face of nature and common sense.

What is needed is a diet with proven long-term benefits that is acceptable, available and achievable to all. And here it is: The latest study[3] of 14 of the most popular diets confirms The Mediterranean Diet is the only one to have long-term benefits, and, oh yes, it also controls weight too.

The Newtrition Micronutrient Diet has researched the "super" foods which are highest in beneficial micronutrients while *also* tweaking the Traditional Mediterranean Diet's amounts of fruit, vegetables, grains, seeds, nuts and protein in the light of the latest, best research.

There are these foods that provide benefits, there are foods that damage us, but Big Business and the Fast Food Industry also want a slice of the pie, and all are peddling misinformation. Sadly, it would seem, even the Researchers and Dieticians have been now been infiltrated, bribed and corrupted.

Here, by contrast, is the best independent sensible, advice based on the world's best studies and the experience of my 50 years of clinical medicine.

It has obviously worked for me, my (older) physician Sister who is now 87 and "with it" and for my Father who practised medicine until he was 84 and who first alerted me as to beneficial and damaging foods. Genetics account for only some 6% of our health – the rest is up to you and it starts with what you eat (and don't eat).

[3] BMJ 2020;369:m696

COVID-19: ANTI-VIRUS ADVICE

Firstly, there is no diet or food that will kill a virus.

The best defence against them is to build up your own resistance and keep fit.

This is best done with the (Super)-Mediterranean Diet which is also anti-*inflammatory* and *boosts our immune system* as much as any diet can.

The next most practical measure is personal hygiene:

- Wash hands (Doctors have to do it for a minimum of 2 minutes pre-op and most do it longer up to the elbows)
- Or use alcohol-based hand cleanzer
- Air dry hands (no blowers) or use throw away paper towels
- Avoid people breathing, let alone coughing or sneezing at you
- Masks, unless high-grade medical standard, are just to diffuse such droplet infections reaching you
- Droplets, carrying the virus, can travel up to 8 meters.
- So, keep your distance, avoid crowds, get the flu shot

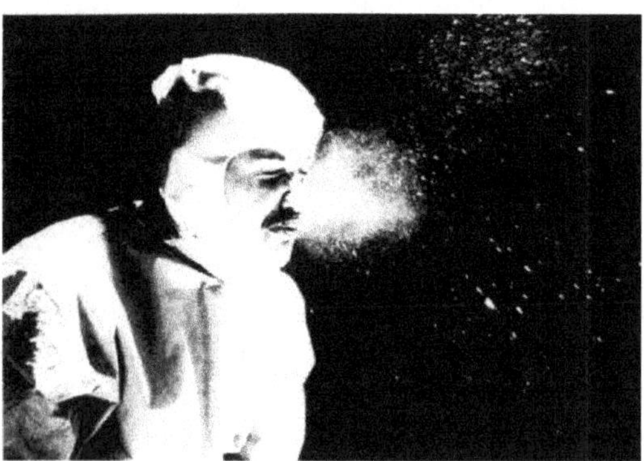

Potential Drugs[4]: Some promising 50 drugs are under investigation.

[4] Nature, online April 30, 2020.

CONTENTS

A NOTE ON OBESITY

Think on This

Obesity is a profound medical problem. But there are many of us who are overweight when we were previously slim.

Previous generations were slim: We are now the fattest people in history.

What has happened?

Up to the age of 17 to 25years we are in 'negative-nitrogen balance' wherein we are growing (taller - bones and filling out - muscle) and fat is hard, but obviously not impossible, to put on. We need to eat to feed this growth and thus we can eat more than when we stop growing.

Thereafter, it becomes progressively difficult to not gain weight, if we eat the same amounts.

But a new villain has entered to cause unprecedented problems: Processed foods.

What we eat has changed. It changed after World War 2 when scientists invented chemicals to make flavorings, aromas, textures, and every possible inducement to make eating this new synthetic food irresistible.

Welcome the Fast Food Industry.

The food that is now paraded in front of us 24 hrs a day, 7 days a week and home delivered. It is three times cheaper than fresh food, it is delicious and we don't have to cook.

There have been some 100,000 new chemicals invented since WW2 and many of these have entered our food chain and whereas before it took thousands, hundreds of thousands even millions of years to evolve enzymes so as to digest, absorb and metabolize the fresh different foods, we have now been presented with brand new chemicals in less than a mere 80 years.

And it is difficult to conceive our evolutionary processes can keep up with them. It would be logical to think that we simply cannot metabolise these new chemicals.

So, there are now two sources at work here to make the fat generation:

1. Cheap, delicious, available synthetic (processed) foods
2. Our inability to metabolize them

As noted these processed fast foods began in 1946. The first McDonald's with fast food was opened in 1948. Burger King and Taco Bell opened in the 1950s.

The fact that Americans were becoming “heavier’ was noted in the mid 1980s and obesity declared and epidemic in the 1990s.

This pandemic of weight gain follows the introduction of fast, processed foods.

Many diets advocate low fat or low carbs or some such and most of these are focused on losing weight and all of these are successful to a greater or lesser degree, if adhered to.

Many, if not most, rail against “calorie-counting”.

But, “think on this”, there was never a fat prisoner-of-war.

Newtrition does not advocate counting calories (until you know how much you eat), nor one food group in preference to another.

Simply, we are eating too much, and too much of the wrong foods.

Newtrition provides the correct foods but you must also restrict your intake.

PART A

The NEWTRITION MICRONUTRIENT REVOLUTION DIET

MICRONUTRIENT BALANCED DIET

CHAPTER 1

The NEWTRITION MICRONUTRIENT DIET

Easy! Just some from each 5 groups:

20% Fruit
20% Vegetables
20% Grains, Seeds and Nuts
20% Protein - mostly plants - from the above or below
20% Superfoods (Micronutrients)

NO added sugar, NO added salt, NO Processed Foods

Fish 2 to 3 times a week. Some lean meat if you want

The Newtrition Micronutrient Superfoods:

Some foods are richer in micronutrients and which donate greater benefits

Apples/pears (white fruit), Apricots (dried), Beans, Beetroot, Berries*, Celery, Chillies, Chocolate-dark/cocoa, Citrus, Coffee, Egg plants, Food Fiber, Fish, Garlic/onion family, Grains, Green Leafy Vegetables-Bok Choy, Inulin vegetables (chicory, leeks, asparagus, Jerusalem artichokes), Legumes, Nuts (all), Oats (barley) (rolled/cut), Olive Oil, Peppers Orange (Men), Prunes, Sweet Potato (purple), Vegetables green-yellow-cruciferous), Purple/red veg

Maybe: Magnesium, Curcumin, Cinnamon, Pomegranate Juice with Dates, Rosemary, Sage, Shitake mushrooms, Vinegar, Vitamin D, Chamomile, Peppermint and Kombucha teas, Kifir (fermented milk)

Always use only cold-pressed oils.

In a 2020 published study of 68 946 French adults, a significant *reduction in the risk of cancer* was observed among high consumers of **organic food** (ie, a diet less likely to contain pesticide residues). This has to be confirmed.[5]

---

[5] *JAMA Intern Med.* 2018;178(12):1597-1606. doi:10.1001/jamainternmed.2018.4357

EVERY DAY – Variety is the key

1. **Fruit variety, ensure berries, apples (skin), citrus**
2. **Veg: esp. green leafy, purple, legumes and lentils**
3. **Nuts. 20g two handfuls. Walnuts, pecans, peanuts, almonds - any**
4. **Grains**
5. **Berries**
6. **Beans: at least half a cup per day.**
7. **Chilies**
8. **Cocoa, Chocolate (dark)**
9. **Tea, coffee, red wine, water**
10. **Extra Virgin Olive Oil (EVOO)**
11. **Fish (2 to 3 times a week).**
12. **Fiber**
13. **Leave something on your plate: Never get full**
14. **Calm, pleasant meals. Happy people only**
15. **Superfoods**

NO!

1. **Processed foods or meats**
2. **Butter, cream**
3. **Added sugar**
4. **Sugar Sweetened Beverages (SSB)**
5. **Added salt**

FOODS THAT SOUND HEALTHY BUT AREN'T

1. **"Light" Products**
2. **Flavored Yogurt**
3. **Veggie Chips or Straws**
4. **Meatless Meats**
5. **Granola Bars**
6. **Fruit Leather**
7. **Vitamin Water**
8. **Dairy-Free Cheese**
9. **Diet Soda**
10. **High-Protein Snacks**

Do not worry about the occasional lapse or treat. It is the long-term every-day ingestion of junk food that is harmful.

NEWTRITION'S WORLD'S BEST BREAKFAST

1. **Blueberries - for brain health**
2. **Granny Smith (skin) - gut health and stroke prevention**
3. **Walnuts, pecans - anti cancer, heart health.**
4. **Oats or Bran - lowers cholesterol, better microbiome**
5. **Grains - reduce All-Cause-Mortality, CVD and cancer**
6. **Flax (ground) - richest source Omega-3 ALA**
7. **Inulin - reduces visceral fat (see Notes Part D)**
8. **Dried apricots. High potassium - lowers BP**
9. **Green bananas: Fiber speeds gut transit. Potassium**
10. **Biodynamic unsweetened yoghurt (< 4g sugar / 100g)**
11. **Fruit in season**
12. **Prunes - fiber / microbiome gut health**
13. **Coffee - Super-food**

Breakfast is not necessary unless you feel you need it to function better.

WORLD'S WORST BREAKFAST FOODS

1. **Cereals high in sugar and salt (processed), "fortified/enriched"***
2. **Sausages**
3. **Bacon/ham**
4. **Eggs**
5. **Hash browns**
6. **Butter**
7. **Crumpets**
8. **Waffles / Pancakes**
9. **Golden / Maple Syrup**
10. **Muffins**
11. **Sugar in your tea or coffee**

* A whole grain contains the nutrient-vitamin rich endosperm, germ, and bran, in contrast to refined grains, which retain only the endosperm. Corn Flakes, Special K and similar flake breakfast cereals are not whole grains despite their (false) advertising as the nutritious, natural bran and germ have been removed such that synthetic vitamins, flavoring and such have to be added. They are arguably the most insidious ultra-processed of all foods as intensive advertising has given them a false 'health-halo'. A serving of Corn Flakes includes about 24 grams of carbohydrate and 1 gram of fiber, a less-than-ideal ratio. Then there is the sugar and salt content and, of course, we then add sugar on top. Bran, however, is whole grains just crushed.

BREAKFAST

NOT THE MOST IMPORTANT MEAL OF THE DAY

At the outset, if you feel like breakfast, or need it to function, then have it!

This is not an historical treatise. It is to reassure you that breakfast is not necessary and was never "the most important meal of the day".

In the European Middle Ages, breakfast was not considered a necessary or important meal and was practically nonexistent during the earlier medieval period when only two formal meals were eaten per day—one at mid-day and one in the evening.

If having breakfast suits your metabolism then go ahead and eat it. However, rather than sugar-loaded cereals or the incredible load of bacon, sausages, hash-browns and eggs, all of which are bad for our cardiovascular and gut health, there are better choices. Newtrition's 'World's Best Breakfast' has all the best ingredients.

The emphasis on health within the Seventh-day Adventist (SDA) movement led to the development of sanatoriums in mid-nineteenth century America. These facilities, the most notable being that of the Kellogg Brothers in Battle Creek, Michigan, initiated the development of vegetarian foods, such as breakfast cereals and analogue meats.

Cereals were popularized by Dr John Harvey Kellogg, who co-invented the Corn-Flake in 1894, in the hope it would cure the curse of masturbation. It is said he never consummated his marriage and he and his wife slept in separate rooms. The SDAs do seem to have problems with sex – see the longer chapter on the History of Diets – but their most influential founder claimed that meat "*Stimulates lustful propensities, Strengthens the lower passions, Animalizes you, Strengthens the animal appetites…*"

However, John, being more an astute businessman than a medical brain, saw a way to sell his Corn Flakes so, in the issue of Good Health magazine of 1917, which was edited by John Kellogg himself, he wrote, "In many ways, the breakfast is the most important meal of the day, because it is the meal that gets the day started".

The breakfast cereal boom began! Prior to that it was oatmeal or coffee and toast.

John’s brother and co-inventor, William, both SDAs, then argued over whether to make the cereals more palatable by adding sugar – the addition was anathema to John who saw sugar as an adulterant and a scourge, but William reckoned it was needed to stop the products tasting like 'horse-food'.

William won. And it has been observed, ‘the road to nutritional corruption opened up’.

Cornflakes are ultra-processed, generally made by breaking corn kernels into smaller grits which are then steam cooked in batches of up to a tonne under pressure of about 20lbs per square inch. The nutritious germ with its essential fats is first removed because, as the Kellogg brothers discovered all that time ago, it goes rancid over time and gets in the way of long shelf life. Flavorings, vitamins to replace those lost in processing and sugar may be added at this stage. It then takes four hours and vast amounts of energy to drive the steam out of the cooked grits before they can be rolled by giant rollers into flakes.

Many of the health benefits claimed for breakfast cereals depended on fortification rather than micronutrients from the raw ingredients, most of which were either destroyed by the process or stripped away before it.

The earliest fortification was with vitamin D, the so-called sunshine vitamin, and acted as a marketing tool. Today a new wave of fortification is coming, and once again its principal purpose is marketing. Inulin, a form of fiber from plants, known to the food industry until recently as a cheap bulking agent thanks to its ability to retain water and mimic the mouthfeel of fats, is now added as a 'prebiotic'. They have coined this word for it because it resists digestion in the upper gastrointestinal tract and reaches the large intestine almost intact where it is fermented by bacteria, encouraging the production of friendly microflora, which the industry markets too, as probiotics. The inulin, in other words, does what the fiber naturally occurring in whole grains would do if it hadn't been stripped out by over processing.

The breakfast cereal promotion was followed by another commercial scam, in 1927 – ‘Bacon and Eggs’.

Edward Bernays, Sigmund Freud's nephew, who knew a thing or two about psychology, if not psychiatry, became the guru of public relations and advertising, even being hired by the President of the USA in 1924 to get re-elected.

He was then hired by the Beech-Nut Packing Company who wanted to boost their sales of bacon.

By a skillful seduction of the companies physician who, knew not only on what side his bread was buttered, but that it should be accompanied by bacon, Bernays got him to write to some 5,000 USA physicians to endorse his 'study' to encourage the American public to eat a heavier breakfast – namely "Bacon and Eggs".

An advertising campaign then urged "Eat a Good Breakfast—Do a Better Job", and grocery stores handed out pamphlets that promoted the importance of breakfast while radio advertisements announced that "Nutrition experts say breakfast is the most important meal of the day."

The Pig farmers of Idaho and the Beech-Nut Packing Company were delighted as sales of hogs boomed.

But this advertising confidence trick is still endorsed by doctors, dieticians and nutritionists today, much to their discredit. Advertisements for commercial profits, and not nutrition, were key to the rise of cereals and bacon and egg breakfasts.

I must admit I love bacon and eggs but, sadly, bacon and other processed meats, such as sausages, are associated with cancer of the colon and are our number two and even number one killer, so I minimize it to being a rare treat.

GOLDEN RULES

1. **Ensure great variety of freshest, local, ripest produce Benefits exceed any residual pesticides but wash**
2. **Pleasant, calm environment; enjoy your food and company**
3. **No eating in cars. No Gas Station foods**
4. **Don't eat until you feel full. Leave some food**
5. **"It's not what you cut out, it's what you replace it with". Do not replace fat with refined carbohydrates**
6. **Avoid all processed foods. Anything in a package is processed. All processing is bad until proven otherwise**
7. **No smoked, preserved (processed) meat (bacon, ham, sausages) and processed cheese**
8. **Think more vegetarian - but a little lean grass-fed meat is fine.**
9. **Vegetables every day esp. purple and dark green leafy "cabbage"**
10. **All fruit and vegetables are good, full of antioxidants. Variety of fruit every day. Eat whole fruit, not just juice**
11. **The skin contains over 90% of the nutrients**
12. **Orange capsicums / peppers reduce Ca prostate**
13. **Berries x 3 times a week (slows cognitive decline)**
14. **An apple a day can reduce all-cause mortality, heart attacks and strokes. Oranges, pears too**
15. **Reduce potatoes (associated with hypertension)**
16. **Purple Sweet Potato / purple vegetables good**
17. **20 g nuts every day. Stroke & prostate cancer risk reduced.**
18. **Grains 70g/day lowers risk all-cause death, cancer, CVD**
19. **High-fiber reduces heart attacks, colorectal Ca (CAC)**
20. **Olive oil (EVOO) 20 ml / day. Reduced risk of stroke and CAD**
21. **Polyunsaturated oils (cold pressed) the best for heart protection**
22. **No butter, no cream. Fermented dairy OK**
23. **Skim or "heart healthy" milk**
24. **Milk 200g, 50g cheese or 400 g dairy reduces risk Cancer of Colon (CAC)**
25. **Every 300 mg Calcium (to 1900mg) reduces risk CAC**
26. **Eat fish x3 / week (anti-cancer, heart protective). No capsules.**
27. **Less red meat. All-cause mortality, Ca and CVD higher in meat eaters**
28. **No processed meat (bacon, ham, sausage)**
29. **Eat only organic poultry and eggs**
30. **More vinegar. Maybe a secret of the Mediterranean Diet**
31. **More fresh herbs, garlic**

32. **Chilies lower risk of total mortality and Ca risk**
33. **Breakfast cereals of oats best. Avoid commercial processed brands. Breakfast is not necessary**
34. **A glass of red wine with food daily. Women with family history of breast Ca or men who smoke should abstain**
35. **Coffee 4 cups a day. Green or no-milk tea**
36. **Vitamin D 1000 IU /day. Some recommend 4000 IU/day if no sun**
37. **Dark chocolate or 2 heap teaspoons cocoa, daily**
38. **Salt: Current guidelines are for 2.3g / day. Check labels**
39. **Taste before you add salt; break the "autopilot" habit**
40. **Increase potassium: fruits (dried apricots)**
41. **Reduce sugar intake < 4 g sugar per 100 g in any serving**
42. **Avoid HFCS (High Fructose Corn Syrup in many drinks)**
43. **Micro-filtered water (to avoid *Giardia* & *Cryptosporidium*).**
44. **Don't shop hungry. No portion distortion, small, no 2nds**
45. **Dry bake vegetables or microwave.**
46. **Avoid soya bean oil may increase obesity and diabetes.**
47. **Microwaving veg best preserves vitamins and minerals**
48. **Avoid the middle aisles in supermarkets.**
49. **No very hot beverages (carcinogenic)**
50. **Intermittent Fasting Diets for health and weight loss**
51. **Pomegranate juice + 3 dates**
52. **Wash all fruit and vegetables**.
53. **Residual pesticides: while** the benefits of fresh fruit and vegetables may exceed any residual pesticide. Organic food is associated with less cancers.
54. **Olive oil use** decreases the use of vegetable oils (corn, safflower) while increased fish (especially), soy, walnuts, green leafy vegetables will increase the supersaturates and optimise the Omega 6 : 3 ratio.
55. **Extra Virgin olive Oil (EVOO)** is the first pure pressing of an olive whereas thereafter it is may be extracted with heat and chemicals and thus the basic beneficial qualities may be altered detrimentally.
56. **Beware Italian EVOO**, it was often adulterated.
57. **All oils are fats** so minimise. Use Spray EVOO.
58. **Substitute good for bad** e.g. olive oil for butter and is user friendly
59. **Saturated fats are minimised** if less meat, fat, skin and processed foods
60. **Do not cook in meat tailings** in the baking dish but dry bake or spray lightly with EVOO.
61. **Enough fruit & vegetables,** 5 serves each, per day, for adequate fiber, vitamins and essential co-factors. Become a 'fruit-Bat' by making whole fruit your snacks. Eat the pulp for fiber and avoid bought juice (fructose).

62. **Prolonged boiling** destroys the water-soluble vitamins (B,C,A). Short microwaving is OK.
63. **All vitamins and minerals** should come from foods: Calcium, folate, Vit E, other vitamins, minerals and anti-oxidants from dairy, fruit and vegetables so there is *no need for supplements* except Vitamin D.
64. **Women with higher bone-mineral** got most of their calcium from food had densities than from supplements[6]
65. **Whole grain cereals** also appear beneficial reducing All-Cause Mortality[7]
66. **Tail off junk:** If you like junk food, you may feel that this diet is restrictive and even punitive. If, however, you do yourself the biggest favour in your life and stick to it, you will look back in disgust at the awful junk you were eating and wonder how you could ever eat it.
67. **Reducing cream and sugar** should be done *gradually*
68. **Salt:** Higher dietary salt is an independent risk factor for heart disease in overweight adults (BMI > 27.7 for men and 27.3 for women. Salt may be a preventable cause of high Blood Pressure. Reduce its use.
69. **Salt is mostly 'hidden'** in 'healthy' foods such as bread, breakfast cereals.
70. **Restrict Calories**:<2,000-2,500(10,500Kj) men, 1600-2000(8,400Kj) women
71. **Eat less.** There would seem a straight-line improvement in longevity and health with calorie restriction. Leave a third of food on your plate.
72. **Insensible calories**: We do not notice eating 400 more calories a day so we shouldn't notice eating 400 less and 600 cals a day less loses weight.
73. **Eat food, not food products.** Don't eat anything your Great Grandmother wouldn't recognise as food e.g. processed or sweetened yoghurt
74. **Shop at markets** - eat foods in season.
75. **Follow 'Granny's' rules:** Eat moderate portions, don't have seconds, don't eat between meals, eat at the family table (not alone), enjoy and make the family dinner pleasurable.
76. **Avoid foods with high-fructose corn syrup (HFCS).** Only introduced in 1975 and now in cereals, soft drinks, tomato sauce, baked goods, soups and salad dressings contributing 200 Cal /day or 20 kg pa to each of us = Empty Calories.
77. **Spend more on quality**. Americans spend less income on food (9.7%) than any other nation. It is also the fattest and spends more than any other nation on healthcare (16%). Buy better quality food.
78. **Pay little heed to health claims on packages** - the healthiest food is the fresh produce with no health claims!
79. **Don't become obsessed with the minutiae.** Variety is all-important such that the highest anti-oxidant fruit may not have a beneficial ingredient another has. Get the broad plan. Know what's good and what's bad.

---

6 Am J Clin Nutrit 2007;85:1428-33

7 Am J Clin Nutrit 2003;77:594-9, 2014

80. 100% Whole Wheat or Whole Grain Bread better than “Multi Grain”.

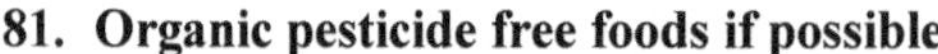

81. Organic pesticide free foods if possible

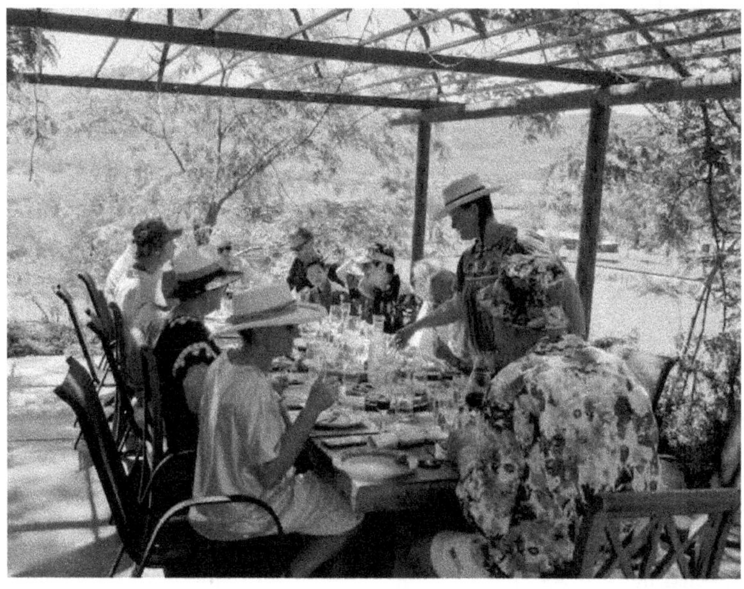

Ensure great variety of freshest, local, ripest produce, pesticide free if possible, in a pleasant, calm environment; enjoy your food and company.

CHAPTER 2

THE MICRONUTRIENT REVOLUTION

MICRONUTRIENTS: Chemical elements required in trace amounts for the normal growth and development. Some are "essential" for life.

Classification

Vitamins
Minerals
Amino Acids
Phytochemicals or nutrients

MICRO-PHYTO-CHEMICALS

The importance of the *MICRO*-chemicals became evident with the discovery of *vitamins, minerals and amino acids* many of which are essential. Even then, we do not know the full spectrum of what some contribute. But as well as these vitamins and minerals about which we know a great deal, there are also thousands and thousands of Microchemicals in our foods, about which we know very little.

Some are toxic and poisonous, as with cyanide, others can cause allergic reactions, make us ill or take 'trips'. But there are others which though not essential for life, are being progressively recognized as contributing a number of dietary benefits.

These are the Micro-*nutrients.*

MICROCHEMICAL CLASSIFICATION

1. **Animal:**
   There are only five micronutrients that are animal based
2. **Plant or Phyto: Over 5,000 and probably 10,000 (+)**
   Phyto is Greek for "plant" and these thousands of micro-chemicals are mostly plant based. As a whole plant family they are grouped as phytochemicals but the beneficial ones are classified as *phyto-nutrients.*

While the lack of a vitamin or a mineral may result in a devastating disease, which makes its function obvious and essential to life, the phytochemicals and other micronutrients are not essential to life and are an evolving mystery.

A mystery, however, that is just being unlocked.

Protein, carbs and fat are essential, but other preventive benefits do not seem to be derived from them, nor from the vitamins, minerals or the amino acids, which contribute to our health in more dramatic "essential" ways (no vitamin B12 etc - we die).

However, while not "essential", these micro-nutrient's benefits are profound and include: Improved All-Cause Mortality, Less Heart Attacks and Strokes, Prevention of Cardiovascular Disease, Halving the Metabolic Syndrome, Slower Aging, Less Total Cancer, Less Diabetes, Less Dementia/ Alzheimer's, Less Depression, Improvement of erectile dysfunction, Further, Reduction of Premature Death and much more.

Caution: However, when synthetic vitamins, minerals or phytonutrients are then added (replaced) to processed or junk foods, they don't provide the same benefits, nor do they when taken as a pill or supplement (unless you have a diagnosed deficiency or need).

As before it was documented how not one plant supplied all the necessary amino acids and the need, therefore to eat a variety, but more than this it would seem these micro-nutrients also need not only to come from a variety of plants but then, arguably, to form beneficial metabolic chemical reactions.

It must be the amalgamation, the variety, the diversity, the array, the complete spectrum and combination *of all the ingredients from different foods* working in a symbiotic partnership.

It must therefore be necessary to consume a variety of plants (fruit and vegetables).

All the best diets were based on the Traditional Mediterranean Diet. And recent research of some 2,000,000 people, has found yet even more benefits if we eat more of certain food groups which provide these phytonutrients.

It should be understood that there was no single "Mediterranean Diet" but each nation from Greece, Crete to Spain and probably those of the north coast of Africa, shared common ingredients and an approach which proved healthier than those of the colder Northern Europe.

They favored Olive Oil rather than butter or lard and they had greater access to fish and seafoods which probably saw them eat less red meat. It may be that the warmer climate also slowed the pace of meals to make them more pleasant and it allowed for all year-round physical activity. Other than that, the emphasis was on fresh fruit and vegetables and possible nuts and grains. Rather than milk, cheese seemed to be preferred.

But the benefits from eating as well as possible via the **Newtrition Micronutrient Diet** will nevertheless be nullified if processed food is also eaten. My analogy to this is that "By breathing fresh mountain air you cannot continue to smoke...by eating the beneficial foods you cannot continue to eat processed foods".

There are also some single foods or family of foods, not in the Traditional Mediterranean Diets, that do seem to have "super" qualities: "Green leafy vegetables" seem to be good for our gut and reduce cancer of the colon. Coffee has been called the "ultimate super-food" reducing all-cause-mortality, cardiovascular disease, diabetes, cancers, depression and many more. Coffee contains more than 1,000 chemical compounds yet, despite it being the most consumed beverage in the world, less than 30 of these 1,000 compounds have been subjected to juried, health related research.

As far as is now known I have listed these in the **Newtrition "Super" Foods**, and it is these that upgrades and updates Newtrition from the Traditional Med Diet.

As it took centuries for the vitamins to be recognized and their every-day ingestion to be recognized as essential, this is where we are at today with the phytochemicals. Eventually, but a long way away, no doubt a specific phyto will be found to provide specific benefits such as prevention of atheroma- heart attacks or prevention of cancer of the colon or even Alzheimer's Disease but, until then it doesn't really matter, because all we have to do is eat them now - we don't have to know how they work!

The orange has more vitamin C than any other citrus, but it also has some 69 other ingredients or phytochemicals. We humans have been evolving on this planet for some 2.7 million years. We can't make vitamin C, so we had to find foods that did. Now, you don't have to be Einstein, who didn't know much or anything about vitamin C or Linus Pauling who invented the Pill and thought he did, to wonder, as I have, "what are these other 69 nutrients doing?" They are not just there to give color or flavor, although some do. What then? Surely, it is just plain common sense that they help our gut better absorb the Vitamin C and then speed it more efficiently throughout our bodies' metabolic chains? And, in fact, this has already been shown to be the case. So, what are the other 5,000 flavenoids and the thousands of other micro-nutrients doing? We need them from different foods to mix with each other to provide this amazing protection and enhancement to our health.

There are only 13 vitamins and the drug companies push "multivitamin" supplements unmercifully with no evidence as to benefit. There are only 13 vitamins but there are over 5000 phytochemicals.

Welcome to the Micronutrient Revolution

1. ANIMAL MICRONUTRIENTS

These are very important for the brain and only found in animal foods.

i. Vitamin B12

The most well-known vitamin that the body can't produce and that can only be obtained from animal foods, is Vitamin B12.

The only good food sources of B12 were animal foods like meat, fish and eggs. Deficiency is widespread among vegans and vegetarians, who need to supplement with Vitamin B12 or eat foods that have been fortified with it. B12, however, comes from bacteria in raw water or soil and today with pesticides and antibiotics the grazing animals get far less. But further, most animals today are factory fed and hence they too need supplements and it is not only vegetarians who may be B12 deficient.

ii. Creatine

Creatine is actually not an essential nutrient, because the liver can produce it out of other amino acids. However, this conversion process appears to be inefficient.

Creatine supplements are used by athletes, bodybuilders, wrestlers, sprinters and others who wish to gain muscle mass. It is the most popular muscle-building supplement. It forms an energy reserve, where it is able to quickly recycle ATP - the energy source in our cells. About 95% of the creatine in the body is stored in skeletal muscle. However, creatine is also concentrated in the brain.

Vegetarians who take creatine supplements see improvements in cognitive performance, especially in more complex tasks, while there is no difference in non-vegetarians. This implies that vegetarians have a deficiency of creatine that is adversely affecting their brain function. Vegetarians also have a lower amount of creatine in skeletal muscle. Creatine supplements are particularly effective at improving athletic performance in this group.

Many meta analyses found that creatine treatment resulted in no abnormal renal, hepatic, cardiac, or muscle function. While some research indicates that supplementation with pure creatine is safe, a survey of 33 supplements commercially available in Italy, found that over 50% of them exceeded the European Food Safety Authority recommendations in at least one contaminant. Extensive research has shown that oral creatine supplementation at a rate of five to 20 grams per day appears to be very safe and largely devoid of adverse side-effects, while at the same time effectively improving the physiological response to resistance exercise, increasing the maximal force production of muscles.

Creatine also has a critical role in brain bioenergetics, and small studies have hinted that dietary supplements might protect against depression.[8]

Creatine is probably the most well-researched supplement on the market today. Numerous studies have found positive adaptations in strength, power and muscle mass thanks to creatine supplementation—especially when it's combined with resistance training.[9] And the timing of creatine ingestion plays a role in getting bigger and stronger. Supplementation before resistance training increases muscular strength and lean muscle mass. Taking creatine immediately *after* lifting weights results in greater muscle growth than taking it immediately before. However, in terms of strength gains, no difference between pre- and post-workout ingestion was observed.

Advocates feel that taking creatine is better than not taking it. It's one of the few legal supplements out there that has been shown to produce notable strength and size gains time and time again in controlled studies. There are two equally effective options:

1. Load up on creatine with around 20 g/day for 5-7 days, or
2. Take a standard dosage of 3-5 g/day for a month

---

[8] *Transl Psych* doi:10.1038/s41398-020-0741-x

[9] "Effects of Creatine Supplementation on Muscle Power, Endurance, and Sprint Performance." *Medicine and Science in Sports and Exercise.* 2002 Feb; 34(2):332-343; "Performance and Muscle Fiber Adaptations to Creatine Supplementation and Heavy Resistance Training." *Medicine and Science in Sports and Exercise.* 1999 Aug; 31(8):1147-1156; "Creatine Supplementation Enhances Muscular Performance During High-Intensity Resistance Exercise." Journal of the American Dietetic Association. 1997 Jul; 97(7):765-70; "Effect of Creatine Loading on Anaerobic Performance and Skeletal Muscle Volume in NCAA Division I Athletes." Nutrition. 2002 May; 18(5):397-402; "Effects of Creatine Supplementation on Performance and Training Adaptations." Molecular and Cellular Biochemistry. 2003 Feb; 244(1-2):89-94. "Timing of Creatine Supplementation and Resistance Training: A Brief Review." Journal of Exercise and Nutrition. 2018; 1(5); Persky, "Clinical Pharmacology of the Dietary Supplement Creatine Monohydrate." Pharmacological Reviews . 2001 Jun; 53(2):161–176.

Both produce similar outcomes. It takes about 30 days of regular doses to reach muscle creatine contents that can be achieved in five days of high loading. If you plan to use creatine long-term, high loading is not necessary. With that in mind, to optimize muscle gains, add 5 grams (or 20 grams if you're high loading) of creatine into your post-workout shake or water.

iii. Vitamin D3

Vitamin D is produced out of cholesterol in the skin when it is exposed to ultraviolet rays from the sun and actually functions as a steroid hormone in the body.

There are two main forms of Vitamin D in the diet: Vitamin D2 (ergocalciferol) and D3 (cholecalciferol). D2 comes from plants, D3 from animals. D3 is much more effective than the plant form.

There are few good sources of Vitamin D3 in the diet. Cod liver oil is the best source. Fatty fish also contains some D3, but you'd have to eat massive amounts of it to satisfy your body's need. If getting enough sun is not an option, the only way to get D3 from foods is to take cod fish liver oil or eat lots of fatty fish.

Get tested. If deficient take a D3 supplement 1000 iu a day but check.

Today, a large part of the world is deficient in this critical nutrient. Many people live where sun is basically absent throughout most of the year. But even in countries where sun is abundant, people tend to stay inside and cover up when they go outside.

iv. Carnosine

Carnosine is a very important nutrient of two amino acids, alanine and histadine, and is highly concentrated in muscle tissue, brain and the lenses of the eye. It is very protective against various degenerative processes in the body. It is a potent antioxidant, inhibits glycation caused by elevated blood sugars and may prevent cross-linking of proteins. For this reason, it has become very popular as an anti-aging supplement. It may help preventing and improving cataracts. Levels are significantly lower in patients with various brain disorders, including Parkinson's and Alzheimer's

Many researchers have speculated that animal foods may protect the brain and body against aging due to their large amount of carnosine. It acts as an antiglycating agent, reducing the rate of formation of advanced glycation end-products (AGEs) that can be a factor in the development or worsening of many degenerative diseases.

There's no set dose for carnosine supplementation, since the benefits have not yet been established through trials. It has no significant side effects.

v. Docosahexaenoic Acid (DHA)

Omega-3 fatty acids are extremely important. The human body cannot make them, which is why Omega-3s (and Omega-6s) are termed "essential" fatty acids therefore we must get them from the diet.

There are two active forms of Omega-3s in the body, EPA and DHA.

DHA is the most abundant Omega-3 fatty acid in the brain and it is critical for normal brain development.

Many people who avoid animal products supplement with flax seed oil instead, which is a great source of ALA… a plant form of Omega-3. However, ALA needs to be converted to DHA for it to work. Studies show that this conversion process is notoriously ineffective in humans. For this reason, vegans and vegetarians are very likely to be deficient in this very important fatty acid.

The best source of DHA is fatty fish. Other good sources include grass-fed and pastured animal products. There are also some algae that can produce EPA and D

Addenda:

The primary driver of muscle loss with is a reduction of muscle proteins being built from amino acids. These amino acids come from protein that we eat and are also formed when we exercise. Research from The Physiological Society's Future Physiology 2020 conference about soy and wheat proteins showing that a larger dose of these plant proteins is required to achieve a comparable response of building muscles or meat is a better or more efficient source.

2. PHYTO: PLANT MICRONUTRIENTS

Phyto is Greek for plant. It is considered that we needed to eat more of these phytonutrients in beneficial phyto-rich foods.

Newtrition has recognized the emergence and importance of the micronutrient phytochemicals and the foods recommended incorporate the latest and best research and beneficial plan. Most, if not all, countries fall way short of even the best Official Guidelines. These invariably recommend only some 10% when the evidence now is that we need twice this amount - 20%.

As noted, we are entering the "Age of Micronutrients". Phytonutrients are the thousands and thousands of chemicals in plants which seem to have increasingly recognized benefits for our health, yet only 200 or so have been studied and many more remain to be discovered.

There is, however, now a great deal of medical research investigating whether these health effects are due to one specific micronutrient but while these individual nutrients will inevitably be discovered, **Newtrition** takes the position that here and now, at a practical level, we can all enjoy these benefits by adopting a diet that includes all these "secret" ingredients. This is much in the same way that people knew that eating citrus fruits prevented scurvy, brown rice prevented Berriberri and Cod Liver Oil prevented Rickets. We then didn't know it was the vitamins let alone which vitamins prevented these Deficiency Diseases; we only knew that by eating certain foods it prevented them.

There are, however, some single phytochemicals that are incredibly powerful but not all "phytos" are beneficial, some just add color or smell but others are toxic and cyanide is an outstanding example of a singly powerful but toxic phytochemical found in substantial amounts in certain seeds and fruit stones, e.g., those of apricots, apples, and peaches. Never underestimate a phytochemical!

Newtrition, however, just concentrates on those that are beneficial - the phyto-nutrients. *Primary constituents include*: The common sugars, amino acids, proteins, purines and pyrimidines of nucleic acids, chlorophyll's etc.

Secondary constituents are: The remaining plant chemicals such as alkaloids, terpenes, flavonoids, lignans, plant steroids, curcumins, saponins, phenolics, flavonoids and glucosides.

The major classes of phytochemicals with disease-preventing functions are *dietary fiber, antioxidants, anticancer, detoxifying agents, immunity-potentiating agents and neuro-pharmacological agents.* Each class of these functional agents consists of a wide range of chemicals with differing potency. Some of these phytochemicals have more than one function.

Classification is difficult because of the wide range of different chemicals and the existence of different classifications. The simplest is provided here. But if you want to be overwhelmed, and find out more, see Wikipedia. It is worth a look if only to be astounded as to how many of these "secret ingredients" are in our fruit and vegetables.

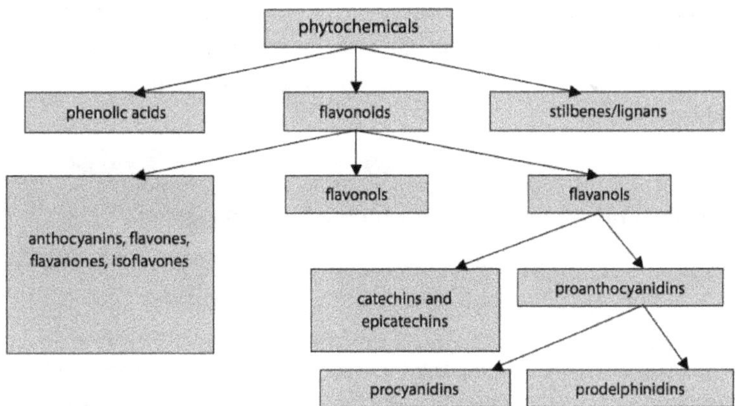

Flavonoids are a class of polyphenolic compounds found in abundance in plant-derived foods and beverages such as fruits, vegetables, dark chocolate, tea, and red wine. Flavonoids are categorized into six main subclasses based on their chemical structure: flavonols, flavan-3-ols, flavanones, flavones, anthocyanins, and isoflavones. Structural differences bring about variations in metabolism and bioactivity which may result in varying effects on health outcomes.

Flavonoids are the most diverse group of phytochemicals. Research suggests that they, in particular, may be an important phytochemical group that contributes to the reduced mortality rates observed in people consuming high levels of plant-based foods.

One Study[10] revealed a significant inverse association between flavonoid intake and myocardial infarction. Similarly, findings from the Seven Countries Study[11] suggested that consumption of flavonoids was responsible for 25% of the observed difference in mortality rates in the various countries studied. Once

---

[10] 1993. Dietary antioxidant flavonoids and risk of coronary heart disease: The Zutphen Elderly Study. Lancet 342(8878): 1007–1011.

[11] 1995. Flavonoid intake and long-term risk of coronary heart disease and cancer in the seven countries study. Arch Intern Med 155:381–386.

consumed and absorbed, flavonoids act favorably in the body through actions such as inhibiting xanthine oxidase and arachidonic acid metabolism.[12]

A plant-based diet feeds the microbiome bacteria in the gut that appears to play a tremendous role in our overall health. Plants are also very "nutrient dense," so they have more nutrients per calorie.

Phytochemicals are some thousands of compounds produced by plants and include antioxidants, flavonoids, phytonutrients, flavones, isoflavones, catchechins, isothiocyanates, carotenoids, allyl sulphides, polyphenols which contribute different effects and benefits to body metabolism. The flavonoid group also includes over 5,000 anthocyanins, flavanols, flavones, flavanones, flavan-3-ols, and isoflavones

Better-known phytonutrients and proposed benefits include:

Beta carotene	Orange and dark green leafy vegetables Immune system, vision, Skin and bone health
Lycopene	Red fruit and vegetables, Prostate and heart health
Lutein	Green leafy veg. Eye, heart health, ? anti-cancer
Resveratrol	Red wine, grapes, peanuts Heart, lung health, possible anti-cancer
Anthocyanins	Red, purple, blue pigment berries, vegetables, fruits Blood vessel (CVS) and brain (cognition) health
Isoflavones	Soya beans, Menopause, Breast cancer, Bone, Lower cholesterol

[12] 2001. Flavonoids: A review of probable mechanisms of action and potential applications. Am J Clin Nutr 74(4): 418–425.

Other Attributed Benefits

Phytonutrient	1	2	3	4	5	6	7	8	9
Carotenoids	+		+		+	+		+	
Flavonoids	+	+	+	+	+	+	+	+	+
Glucosinolates	+	+						+	
Monoterpines	+	+				+		+	
Phytosterols	+							+	
Phytoestrogens	+		+		+				
Phenolic Acids	+	+	+		+	+			+
Phytic acid	+		+		+				+
Protease inhibitors	+		+						+
Saponins	+	+			+			+	
Sulfides	+	+	+	+	+	+	+	+	

1 = Anticarcinogenic
2 = Antimicrobial/viral
3 = Antioxidant
4 Antithrombotic
5 = Immunomodulatory
6 = Anti-inflammatory
7 = Blood pressure modulator
8 = Cholesterol lowering
9 = Blood Glucose modulator

Synthetic vitamins and supplements can't make the range and exquisite ratio and the biological-metabolic inter-action they then confer. We are much better off eating a variety of fruit and vegetables than taking man-made vitamins or supplements. A more complete list of plant phytochemicals may be seen via Wikipedia. This is worth a look to show the incredible array of micronutrients and how no vitamin pill or supplement can match this range and how, surely, they are essential for our best health and why we should eat a variety of fresh foods.

One medium Orange (131g) Phytonutrient Content:

Other fruits and vegetables have other micronutrients and phytochemicals and **Newtrition,** and now research, contend that it is by mixing and amalgamating these different micronutrients from these different sources, by eating a variety of fruit and vegetables, that the combined benefits of fruit and vegetables are optimized.

The Micronutrient Content of Just One Orange

Vitamins		
Water-Soluble Vitamins	Vitamin B6	Pantotenic Acid
B-Complex Vitamins	Choline	**Vitamin C**
Vitamin B1	Folate	*Fat Soluble Vitamins*
Vitamin B2	Folate (DFE)	Vitamin A
Vitamin B3	Folate (food)	
Minerals		
Boron	Iron	Selenium
Calcium	Magnesium	Zinc
Chromium	Maganese	
Copper	Phosphorus	
Individual Fatty Acids		
Omega-3	Monosaturated	Oleic
Omega-6	Myristoleic	
Polyunsaturated Fatty Acids		
Conjugated Linoleic		
Linolenic		
Saturated Fatty Acids		
6:0 Palmitic		
INDIVIDUAL AMINO ACIDS		
Anine	Soleucine	Erine
Aspartic Acid	Eucine	Cryptophan
Cysteine	Lysine	Cyrosine
Glutamic Acid	Methionine	Yaline
Glycine	Phenylalanine	**Other**
Histidine	Troline	Ash

Hands up those who knew the simple orange contained all these amazing ingredients? I certainly didn't until I started this research but, more's the point, we don't have to know. All we have to know is to eat more fruit and vegetables - say 20% (each) of our daily intake. By the way, I counted ‘only’ 46. Should I ask for a refund?

Can one vitamin tablet match this orange's content? I think not.

This and other citrus contain an enormous variety of micronutrients. We all know they are an excellent source of vitamin C, but their micronutrients make their vitamin C work better in our bodies. Goodness knows what other beneficial effects they have but it stands to reason they enhance our health. As such they are far superior to vitamin supplements / pills. This was just for an orange, but each fruit and vegetable contain their own array of micronutrients, which, again, would seem beneficial to our health. It was only documented for your interest to show you that it isn't just vitamin C an orange provides.

Flavonoid levels are highest in ripe, fresh-picked fruit. If they were picked unripe, or they have been in storage, their health benefits will be lower. The antioxidant content decreases within days.

As noted elsewhere, research has found that diets rich in fruits and vegetables (FV), which contain polyphenols, protect against age-related inflammation and chronic diseases by reducing cytokines and how In this study thirty-one polyphenols and six polyphenol mixtures were compared for their effects and results suggest that polyphenols derived from onions, turmeric, red grapes, green tea and açai berries may help reduce the release of pro-inflammatory mediators in people at risk of chronic inflammation.[13] Most of these polyphenols were flavonoids.

Citrus flavonoids are found in the fruit's tissue, juice, pulp and skin and are the main reason that eating the whole fruit is much more healthful than just drinking the juice. Two of the flavonoids in citrus—naringin in grapefruit and hesperidin in orange— occur only rarely in other plants and are thus essentially unique to citrus but they contain many other nutrients as well as being powerful antioxidants. The most potent of these citrus nutrients are a group of bioactive flavonoids also known as vitamin P. They include diosmetin, diosmin, hesperidin, naringin, narirutin, neohesperidin, nobiletin, quercetin, rutin and the flavone tangeritin, carotenoids, isohesperidin, terpeniol, limonin, flavonoids, limonene. *They are essential for the proper absorption of Vitamin C and enhance and prolong the action of vitamin C.*

Citrus flavonoids are antioxidant and shown to inhibit cancer cell growth: A 248-page report, "The Health Benefits of Citrus Fruits," released December 2003 by Australian research group, CSIRO (The Commonwealth Scientific and Industrial Research), reviews 48 studies that show a diet high in citrus fruit provides a statistically significant protective effect against some types of cancer. Citrus appears to offer the most significant protection against esophageal, oro-pharynygeal / laryngeal (mouth, larynx and pharynx), and stomach cancers. For these cancers, studies showed risk reductions of 40-50%.

---

[13] Br J Nutr. 2016 May 28; 115(10): 1699–1710. Published online 2016 Mar 17.
doi: 10.1017/S0007114516000805 PMCID: PMC4836295
Identification of (poly)phenol treatments that modulate the release of pro-inflammatory cytokines by human lymphocytes

Flavonoids also strengthen capillaries, are anti-inflammatory, antiallergenic and antimicrobial. Flavonoid intake is inversely associated with the incidence of heart attack and stroke as well as a host of other ailments. The Framingham Nurses' Health Study found that drinking one daily glass of orange juice reduced the risk of stroke by 25%.

Summary

Just as vitamins were a mystery and then a miracle, other constituents of fresh, ripe foods would seem to have many beneficial micronutrients as well as many yet to be discovered. Certainly, their deficiency is in no way as dramatic as that of a vitamin, but it would seem reasonable to suggest that they enhance our metabolic pathways.

We need not, and should not, wait to eat better, as did the millions who died from deficiency diseases. They did not have to know it was vitamin C, thiamin or some other vitamin, all they had to do was eat a variety of fresh, ripe foods.

If you do this, you will get all the nutritional goodies in the best and correct bioavailable doses.

As modern research charges on there do seem some foods that bestow particular benefits: If green leafy or nut extracts are dripped on cancer cells growing in a laboratory, the cancer cells are inhibited and stop growing (Bok Choy, walnuts and pecans maybe best), so these micronutrients may have even more profound effects beneficial to human health.

CHAPTER 3

THE PROBLEM

FOOD FOR THOUGHT... and Illnesses and Obesity

Our food has been changed (for the worse).

It has altered more in the last 80 years than the previous 80,000 or even 800,000.

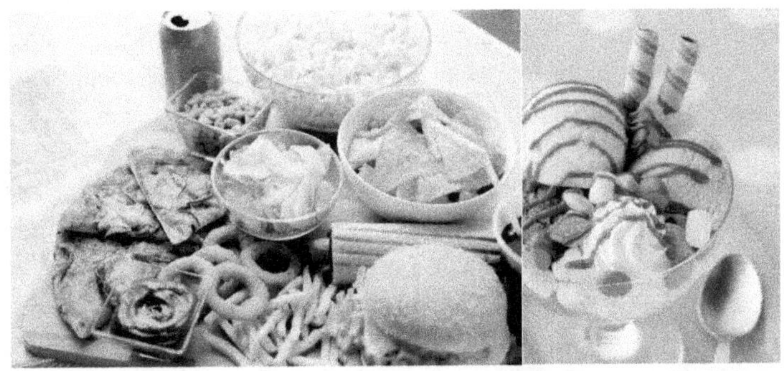

The quite incredible alterations to our food or rather, what we eat, began with the needs of World War 2 (WW2). Since then, probably some 100,000 new chemicals have been introduced, many into our foods, yet they are untested until there is some obvious problem.

Many of these have contributed to the incredible explosion of convenient, fast, processed foods which have been researched to taste delicious, be irresistible, available 24 hours a day, seven days a week and can be delivered to our door.

We don't know or notice the changes to our foods and diet. Only someone from our Grandparents vintage, if they had been frozen in time and brought back now, would see the absolutely incredible rows and rows and rows of supermarket ready to eat packaged foods and meals with a list of ingredients, in small print, that would defy a university chemist to decipher.

And while the onslaught of processed food may be apparent, the sterilization of our land and the factory feeding of our animals, as has been pointed out, has seen the now necessary supplementation of animals with such the essentials as vitamin B12.

The extensive Global Burden of Disease studies show that poor diet is consistently responsible for more disease and death than physical inactivity, smoking and alcohol combined.[14]

Many people follow what they believe to be a healthy diet. But overall dietary habits have changed over the past century, and, generally, not for the better. There has been a large shift from whole foods to processed to ultra-processed foods. In addition, higher sugar consumption, more refined carbohydrates, and more foods with dyes, preservatives, additives and trans fats are being consumed.[15]

Food is becoming more and more unnatural. It would not seem unreasonable, in fact irresistible, to associate this new altered food with the present epidemic of the The Diseases of Affluence (DOAs): Obesity, cardiovascular disease (including heart attacks, strokes, peripheral vascular disease) high blood pressure, type 2 diabetes, osteoporosis, colorectal cancer, acne, gout, depression, and paradoxically, diseases related to vitamin and mineral deficiencies.

While this may just be a coincidence, obesity and its subsequent illnesses, occur for the first time or increase whenever Western junk-food is introduced to previously affluent societies with a more natural diet, such as Asia, or when introduced to primitive tribes. As detailed later, Japanese who moved from Japan to Hawaii and then Los Angeles had greater rates of heart attacks as they consumed more Western processed foods while those in the Blue Zones, the longest living people, also develop these DOAs (how exquisitely appropriate) when they depart from their previous natural foods to eat Western junk.

Obesity is an epidemic: Humans have never been fatter nor these illnesses more prevalent. What else can explain this explosion of these diseases. Perhaps they can also be called the "Diseases of Processed Foods". And they are now shortening our lifespans, killing us prematurely.

Today just some ten companies now effectively control the Western if not the entire world's nutrition. Together they are worth greater than $1 Trillion.

Welcome to the Fast Food Industry (FFI).

Humans have been evolving for some 2.8 million years and our similar eating ancestors for millions of years before that. They ate what they could and soon worked out what they thrived on (and what killed them) and even evolved

---

[14]Global Burden of Diseases, Injuries, and Risk Factors Study 2013. The Lancet, 22 Jul 2014.
[15] American Psychiatric Association (APA) 2016 Annual Meeting: Presented May 17, 2016.

enzymes and alterations in their anatomy to digest a greater variety of natural foods more efficiently.

Humans worked out that certain foods donated benefits, so we ate citrus which provided us with vitamin C, and meat which gave us vitamin B12, both essential for survival, but it was not until 1926 that vitamin C was discovered and B12 in 1948 – less than 100 years ago. And when we didn't eat these we could die from scurvy and pernicious anaemia.

Food science has really only existed in the last 80 years of the previous 2.8 million. Altered processed–ultraprocessed foods have only been developed in these last 80 years.

And that's the problem. While it took centuries, thousands, hundreds, if not millions of years, for humans to evolve enzymes and alter their anatomy so as to absorb and best metabolize the natural foods, we have only had some 80 years to adjust to these new chemicals, additives and processed foods.

And that's simply not enough time.

We cannot process processed foods.

It took centuries for vitamins and minerals to be recognized as essential for our health and now the formerly secret world of the micro-nutrients is being revealed. We knew we needed something in citrus, but until recently we didn't know it was vitamin C nor that there were some 69 other constituents in an orange which make the vitamin C be absorbed and work better.

The science of nutrition didn't really begin until World War 1 in a small way, then World War 2 (WW2) in a big way – but then lapsed by Governments when the war was over. This left the clever, and I do mean clever, food scientists looking for work and the Fast Food Industry (FFI) was born.

The onslaught of the synthetic food and miracle drugs, like penicillin, saw the demise of the doctors, like my father, who had seen and used the miracle of vitamins. They had seen how white rice, with its vitamin husk polished off, caused beriberi (swollen hearts) and peripheral neuropathy (nerve damage) only to be cured as if a miracle by natural brown rice with its husk on containing thiamin (vitamin B1). Bandy legged kids with the "Rachitic Rosary" of bony chest nodules where their little bones failed to form properly cured by Cod Liver oil (vitamin D) and Dr Goldberg chased out of town for daring to suggest Pellagra, which was killing the Good Ol' Boys and Slaves of the South, was due to a nutritional deficiency in their Sick American Diet (SAD). They insisted it was from a germ.

Now all we need are some anti-biotics and some vitamin pills – well maybe some anti-depressants too.

People, understandably, only go to the doctor when they are ill and not for preventive-nutritional advice and doctors were not reimbursed for such. Nutrition lapsed from the medical curricula and, of course, this opened the door to 'health' gurus, the vitamin scammers, who sold useless vitamins, totally excreted in our urine, at inflated price-fixed mark-ups that, only a few years ago, saw the biggest drug-vitamin companies in the world fined $billions for profit gouging.

It was (and is) a case of "fresh food out, vitamin pills and processed foods in".

Think About This

WW2 saw the development of food science for compressed / processed foods to feed the troops. Thereafter, these food scientists moved into private enterprise and the Fast Food Industry was established and our food progressively altered.

It obviously would take some time for processed-ultraprocessed foods to become the established Western Diet, but they did and by the early 80s it was noticed people 'were heavier' and by 1997 the WHO declared obesity an epidemic. It would seem that, as our genes had not changed and as our microbiome had not changed, the only thing that had changed, and therefore the most likely cause of this new phenomenon of obesity, was this change in our food.

Obesity, in other words, increased lock-step with the increase in processed foods. We now spend nearly 20 times more of fast food than we did 30 years ago which is just about when the obesity epidemic began.

The more processed foods were available, such as the USA, the higher the rates of obesity and the downstream Diseases of Affluence.

Processed Food 60% of Our Diet

Ultra-processed foods now make up nearly 60% of total calorie intake consumed in the US diet, contributes almost 90% of energy calorie intake from added sugars and 70% of our salt intake.

Ultra-processed foods include substances not generally used in cooking, such as *flavorings, emulsifiers*, and other *additives* designed to mimic the qualities of 'real foods' and include mass produced *soda/soft drinks*; *sweet or savory packaged* *snacks; confectionery and desserts; packaged baked goods; chicken/fish nuggets and other reconstituted meat products; instant noodles and soups.*[16]

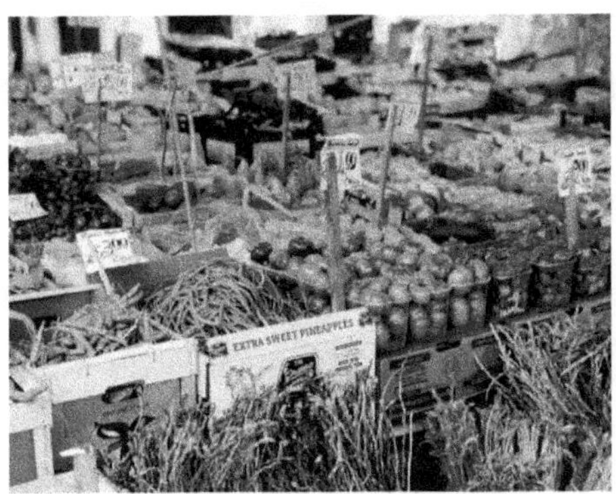

Shop here- fresh fruit and vegetables

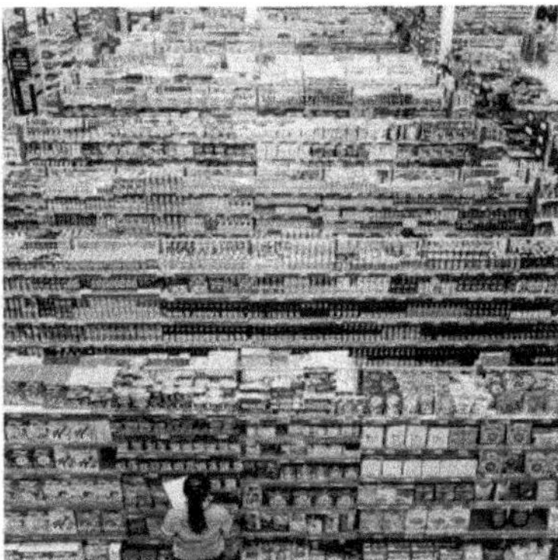

Avoid the central packaged aisles

Fast Food Exceeds All Other Expenditure Combined

Americans, and therefore the rest of the first world, now spend more on fast food than on higher education, personal computers, software or new cars and more on fast food than on movies, books, magazines, newspapers, videos and recorded music – *combined.*[17]

Fast Food Advertising

The Food Industry spends $1million a day advertising processed ($36 billion pa $10 billion directed to kids).[18] There is deliberate targeting of small children from 52 new products in 1994 to more than 500 in 2004. Foods advertised are high-calorie, low-nutrition. Since 1994 it has only become worse. Obesity rates have tripled in this age group in the last 40 years.

Food Cues Undermine Healthy Choices19

Health warnings for healthy food choices only seem to be effective where there are no advertisings /displays or 'food cues". Whenever such stimuli are present people are triggered (conditioned by previous advertising) to choose the unhealthy

[16] Ultra-processed foods and added sugars in the US diet: evidence from a nationally representative cross-sectional study. *BMJ Open*, 2016; 6 (3): e009892 DOI: 10.1136/bmjopen-2015-009892
[17] Fast Food Nation: The Dark Side of the All-American Meal (2001) by Eric Schlosser
[18] Time 4/6/06
[19] Failing to pay heed to health warnings in a food-associated environment. Appetite, 2018; 120: 616 DOI: 10.1016/j.appet.2017.10.020

food product, even when they know it is unhealthy or aren't really craving that food product. It didn't matter whether they were alerted the subjects before or after they learned the associations with food cues.

Non-Hungry Shopping

Hungrier shoppers spent 64% more money than those less hungry.[20] Sugar Sweetened Beverages (SSB) – soda/soft drinks, add an average 213 calories per day to their diet. Discretionary foods (foods and drinks not necessary to provide the nutrients the human body's needs) add, on average, 439 calories per day. [21]

Most Popular Fast Food: Big Mac + Fries + Large Coke =1360 Cals

Accept Responsibility

If you want to optimize your health, it is up to you and you alone as all Governments don't have the money to match the FFI's advertising budget but, what is more, throughout the World, the FFI had nobbled the politicians as they employ so many people, build so many factories and sponsor so many sports organizations that they can, and do, point out how any interference with their profits will see factories close and that politician lose his or her seat.

Then there are those who, no matter how ill, prefer their instant pleasures:

A survey of 1127 patients who had myocardial infarction (80%) or angina (20%) showed that 90% had been through complex procedures. But, despite all this, 56% of the smokers were still smoking, 57% of those taking statins still had high LDL cholesterol, 46% of those treated for hypertension were outside target, and 59% of those with diabetes had suboptimal glucose control. Obesity was found in 34%, and 60% were physically inactive.[22]

---

[20] University of Minnesota. "An empty stomach can lead to an empty wallet." ScienceDaily. ScienceDaily, 18 February 2015.

[21] Consumption of sugar-sweetened beverages and discretionary foods among US adults by purchase location. European Journal of Clinical Nutrition, 2016; DOI: 10.1038/ejcn.2016.136

[22] *BMC Cardiovasc Disord* doi: 10.1186/s12872-016-0387-z

Junk Food is for The Poor - and They Prefer It

Over an 18-year period the number of takeaway food outlets rose by 45%, with the highest increase in density of outlets found in areas of highest deprivation.

The upgrading local corner stores in East Los Angeles, by a team who poured more resources into a healthy eating intervention through adding fresh fruits and vegetables, improved shelving, training and social media marketing, resulted in no real changes in food purchasing or diet at the community level.[23].[24]

Overweight & Obesity

Body Mass Index (BMI) of over 25 defines 'overweight' and a BMI of 30 or more defines 'obese'. The figures increase each year.

USA: 69.0% (2011-2012); Overweight, including obesity: 71.6% (2015-2016)

UK: 67% of men and 57% of women are overweight or obese;
Australia: 55.7% of women and 70.3% of men are overweight

Your waist circumference is a better measure: Men < 102 cm; Women < 88 cm.

Children

We now have the fattest and most unfit kids in world history. The average child spends 21 hours a week or one and a half months a year watching TV. 95% European TV ads encouraged kids to eat foods high in sugar, salt and fat' 31.8% of children in the USA takes vitamin and mineral supplements (48.5% aged 4 to 8 yrs.).25

Food Indexes

Food Indexes are measures of the diet quality and assess conformance to their various Guidelines. One of the early dietary index was the Healthy Eating Index (HEI), which was created by the US Department of Agriculture to describe adherence to the 1995 US Dietary Guidelines.

---

[23] Substantial improvements not seen in health behaviors following corner store conversions in two Latino food swamps. *BMC Public Health*, 2016; 16 (1) DOI: 10.1186/s12889-016-3074-1

[24] Area deprivation and the food environment over time: a repeated cross-sectional study on takeaway outlet density and supermarket presence in Norfolk, UK, 1990 – 2008. *Health & Place*, 2 April 2015

[25] Arch Paed Adolesc Med 2007;161;978-8

Dietary indexes, Food Quality and Improved Mortality[26]

FYI only. The Mediterranean Diet exceeds all these.

The original Healthy Eating Index (HEI) was designed to assess adherence to the Dietary Guidelines for Americans and the Food Guide Pyramid, but only resulted in a small reduction in major chronic disease risk in US adult men and women.

In contrast with the original HEI, the AlternativeHEI was developed and distinguished quality within food groups and acknowledged health benefits of unsaturated oils.

Dietary indexes scoring was based on food groups from the MyPyramid Equivalents Database.

- The HEI-2010 includes 12 components (total fruit, whole fruit, total vegetables, dark green vegetables and legumes, whole grains, dairy, total protein foods, seafood and plant proteins, ratio of PUFAs and MUFAs to SFAs, refined grains, sodium, and empty calories) and reflects the 2010 Dietary Guidelines for Americans, with higher scores reflecting better adherence to federal dietary guidelines.
- The AHEI-2010 includes 11 foods and nutrients
- The aMED score includes 9 components
- The DASH index includes 8 components

A large study found consistent associations between improved diet quality over 12 years as assessed by the Alternate HEI, Alternate Mediterranean Diet, and DASH scores and a reduced risk of death in the subsequent 12 years with an estimated 17%-26% reduction in risk of all-cause mortality.

The Newtrition Diet is not a slavish measuring of 20% of each of the five groups but rather an easy reminder to eat some of each every day and this is an optimum diet.

The Newtrition Micronutrient Revolution Diet improves on these Food Index Diets.

Nutrient Deficiencies in Western Diets13

Affluent Nations often have poor nutrition because of availability of junk foods.

Although the following nutrients are key to brain function, statistics from the US Department of Agriculture show that most Americans are not getting enough of

[26] Liver International. 2020;40(4):815-824.

them (due to reliance on Fast Food). For example, the percentages of the U.S. population that do not meet the recommended daily allowances for these key nutrients are as follows: Vitamin E: 86%, Folate: 75%, Calcium: 73%, Magnesium: 68%, Zinc: 42%, Vitamin B6: 35% Iron: 34%, Vitamin B12: 30%.

But we don't know this as we have plenty of food, eat till we are full and most of us are overweight if not obese. The problem is that it is low quality processed food, lacking in these essential nutrients and certainly not enough fresh foods.

First World Nations Poor Quality Diets

People living in many of the wealthiest regions (e.g., the USA and Canada, Western Europe, Australia and New Zealand) still have among the poorest quality diets in the world, because they have some of the highest consumption of unhealthy food worldwide.[27]

We cannot mix bad food with good, in the same way breathing fresh air will not allow us continue to smoke. And so it is that the affluent but busy person eats well but then destroys it by grabbing some fast food.

Lack of Variety

Around 15,000 years ago humans ate around 150 ingredients a week.

Today for the Western diet we mostly only eat 20, most of which are processed. Most come from just four sources: corn, soy, wheat or meat[28] or milk.

Italians select from 60 foods. The Japanese have a saying that eating from less than 30 different foods a day leads to ill health.

The Western Diet

It has been reported that less than 1% of U.S. adults age 50 and over has an ideal dietary score.[29] With the universal influence of American fast food this startling depressing trend is now applicable to most countries.

---

[27] Dietary quality among men and women in 187 countries in 1990 and 2010: a systematic assessment. *The Lancet Global Health*, 2015; 3 (3): e132 DOI: 10.1016/S2214-109X(14)70381-X

[28] The Diet Myth by Tim Spector Ch 1

[29] Reported at the annual meeting of the International Stroke Conference / the American Heart Association/American Stroke Association. Feb 2015.

Worldwide: Bad Food Outstrips Good

While the worldwide, consumption of healthy foods such as fruit and vegetables has improved during the past two decades, but this has been outpaced by the increased intake of unhealthy foods including processed meat and sweetened drinks.

Bad nutrition is now the greatest health problem of the Western World (where there are adequate public health measures of clean water, sewerage, waste disposal etc.). The DOAs (*'Diseases of Affluence),* obesity, diabetes 2, hyperlipidaemia, hypertension and coronary artery disease, are now epidemics. Their downstream effects of heart attacks, strokes, arthritis and depression only add to the problem and the incredible burgeoning of health costs.

The Big Primate Brain

There are two theories as to why humans are big-brained: Sociality or diet.

Sociality: One theory is because of social pressures and the need to think about and track our social relationships. Complex foraging strategies, social structures, and cognitive abilities are likely to have co-evolved throughout primate evolution.

Diet: However, as to the more important when it comes to determining the brain size of primate species, new research suggests that factor is *diet*.[30]

The Human Brain - Meat and Grains

Human diets have changed through millions of years of evolution. Originally, it is alleged we were vegetarians but around 2 million years ago we began incorporating meats and cooking (unlike other animals). Cooking speeds up absorption of food. It also tends to increase nutrient availability and decrease toxins. This increased efficiency allowed the shortening of the human gut by 20% and development of the advanced human brain.

Around 6000 - 10,000 years ago, agriculture was developed and added grains, dairy, and legumes to our diets. Humans developed salivary amylase which allowed the digestion of grains and the extraction of their essential vitamins which

---

[30] Primate brain size is predicted by diet but not sociality. *Nature Ecology & Evolution*, 2017; 1: 0112 DOI: 10.1038/s41559-017-0112

saw the second boost to make the human brain the biggest. This is discussed later in detail.

It is odd that if humans were vegetarians, how and why did they never gain the ability to metabolize cellulose (eat grass/leaves) and why did we come to depend on meat for vitamin B12 and, to a lesser extent, iron.

(I still remember the 1:4 beta-bonds of Knoop in cellulose, from my biochemistry studies. These β 1-4 linkage cannot be broken down by human digestive enzymes, but herbivores such as cows, koalas, buffalos, and horses are able, with the help of the specialized flora in their stomach, to digest plant material that is rich in cellulose and use it as a food source).

It is alleged that 'no tribe voluntarily adopts a vegetarian diet' as B12 was essential for life and humans would have died out.

People cherry pick and use only that information that favors their bias. Vegetarians will claim proof positive we started as vegetarians while meat eaters will claim we were always omnivores, eating both plants and meat.

I shall leave this to the nutritional anthropologists. But what we have ended up being are omnivores, able to eat both meat and plants (except cellulose), and this suits us metabolically more than being vegetarians who need artificial supplements (B12, Vit D and iron). But because of these supplements are now available people now can easily be vegetarians.

Modern Mush and Processing

Only in the past 100 years, and especially since World War 2, has our diet drastically switched from whole foods to one that is more processed and high in refined carbohydrates that include more vegetable fats rather than meat fats, preservatives, emulsifiers, and other additives, which appear to have contributed to a decline in our collective health. Nutritious kernels were stripped of their nutrients as new refining practices emerged, only to have specific vitamins added back artificially, due to the health problems associated with overly refined grains. Grains and other foods had been processed and preserved for thousands of years by much healthier means. For example, fermentation of grains—and letting them sprout—increases nutrient availability.

We now have food that is mostly processed but we also have a glut of it available 24 hours a day, 7 days a week and can even be home delivered. Whereas when the UK was rationed to a minimal sustainable diet in World War 2, the health records reveal that the population has never been healthier; as was also the case in Cuba when the US embargo saw food being rationed; and those who starved, in the USA's Dust-bowl famine of the 30s, lived six years longer.

When food is restricted due to famines, droughts, wars, embargos or whatever, peoples' longevity improves.

CHAPTER 4

WHAT NOT TO EAT

PROCESSED, REFINED FOODS, ADDITIVES

Coca-Cola started in 1892. It was, as we all know, a soda/soft drink product, and not food, but arguably set the business example for all to follow.

Henry Ford invented the assembly line and it was enthusiastically copied all across America such that a restaurant White Castle adopted this model in 1921. They had food that was prepared quickly in a very highly mechanized, highly systematized way. Every inch of the grill was dedicated for either the bread or the beef in small, square patties.

Walt Anderson, a short-order cook in Wichita, Kansas, liked to experiment with the size and shape of the hamburger patties. One day he became so frustrated when the meatballs he was cooking kept sticking to the griddle that he smashed one with a spatula. And thus, the flat patty was born.

In 1916, he opened a hamburger stand and quickly expanded to four locations with W.E. "Billy" Ingram, a local real estate broker who would eventually become the company's CEO, buying in, and in 1921 they established a chain of small, efficiently run restaurants selling five-cent burgers by the sack. White Castle is widely credited as the first fast food concept in America.

To feed the troops in WW2 'compressed' foods, 'rations', were necessary and food science burgeoned. In addition, the modern age of ice cream history started shortly after the end of World War I when refrigerators became available. Ice cream, arguably, became the first commercial Fast Food when flash frozen and dried ice creams became part of the official US Army rations of World War II, and was distributed on all fronts across Europe, North Africa, East Asia and Pacific. And this set up an established example to be followed.

After WW2 these war food-scientists were stood down and went to work for private firms and the Fast Food Industry (FFI) was born and fast food was progressively synthesised along with expansion of fast food restaurants which became progressively popular during the 1950s as women had joined the workforce and girls no longer learned cooking at their mothers' apron strings. It was alleged some years ago that most people under the age of 30 years 'couldn't cook an egg'. Families were busier and they needed a place where they could quickly pick up food. People also wanted to be able to get quick food that they could eat in front of their new TVs.

The first McDonald's with fast food was opened in 1948. Burger King and Taco Bell opened in the 1950s. It is also alleged that fast food took off in large part because of the American highway system built in the 1950s and the1960s and cities, like Los Angeles, were based on car travel.

As Anna Diamond points out "And then there's the food. The food is terrible, and it's delicious, and it's completely ridiculous and we love it. I mean, not everybody loves it, but it has this element of hucksterism to it, these insane ideas that get made. It's a very American idea to just have the biggest, craziest burger or the wildest thing".

This 'American Dream' spread world-wide and with it then came Pre-prepared "Heat and Eat" meals, Instant Noodles, complete packaged meals and, all of which now had preservatives, additives and a list of chemicals none of which we knew but accepted as being OK.

But are they?

We became more and more accustomed to picking packets off the Super-Market shelves and the food scientists simply responded to a commercial demand.

This was no sinister conspiracy, just a response to the demand, but what has happened since, is, if not sinister, then detrimental, with the content and our food being progressively altered to processed, then ultra-processed with some 100,000 new chemicals being invented many of which, as noted, have found their way into these processed foods and most are untested.

The Genie is now out of the bottle and it is impossible for it to be put back. The Fast Food Industry (FFI) is simply too powerful and with our modern lifestyle we now don't cook much and, even if we do, we buy some commercial sauce or dressing. We don't grow our own fruit and vegetables at all...and we are overweight and dying before we should.

The FFI has become so big and competitive it is now a self-perpetuating monster that uses every trick, bluff, bribe, false advertising, advertising focused on the vulnerable (such as kids), infiltration of every health, nutrition organization and political parties it can, as it ruthlessly pursues profits.

Everyone should read Eric Schlosser's book *Fast Food Nation.*

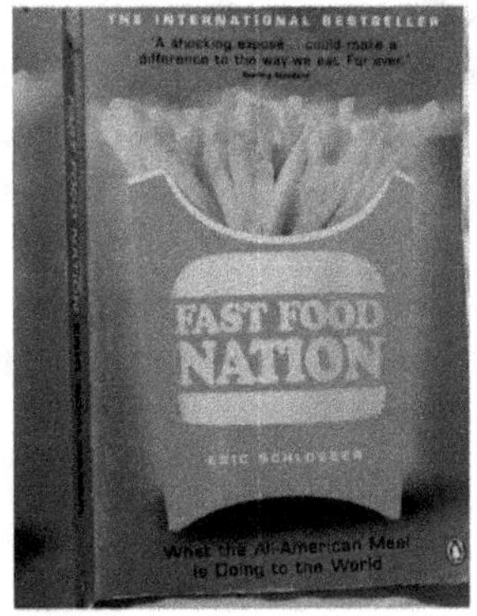

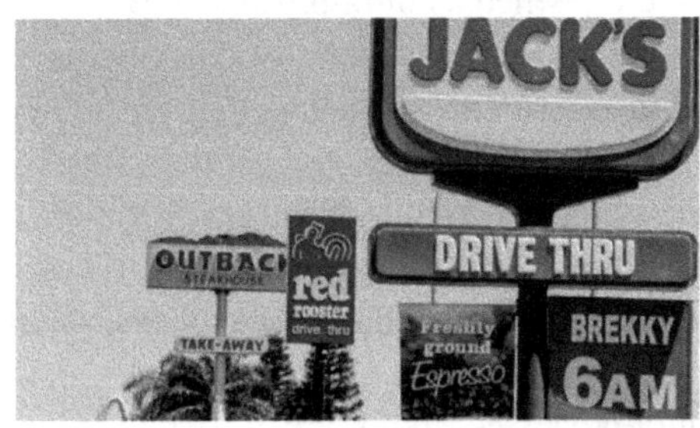

Warning: "Refined" sounds elegant, sophisticated and therefore preferable but when it comes to food, we must recognise it as "unnatural and bad".

0.5 million deaths per year are attributable to poor diet in the USA, which now represents the leading cause of death.[31]

In 1997, much to the delight of the Fast Food Industry, they found that '*consumers (had) dropped all pretence of wanting healthy food'*.

There would seem to be a distinction between 'ultra-processed' and 'processed'

'Processed' can mean something as simple as pounding meat to tenderise it whereas 'Ultra'-processed food is a concept devised by the Brazilian nutrition researcher Carlos Monteiro. As of 2018 the concept is loose and evolving.

The NOVA Classification

The NOVA Food Classification System was developed at the University of Sao Paulo in Brazil and is now the reference standard. "Ultra-processed food and beverages are industrial formulations made entirely or mostly from substances extracted from foods (oils, fats, sugar, starch and proteins). They are derived from hydrogenated fats and modified starch and synthesized in laboratories".

[31] Global improvement in dietary quality could lead to substantial reduction in premature death *J Nutr* 2019;149:1065–74.

Scientists analysed 230,156 products and found 71% of products such as bread, salad dressings, snack foods, sweets, sugary drinks and more were ultra-processed. Among the top 25 manufacturers by sales volume, 86% of products were classified as ultra-processed. Bread and bakery products were consistently among the highest. Even food like olive and other oils are heated then chemically extracted with hexane unless they are 'cold pressed'.

Ultra-processed foods, Nova classification, are industrial formulations with five ingredients, but usually many more. These ingredients include casein, lactose, whey, gluten and hydrogenated or inter-esterified oils.

Ultra-processed foods are also defined as "ready-to-eat" or "ready-to-heat" formulations made mostly from ingredients usually combined with additives.

Ultra-processed foods don't just include obviously unhealthy things like fast food, soda, sugary soft drinks, chips, and hot dogs but what appear to be, ostensibly, 'healthy' or 'harmless' foods like flavored yogurt, energy bars, baby formula, and cereal can also be, and mostly are, ultra-processed, as well as fast food, lunch meat, packaged bread, and most energy bars.

Fast Foods now include processing of substances derived from baking, frying, extruding, moulding, hydrogenation and hydrolysis and several transformation processes including heating at high temperatures and the presence of additives, emulsifiers and texturisers. Many ready-to-heat products that are rich in salt or sugar and low in vitamins and fiber fall under this category.

They generally include a large number of additives such as preservatives, sweeteners, sensory enhancers, colorants, flavors and processing aids, but little or no whole food. They may be fortified with synthetic micronutrients. The aim is to create durable, convenient and palatable ready-to-eat or ready-to- heat food products suitable to be consumed as snacks or to replace freshly prepared food-based dishes and meals.

Many of the packaged foods on our supermarket shelves are made "hyper-palatable" through chemical processing and "cosmetic" enhancement, such as the addition of colors, flavors and emulsifiers. The clever food scientists can make a mouth texture that hits 'the Bliss Point'. High in added sugar, fat and/or salt but with little, if any, nutritional value, they include confectionery snacks, fizzy drinks, cakes, sports drinks, many breakfast cereals, pastries, dehydrated vegetable soups and reconstituted meat and fish products.

Globally, these foods are believed to account for up to 60 per cent of daily energy intake (in Australia they account for about 35 per cent) and are already associated with obesity, high blood pressure, cholesterol and some cancers.

Even the much promoted 'Veggie Burger' and meat substitutes as 'healthy' may have damaging contents and may take more to manufacture with respect to global warming than real meat.

We simply don't know what we are eating when it comes to Fast Foods.

The Bliss Point

The Bliss Point is "that sensory profile where you like food the most."

It depends on just the right amount of saltiness, sweetness, richness and mouth feel as salt, sugar, or fat which optimizes deliciousness. In food product optimization, the goal is to include two or three of these nutrients. The human body has evolved to favour foods delivering these tastes: the brain responds with a "reward" in the form of a jolt of endorphins, remembers what we did to get that reward, and makes us want to do it again, an effect run by dopamine, a neurotransmitter. Combinations of sugar, fat, and salt act synergistically, and are more rewarding than any one alone.

It was initiated by American market researcher and psychophysicist Howard Moskowitz, known for his successful work in product creation and optimization for foods ranging from spaghetti sauce to soft drinks.

The Most Irresistible and Desirable Food

The most irresistible, delicious food is a combination that does not occur in nature.

This 50:50 combination of fat and sugar is a food invented by humans: Ice cream, cheese-cake, doughnut glaze, fudge bars, and other foods made in a factory.

They are the ultimate weight gaining "foods". One study on identical twins found that a sugar diet did not put weight on one, while a fat diet did not put weight on the other, but the combination of sugar and fat did. Rats fed on cheesecake can't resist it and become obese. Susie Maroney who swam Cuba to Miami and the English Channel a record number of times, ate cheese-cake to pile on the fat needed as a protective layer against the cold water.

Refining of Grains

The refining of grains wherein the husk is removed stripping out all the vitamins and micro-nutrients and referred to as 'refining' is ultra-processing.

Refining consists of when the fiber-rich bran and nutrient-vitamin rich germ, are stripped off all that is left is nutrient poor starch in the form of white (Processed) flour. Grains were originally refined/processed to extend its shelf life which the Kellogs soon realised. Breakfast cereals are processed and have to have a few synthetic vitamins put back in. 'Enriching' or 'Fortifying' (sounds so reassuring doesn't it) only chemically adds 5 of the lost 25 nutrients back as synthetic chemicals.

Wheat is the most eaten grain in Western diets and 98% of this wheat is eaten in the form of processed white flour.

% of Nutrients Lost by Refining:

Fiber 95%, Protein 25%, Calcium 56%, Copper 62%, Iron 84%, Manganese 82%. Phosphorus 69%, Potassium 74%, Selenium 52%, Zinc 76%, Vitamin B2 73%, Vitamin B2 81%, Vitamin B3 80%, Vitamin B5 56%, Vitamin B6 87%, Folate 59%, Vitamin E 95%.

OBESITY

It is fashionable to blame our genes, or now our gut microbiome

but these have not changed

only our food has changed.

Obesity is now an official epidemic causing its downstream effects of the 'Diseases of Affluence' of Hypertension, Hyperlipidaemia, Heart Attacks, Strokes, Diabetes 2, Arthritis, Depression and so many more. I also wonder about the new increase in Colorectal Cancers in younger people (<50 yrs) which defies all trends.

But the affordability of junk food (three times cheaper than fruit and veg), it's convenience (24 hrs a day, 7 days a week and home delivered) or its delicious taste designed to hit our 'bliss spot' and with an incredible texture, makes the eating and the over-eating of junk food so much easier.

Americans eat an extra 788 calories a day when only 20 more will make us fat, These then cause an unrecognised 'cascade' corrupting our normal, evolved metabolic pathways, jam them up and divert them to lay down fat.

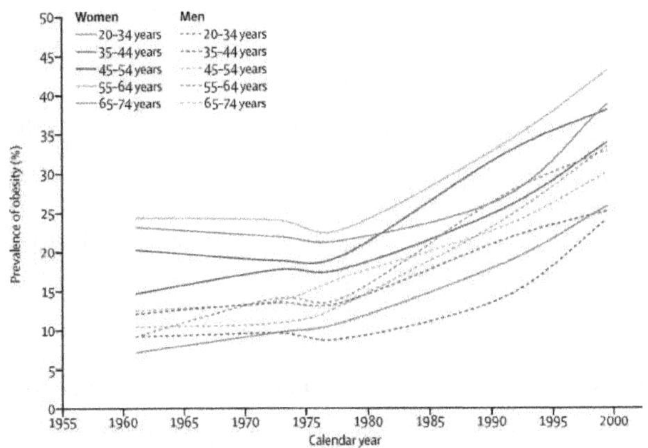

Processed Cascade

The problem with foods that make people fat isn't all caused in that they have too many calories, but also, it's that they cause a cascade of reactions in the body that promote fat storage and make people overeat. Processed carbohydrates—foods like chips, sugar-soda/soft drinks, crackers/cakes/ biscuits, and even white rice—digest quickly into sugar and increase levels of the hormone insulin.

Avoid Food Bloggers[32]

Out of nine leading UK weight management blogs only one was trustworthy. She was an accredited, qualified nutritionist whereas the rest had no relevant qualifications, their blogs lacked integrity and included unhealthy recipes.

[32] *European Conference Obesity 2019.*

PROCESSED POISON: Ready to Eat: Heat and Eat

The cumulative and cocktail effects of eating different processed foods "remain largely unknown". It is suggested that certain food additives may adversely affect cardiovascular health and that certain processing techniques may also be having a detrimental effect on our health.

The first study as to the effects of ultra-processed foods on health was published online February 11, 2019 in JAMA Internal Medicine.

A study of 105,159 French adults found that a 10 per cent increase in the amount of ultra-processed foods in the diet was associated with a significantly higher likelihood of ending up with cardiovascular disease, coronary heart disease and cerebrovascular disease (increases of 12, 13 and 11% respectively). Those with a diet high in unprocessed or minimally processed foods, on the other hand, were significantly less likely to end up with any of these diseases.

Another study published found that participants on an ultra-processed diet gained weight, while participants on a minimally processed diet that contained the same amount of salts, fats and sugars and calories did not.

A second BMJ study, of nearly 20,000 Spanish adults over the course 10 years, found that eating more than four servings of ultra-processed foods a day (which is pretty easy when you consider that one serving of French fries is about 12 to 15 potato sticks) was associated with a 62 per cent increased risk of premature death by any cause, compared with less than two servings per day. Moreover, each additional serving of ultra-processed food was associated with a statistically significant 18 per cent higher hazard of all-cause mortality.

It is estimated that, in the 1960s (before supermarkets became widespread), Australians had 600-800 foods available - very few ultra-processed. Now the average supermarket stocks more than 30,000 items - many ultra- processed. There are now over 100,000 "health" supplements.

Reformulating foods to lower the amount of salt, sugar or fat often meant increasing the amount of processing (such as adding artificial sweeteners to reduce total sugars in a product).

The Occasional Treat

Finally, it is absurd to deny ourselves a treat. But we should now be aware of how we have insidiously come to accept many processed foods as being healthy such as corn chips, rice wrappers, fruits juices and pasta and to recommend minimize eating them and increase or substitute fresh foods. And the scary part is that eating these foods—even just a couple times a week—could up your chances of dying prematurely, according to a recent study.

How to Identify Ultra-Processed Foods

Read the nutrition label. If you see a long list of ingredients you don't recognize, chances are it's processed.

One of my colleagues even goes so far as to say (and the more I think about it the more I like it), "Just don't eat anything with a label on it or in a packet".

POISON: DO NOT EAT! – Well certainly minimise.

REFINED CARBS AND SIMPLE SUGARS (often called "added sugars")

Sugar: Table sugar/white sugar (aka sucrose; may be cane sugar or beet sugar)
Confectioner's sugar
Honey (Even though honey exists in nature and isn't refined, it is a pure sugar.)
Agave syrup
Corn syrup and high-fructose corn syrup
Brown sugar Molasses
Maple syrup Fructose
Brown rice syrup Maltose
Glucose syrup Tapioca syrup
Rice bran syrup Malt syrup

Fruit Juices except for lemon/lime juice. Most fruit juices require special equipment to produce in significant quantities.

All Kinds of Flour including wheat, oat, legume (pea and bean), rice, and corn flours. 100% stoneground, whole meal flours are less refined and not as unhealthy as other types of flours because they are not as finely ground and take longer to digest.

Instant/Refined Grains including instant hot cereals like instant oatmeal, white rice, polished rice, and instant rice

Dextran Sorghum Treacle Panela Saccharose Carob syrup
Dextrose, dextran, dextrin, maltodextrin Fruit juice concentrates

Refined Starches
such as corn starch, potato starch, modified food starch–essentially any powdered ingredient with the word "starch" in it

Soft Drinks / SodFoods High in Refined Carbs and Added Sugars
All desserts except whole fruit Ice cream, sherbet, frozen yogurt,
Most breads
Many crackers (100% stone-ground whole grain crackers are less refined)
Cookies; Cakes; Muffins; Pancakes; Waffles; Pies; Pastries; Candy; Chocolate (dark, milk and white). Baker's chocolate is unsweetened and is therefore an exception.
Breaded or battered foods
All doughs (phyllo, pie crust, etc)
Most cereals except for unsweetened, 100% whole grain cereals in which you can see the whole grains in their entirety with the naked eye (unsweetened muesli, rolled oats, or unsweetened puffed grain cereals are good examples)
Most pastas, noodles and couscous
Jelly (sugar-free varieties exist but it's much healthier to make your own with unsweetened gelatin and fresh fruit)

Jams and preserves Bagels
Pretzels
Pizza (flour in the dough)
Puddings and custards Corn chips
Caramel corn and kettle corn
Most granola bars, power bars, energy bars (unless sugar-free).
Rice wrappers
Tortillas (unless 100% stone- ground whole grain)
Most rice cakes and corn cakes (unless 100% whole grain)
Panko crumbs Croutons
Fried vegetable snacks like green beans and carrot chips (usually contain added dextrin) Ketchup
Honey mustard
Most barbecue sauces Check labels on salsa, tomato sauces, salad dressings and other jarred/canned sauces for sugar/sweeteners
Sweetened yogurts and other sweetened dairy products
Honey-roasted nuts
Sweetened sodas Chocolate milk (and other sweetened milks) Condensed milk
Hot cocoa
Most milk substitutes (almond milk, soy milk, oat milk, etc) because they usually have sugar added–read label first Sweet wines and liquors

CHAPTER 5

THE SOLUTION

The solution is to find an acceptable diet, that you like, that provides all the macro and micro-nutrients in the right ratios, in the right "doses", in the most biologically available form to facilitate absorption, metabolism and utilization by our bodies and brains. This, by far and away, is the Newtrition Micronutrient Diet.

Later in this book there is the 'History of Diets'. This shows 4,600 years of repeating fads and scams or odd diets which was, as one of my patients who visited one such Institute in California, akin to "eating the bottom of a parrots cage".

There is a strong trait, unmercifully also exploited by religions, for humans to want to be punished: If a medicine tastes vile 'it must be good' and the more odd or disciplined the diet, 'the better'.

The other scams, mostly for weight loss, are the incredible measuring, counting and ratios, all of which were to take the participating dupe's attention from the fact they were eating less.

Small Acceptable Beneficial Changes

Newtrition, however, while optimizing weight control, is for our *overall health.*

- It is simple, easy, available and acceptable to all from vegan to meat lover
- It has more evidenced benefits that any other diet in history
- It depends on a variety of fresh foods
- But, equally important, and a distinction Newtrition emphasizes, is what ***not*** to eat viz: Processed foods, sugar and salt.

To make the **Newtrition Diet** acceptable, to all and every one, the key is to *substitute* pleasant but proven beneficial foods for those that may be injurious, such as Olive Oil for butter, wholegrain bread for white bread, nuts or an apple for snacks rather than factory-made 'health' bars or cookies.

Vanderbilt University proposed that *'the idea is to not give up entirely foods that provide pleasure but aren't nutritious. Instead, the focus should be on lowering the portion of the "vice" foods and correspondingly raising the portion of a healthy food to replace it'.*[33] I have found, over 50 years of clinical practice, that reducing 'vice foods' such as sugar, salt, cream and sugary soft-drinks (sodas) by progressive small increments until the new taste becomes the established anticipated pleasure, that new minimal levels of 'vice' are achieved and the former levels become unacceptable. The patient most often wonders how they ever liked what they previously had.

Be that as it may we simply don't know all the answers as to what are bad or 'vice' foods. High cholesterol foods such as eggs and saturated fat, like the fat on a steak, were considered, until very recently, bad. Now we are not so sure. However, above all, common sense prevails. I do, however, think processed foods, with or without the incredible array of additives, are bad and there is very good evidence against them and very good evidence for the **Newtrition foods**.

Modern Life and Fast Food

Most of us these days are working harder, longer and the fast food meals and drive-thrus are much more convenient to most people, certainly those under 30, today.

Britons in 2006 spent more than £52 billion on food every year - and more than 90% of that money was spent on processed food. But the canning, freezing and dehydrating techniques used to process food destroy most of its flavor. During the past two decades the flavor industry's role in food production has become so influential that many children now like man-made, artificial flavors more than the real thing.

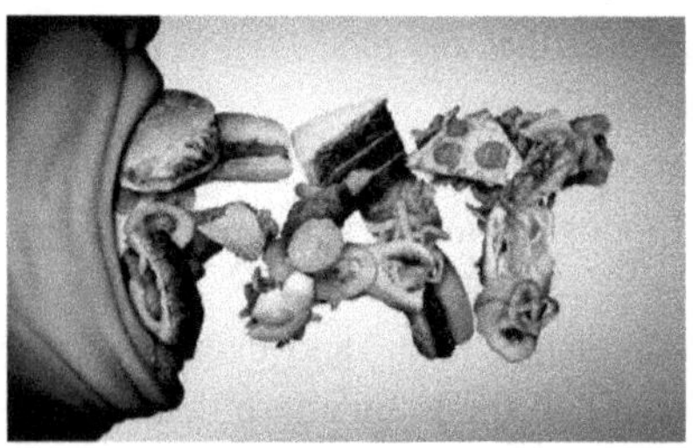 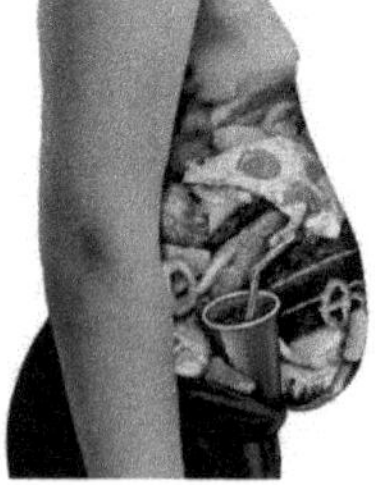

[33] Vanderbilt University. "Size matters when convincing your brain to eat healthier foods." ScienceDaily, 11 August 2014 <www.sciencedaily.com/releases/2014/08/140811180253.htm>

Strawberry Flavoring

It seems ridiculous but a sad fact that we seek strawberry flavoring made from some 59 chemicals when we could buy the actual strawberry. Here are the yummy chemical ingredients of just simple artificial strawberry flavoring:

amyl acetate, amyl butyrate, amyl valerate, anethol, anisyl formate, benzyl acetate, benzyl isobutyrate, butyric acid, cinnamyl isobutyrate, cinnamyl valerate, cognac essential oil, diacetyl, dipropyl ketone, ethyl butyrate, ethyl cinnamate, ethyl heptanoate, ethyl heptylate, ethyl lactate, ethyl methylphenylglycidate, ethyl nitrate, ethyl propionate, ethyl valerate, heliotropin, hydroxyphrenyl- 2-butanone (10% solution in alcohol), ionone, isobutyl anthranilate, isobutyl butyrate, lemon essential oil, maltol, 4-methylacetophenone, methyl anthranilate, methyl benzoate, methyl cinnamate, methyl heptine carbonate, methyl naphthyl ketone, methyl salicylate, mint essential oil, neroli essential oil, nerolin, neryl isobutyrate, orris butter, phenethyl alcohol, rose, rum ether, undecalactone, vanillin and solvent.

The mind boggles at to what the more complex packaged foods contain.

Thanks in large part to the marketing efforts of the fast food chains; Americans now drink about twice the amount of soft drinks as they did 30 years ago. In 1975, the typical American drank about 32 gallons (120 liters) of soft drinks a year. Today, the typical American drinks about 63 gallons (240 liters) of soft drinks a year. That's well over 500 cans of soft drink, per person, every year. Even toddlers are now drinking soft drinks. About 20% of American children between the ages of one and two drink soft drinks every day.[34]

Recent animal tests have linked inflammatory bowel disease (Ulcerative Colitis and Crohn's Disease) to the innocent sounding 'emulsifiers' to be found in nearly every manufactured creamy food.[35] They are preliminary animal tests but it does issue a wake-up call that we mostly don't know what we are eating when we buy junk or processed foods.

There are some 100,000 such chemicals in everyday use which have not undergone any rigorous testing: They are only withdrawn if and when they are found to cause harm. Leeching or even accidental spills into waterways of PCBs has caused falls in human sperm counts while English fish and Florida Alligators, turn into hermaphrodites.

---

[34] The Guardian Tuesday 25 April 2006

[35] Nature 2015. Study Links Common Food Additives to Crohn's Disease, Colitis. *Medscape*. Feb 25, 2015.

Eating a diet lacking in healthy foods and/or high in unhealthy foods was estimated to contribute to more than 400,000 deaths from heart and blood vessel diseases in the United States in 2015.

The Risks from Poor Diets30

The degrees to which dietary risk factors linked to cardiovascular disease deaths are :

1. low intake of nuts and seeds 11.6%
2. low intake of vegetables 11.5%
3. low intake of whole grains 10.4%
4. excess salt 9%

The Mediterranean Diet and Micro-nutrients

People on the Mediterranean Diet didn't get as many heart attacks or much cancer and lived longer. And so, the doctors and scientists started to look at whole foods again and discovered or re-discovered the world of Micro-chemicals. And the hunt was on. Only a few years ago there were very few of these micro-chemicals identified with, even now, only a hundred or so studied. In 2013 there were 4,000, when I first re-edited this book four years ago, in 2016, there were some 5,000 of just one plant sub-group and two years later in 2018, I read they now numbered over 6,000. Now in 2020 I read *"so far, about 10,000 phyto (plant)chemicals have been identified, and still a large percentage remains unknown".*

There are simply thousands and thousands of these phytos belonging to different groups that do everything from coloring your carrots yellow, your egg plants or aubergines purple, your strawberries red and blueberries blue to putting the tannin in your tea and chlorophyll to make plants green.

And as a result of long, high-quality medical trials and studies, certain foods, or rather *their combination*, have been found to confer profound health benefits. Overall, one such combination stands out, *by far and away*, as donating more benefits to our health, than any other:

Evidence and Corroboration

Research done by the Imperial College, London (published in February 2017) was a meta-analysis of *all available research in populations worldwide, included up to 2,000,000 people,* and assessed up to 43,000 cases of heart disease, 47,000 cases of stroke, 81,000 cases of cardiovascular disease, 112,000 cancer cases and 94,000 deaths...so it's a pretty impressive study!

It reported that just eating *more (800g/day)* of this one common food group, fruit and vegetables (FV) resulted in a:

- 4 per cent reduced risk in cancer risk
- 15 per cent reduction in the risk of premature death.
- 24 per cent reduced risk of heart disease
- 33 per cent reduced risk of stroke
- 28 per cent reduced risk of cardiovascular disease
- 13 per cent reduced risk of total cancer
- 31 per cent reduction in dying prematurely

This Study lumped Fruit and Vegetables (FV) as the same one group, but **Newtrition** separates these into two distinct groups to emphasize that we should eat more of each in our daily quota and increase both to 20%.

Superfoods

No specific food has been officially acknowledged by government or health authorities as providing a health benefit. No official definition of a "superfood" exists.

Be that as it may some foods have already been identified as being richer in these micronutrients and which donate greater benefits than others and Newtrition has identified these.

But, what *not* to eat is arguably just as important. My analogy is that 'breathing fresh air will not compensate if you smoke'.

CHAPTER 6

A BRIEF HISTORY of NUTRITION

- Obesity was a problem but not an epidemic (like today) in Roman times
- Henry Viii of England weighed 320 pounds (23 stone or 145 kg). Byron struggled with weight all his life.
- Daniel Lambert, Britain's fattest man in 1806 weighed 50st (700lb or 318 kg) but at December 2016 the world's fattest man, Juan Pedro Franco of Mexico, weighed 500kg (1,102lb).

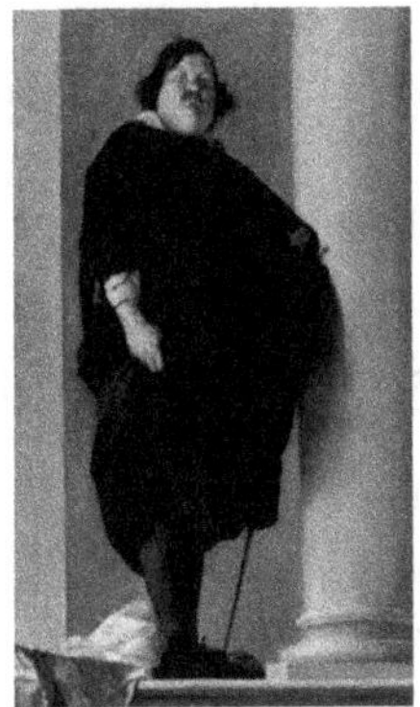

Tuscan General, 1645
Alessandro del Borro

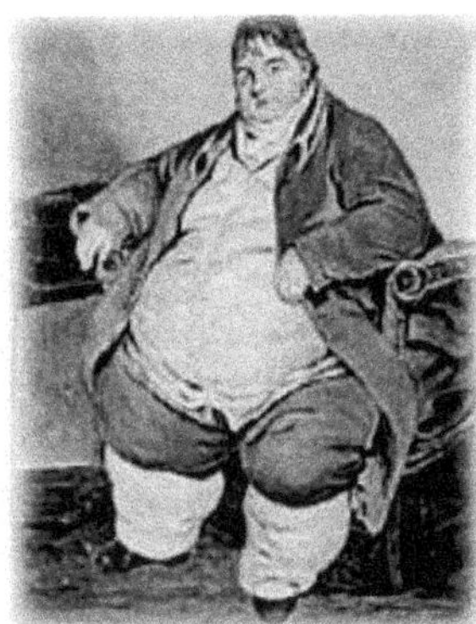

Daniel Lambert, 1806
Britain's fattest man

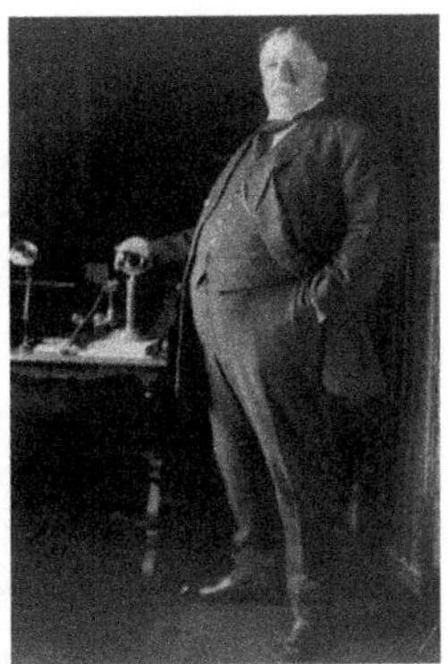

William Howard Taft, 1908
United States President

- Morbid obesity is a complex medical problem. The weight optimisation offered by Newtrition is only for those who were previously not fat but who have insidiously put on weight. However, even for those who are obese Newtrition is still the best diet.
- More sailors died from Scurvy (Vitamin C deficiency) than wars until very recently.
- ***Fats*** were the first to be identified as a separate group when Scheele, a Swedish chemist, discovered in 1779 that glycerol could be obtained from olive oil but it was not until 1815 that the French chemist Michel-Eugène Chevreul (1786–1889) demonstrated the chemical nature of fats and oils.
- ***Proteins*** were first described by the Dutch chemist Gerardus Johannes Mulder and named by the Swedish chemist Jöns Jacob Berzelius in 1838.

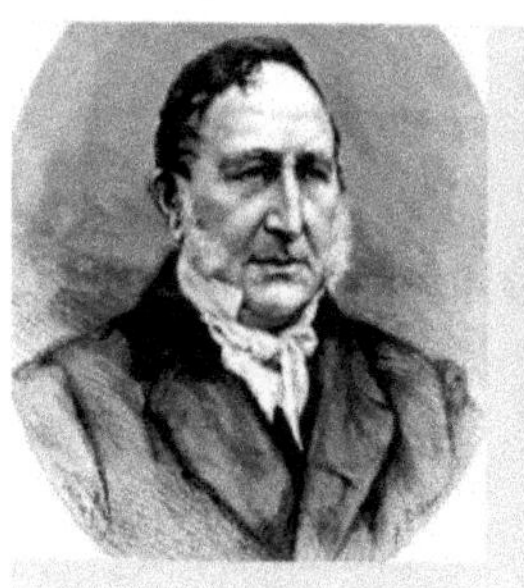

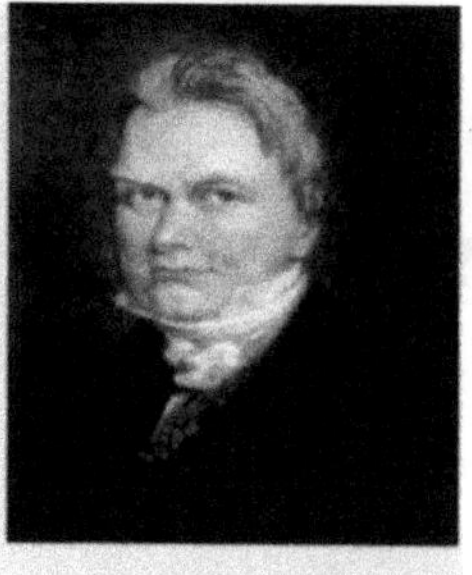

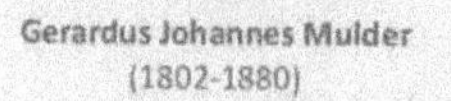

Gerardus Johannes Mulder (1802-1880)

Jöns Jacob Berzelius (1779-1848)

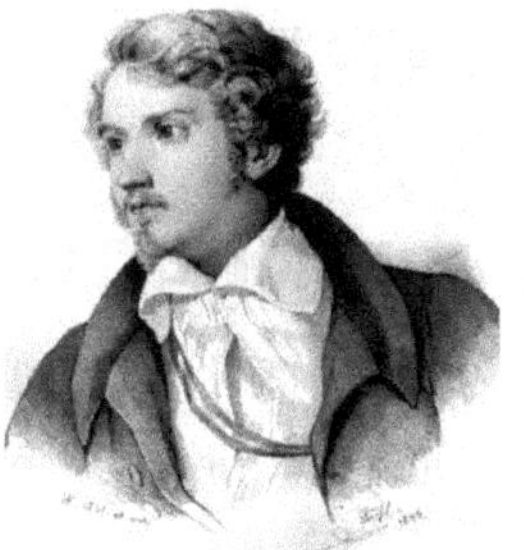

Justus von Liebig (1803 – 1873)

- In the mid-1800s, German chemist Justus von Liebig was one of the first to recognize that the body derived energy from the oxidation of foods we had just eaten. He declared that it was the burning of fats and carbohydrates that fueled this oxidation. To my research it would seem it was he who classified foods into three large groups (fat, protein and carbohydrates), and was the most influential person to establish the science of nutrition.
- The calorie used as the unit measure for food
- 1830s Body Mass Index (BMI) devised and adopted. There are arguably better measures (waist circumference)
- Micronutrients not recognized. Deficiency Diseases attributed to germs
- Gradual recognition that other components in our foods were necessary
- 1912 Funk coins the words "vital amine". Later shortened to Vitamin
- 1914 Dr Goldberg run out of town for suggesting the poor Southern Diet was causing the fatal epidemic of pellagra
- 60% of UK recruits in World War 1 were unfit mostly due to Rickets (vitamin D and Calcium)
- Progressive discoveries of Vitamins - up until 1948
- The dramatic response in patients who were vitamin deficient led to the (incorrect) beliefs that mega-vitamins and supplements are good and prevent other illnesses
- Minerals and other trace micronutrients identified as necessary but more to be discovered
- Vitamin obsession which persists to today
- World War 2 expedited the nutritional research and development of what a nation needed minimally to survive (and, in the UK, they were never healthier with such rationing).
- In 1940, rationing in the United Kingdom during World War 2 developed the first Recommended Dietary Allowances (RDAs) by the National Research Council. (EAR = Estimated Average Requirement).
- Oxford University closed down its nutrition department after World War 2 because the subject seemed to have been completed between 1912 and 1944

- These RDAs have recently been challenged
- 1950 Ancel Keys studies the Mediterranean Diet
- Cholesterol, especially LDL, associated with Heart Attacks
- 1960s, the study of obesity began in earnest, and body fat was defined as an organ, with its own hormones, receptors, genetics, and cellular biology rather than the passive store of energy it had been considered theretofore.[36]
- As the study of fat became an acceptable scientific pursuit, it began to unlock obesity's secrets, each of which, in turn, became the impetus for the growing 30 to 50 billion dollar slimming industry that exists today.
- 1972 North Karelia (Finland) reduces heart attack rate from the worst in the world to the best in Europe largely by lowering cholesterol with a Mediterranean type diet
- 1976 and 1989 The Nurses' Health Studies (Harvard) are long-term epidemiological studies conducted on women's health. The study followed 121,700 female registered nurses since 1976 and 116,000 female nurses since 1989 to assess risk factors for cancer and cardiovascular disease. The studies are among the largest investigations into risk factors for major chronic diseases in women ever conducted.
- Dietary Guidelines issued by most Western Countries
- On-going research especially into fats
- Processed foods need vitamins and minerals added thus ensuring their ongoing sales but at the same time causing the Diseases of Affluence
- 1980s: The more observant Doctors notice the general populace becoming overweight
- 1997 The global nature of the obesity epidemic formally recognized by the World Health Organization
- 1997 much to the delight of the Fast Food Industry, they found that 'consumers (had) dropped all pretence of wanting healthy food'.
- Research documents the emergence of the obesity epidemic among adolescents in the later half of the 1990s, and among young adults in 2000.[37]
- 2011 article in Journal of Nutrition concludes all/most Americans need supplements
- Rich nations undoing good nutrition by feeding on junk / process / fast foods and needing supplements
- Salt and sugar in excess identified as damaging
- Saturated fat does not elevate cholesterol - as Ancel Keys pointed out decades ago
- Move from nutrients (protein, carbs, fats) to whole food variety
- "The Micronutrient Revolution"

---

[36]Wood P.A. How Fat Works. Harvard University Press, Cambridge, MA2006

[37] Hedwig Lee University of North Carolina at Chapel Hill

Obesity

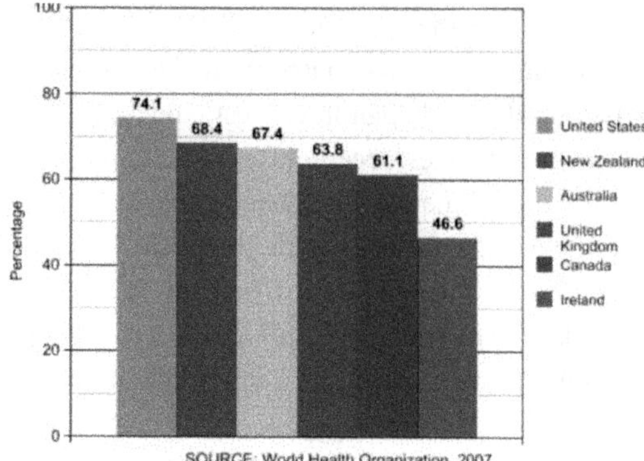
100
80
60
40
20
0
Percentage
74.1
68.4
67.4
63.8
61.1
46.6
United States
New Zealand
Australia
United Kingdom
Canada
Ireland
SOURCE: World Health Organization, 2007

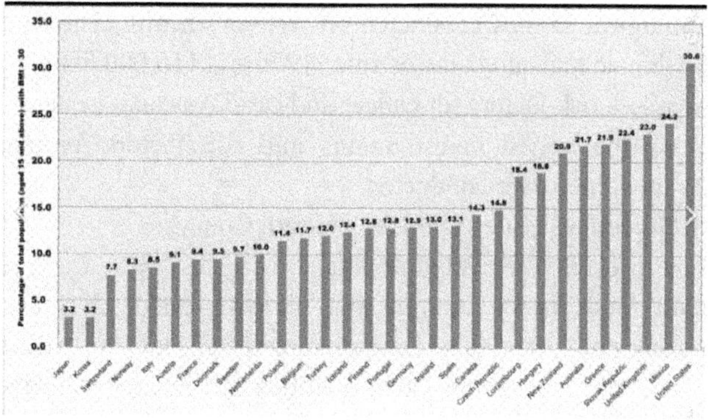
35.0
30.0
25.0
20.0
15.0
10.0
5.0
0.0
3.2
3.2
7.7
10.0
11.7
12.0
12.4
13.0
13.1
14.3
18.4
21.7
22.4
23.0
24.2

CHAPTER 6

THE BRIEF OUTLINE OF DIETS

I have split this History in to two

a) Brief outline, *as here*
b) Complete, for those interested, at the end of the book.

As can be seen in the full version at the end of the book, most of these diets are for losing weight. It is a fascinating romp with all the crazies, zanies, loonies, scam artists, con artists and gurus (which is maybe the collective name for them all) exploiting the vulnerable and the desperate and repeating every generation.

BRIEF OUTLINE: The 4,600 YEARS OF SCAMS and FADS
2,600BC The Daniel Diet (fasting)
500BC The Keto Diet
500BC Olympic Athlete Fad Diets
175BC The Cabbage and Urine Diet:
150BC Venus de Milo
300AD Fasting
600-1000AD Christian "holy anorexia."
1087 Liquid (Alcohol) Diet
1380 Catherine of Sienna self-induced fatal starvation.
1558: The first diet book
1614: "The Fruits, Herbs and Vegetables of Italy" today's "Mediterranean Diet."
17th Century Chocolate, Coffee, Tea and breaking the Vatican's fast
1724 Veganism
1816 The First Celeb Diet and the **Vinegar Diet.**
1825 Physiologie du gout (The Physiology of Taste) Low-carb diet.
Late 1820s The First Fad Diet.
1830 Tapeworms
1856 First Diet Diary
1863 Lo-Carb Diet
1863 Seventh Day Adventist Vegetarianism
1917 Breakfast becomes the Most Important Meal of The Day
1880 High fat, low carb diet
1885 No breakfast and Raw Food
1893: The first weight loss pill

Late 1800s: Arsenic Diet Pills
Early 1900s: The Tapeworm Diet
1895-1919: Fletcherism Diet 'Chew and spit'
1911 Hereward Carrington The Fasting Cure
1911 The Ketogenic diet
1914 The Sun-Kissed diet
1916 "Why be Fat?"
1917 Dr Lulu Hunt Peters "Diet and Health"
1918 Helena Rubenstein's "The Art of Beauty"
1920 The Hay Diet also known as The Food Combining Diet
1920's: Laxative Pills
1926 The "Inuit Diet"
1920s: Cereal, Bacon and Eggs for Breakfast
1925-9 The Cigarette Diet
1930: The first diet drink
1930s: Grapefruit Diet
1930: Dr Stoll's Diet Aid and liquid Diets
1939: Gaylord Hauser's Eat and Grow Beautiful
1939: The Rice Diet Duke University:
1946: "Diet the ice-cream way
1950s: The Cabbage Soup Diet
1950s: Mediterranean Diet
1950s: The Sugar Diet
1952 The Tuna Round the Clock Diet
1954: Tapeworm Diet
1957: Pray Your Weight Away
1958: Dr Jarvis The Alkaline Diet
1960: The Zen Macrobiotic Diet
1961: It's A Sin to Be Fat
1960s: Calories Don't Count -The Vegetable Oil Diet.
1963: Weight Watchers
1964: The Drinking Man's Diet
1968: The Sexy Pineapple Diet1970s: HCG Diet
1970 The Sleeping Beauty Diet
1970s: Ayds
1972: Nutrisystem Low-carbs come into full swing
1973 The Beautiful People's Diet Book
1975 The Cookie Diet
1975 The Stone Age Diet (East African, Inuit and Paleo Diets)
1975 Guzzle milk
1976 The Prolin Diet or Last Chance Diet.
1976 The Master Cleanser
1977 Slim Fast

1977 Help Lord! The Devil Wants Me Fat
1978 The Scarsdale Diet
1979: Dexatrim
1981: The Beverly Hills Diet
1981: The Cambridge Diet
1982: The F Plan
1982: The aerobics craze
1983: Jazzercise
1983: Jenny Craig
1985: Seattle Sutton's Healthy Eating
1985: Fit for Life
1985: The Caveman Diet aka Paleo
1986: The Rotation Diet
1987: Elizabeth Takes Off
1988: Oprah's Liquid Diet
1990s - The Low Fat Diet
1994: The Guide to Nutrition Labelling and Education Act (USA)
1995: The Zone Diet
1995 Diet Pills
1997: Eat Right for Your Type, Blood Type diet
1997: Stacker 2
2000s: The Dukan diet
2002: The Paleo Diet
2002: Eat what Jesus ate
2003: South Beach Diet
2004 Gluten Free Diet
2004: Ephedra Banned
2004: The Biggest Loser
2006: F2
2006: Master Cleanse
2007: Alli
2007: Zantrex
2009: Whole 30
2010s: The Juice Cleanse
2010: The Air Diet
2011: The HCG Diet
2012: Fasting Diets
And then there's
Optavia, Volumetrics, Flexitarian, Traditional Asian, Spark People, HMR, Flat Belly, Engine 2, South Beach, Abs, Eco-Atkins, Aitkins 40, Macrobiotic, Medifast, Supercharged Hormone, Body Reset, Whole 30, The Mono, Pizza (I kid you not), Wild, Disassociated, Military, The Taco (I kid you not again)

and the Golo Diets (to name but a few).
And there will be 100 "new" ones, in name only, on the Internet. Just sign up and pay.

CHAPTER 8

THE GOOD, THE BAD, THE UGLY, THE MAD

WELLNESS vs GOOD HEALTH

"It's funny how Gwyneth Paltrow rarely suggests how to hit a cross-court topspin backhand, Elon Musk doesn't tend to tweet about giving pathos to a portrayal of Richard III, and I'm pretty sure Novak Djokovic hasn't espoused his views about payload distribution for a geosynchronous satellite launch. But yet they all seemed to understand medicine well enough to inform millions of people".[38]

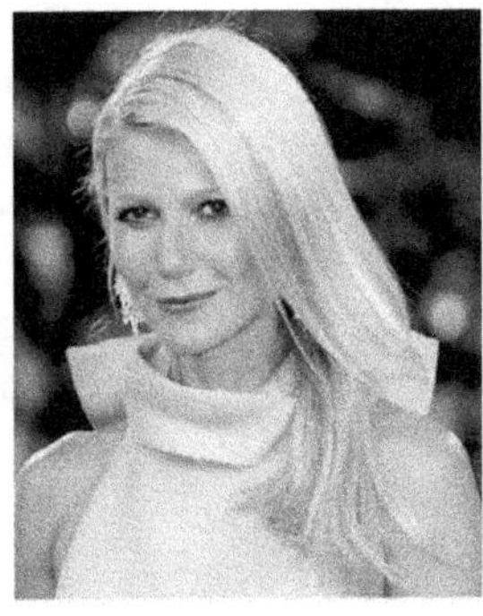
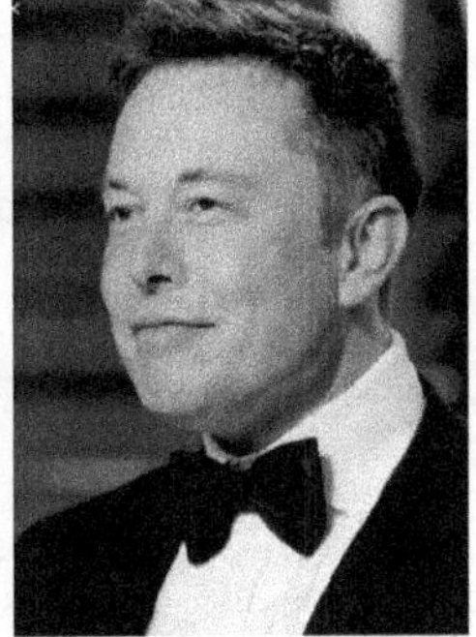
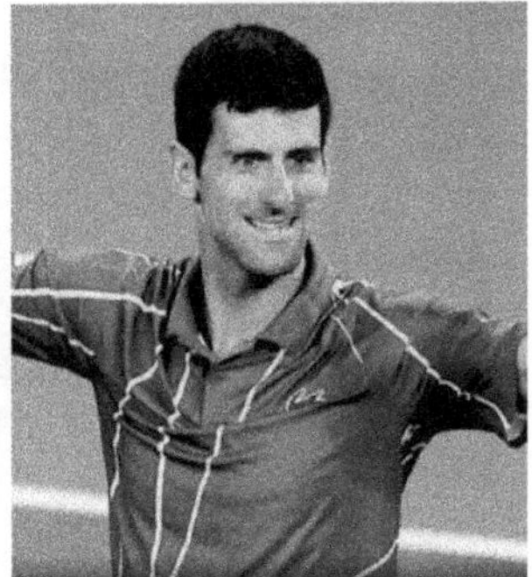

"It is incredible when you became a famous celebrity how you are asked your opinion on matters about which you have absolutely no knowledge and no qualifications. But that's not the incredible part: The incredible part is that you give it!" - *Marlon Brando*

In 1999, two psychologists wrote a seminal paper entitled "Unskilled and Unaware of It" finding that the people who are the most incompetent (their word) believe they know much more than they do and their "incompetence robs them of the ability to realize it." Named after them it is known as the Dunning-Kruger effect.

[38] Rohin Francis, MBBS, Intervention Cardiologist, London

The un-precedented prosperity and exponential technical advances since World War 2, have seen an upwardly mobile migration such that practically anyone without any qualifications whatsoever, can become an "Influencer" and gain a huge following on Twitter, Facebook or some-such. The door has now been opened not only for the unqualified, Gurus, Healers, Snake-oil-Medicine Man, Charlatans and Mountebanks, who have been around as long as humanity, but recently the Self-help authors and now the Celebs, Bloggers and Influencers.

There is now no need to study – just google it – or consult the Internet. The downside is that there is much misinformation, and most is exploitive.

Their followers are identified as "Post-Millennial Narcissists" whose new fad catch-phrase is "Wellness" which seems to have replaced the former generations' "holistic" (which was actually a legitimate medical word until adopted).

This wellness industry is reputedly now worth $4.2 trillion world-wide with their 'recommendations' unusual and ever-more increasingly odd, but the competition is now so fierce that it has now become dangerous as in "extreme wellness" with extravagances of physical endurance, odd diets and supplement scams.

- The jade vagina eggs of Gwyneth Paltrow's Goop brand are now a notorious exposed scam

- Nootropics ('natural' or man-made supplements that are professed to boost memory and mental focus)

- Sweat lodges of hours in extremely hot enclosed spaces 'to purify group bodies and minds'

- Brrrn, the 'world's first cool-temperature fitness studio' in New York where people exercise in freezing conditions, so they lose more calories during a workout as the body shivers

- Flatline UK claims its workout are the hardest and most dangerous fitness class in the world with 45 minutes of high-intensity exercises, such as hoisting 60kg weights and sprinting for 45 metres – all in a 12 kg weighted vest with just 15-second breaks. Paramedics are on hand during classes, and participants are required to sign a death waiver before getting started.

- Raw water, a derivative of the raw-food movement, recommends consuming water from springs or rivers without it being processed; devotees believe it is free of industrial toxins and rich in healthy microbes, which improve gut health. Health experts have stressed how most such water is contaminated from bird or animal dung with harmful bacteria, parasites and pesticides. But it's becoming more and more popular, with 2.5 gallons of untreated water costing $36.99 in the USA.

- Some if not all of these seize on an element of truth; saunas are beneficial, cold showers maybe, grass fed beef preferable and pure water mandatory, but they get it dreadfully wrong as they exploit their lemming followers with progressively bizarre and increasingly dangerous recommendations.

- And on and on and on, as these oh so willingly duped customers seek more and more extreme "wellness" fads to compensate for obvious personality problems and lack of knowledge.

- Also, of concern, are the extreme behaviours under the guise of sports, getting fit or conditioning. It has recently been found that fatalities among high school and college football athletes did not occur while playing the game of football, but rather during conditioning sessions, often associated with irrationally intense workouts, overexertion or punishment drills required by coaches and team staff.

- I thought the Covid-19 pandemic may make these opportunists face their scams but it has only enthused them. There are 126 scams already listed on Wikiepedia.

- A TV 'My Kitchen Rules' cook/judge spruiked his $15,000 BioCharger "light machine" could treat the "Wuhan coronavirus" claiming "is a pretty amazing tool" that will "take me an hour or two to explain it" with "a thousand different recipes and a couple on there for Wuhan coronavirus". The BioCharger is billed as a "hybrid subtle energy revitalisation platform" that uses "four transmitted energies" to "stimulate and invigorate the entire body to optimise and improve potential health, wellness, and athletic performance" but has been labelled as just a 'glorified plasma lamp'. Maybe he should sell it on Goop. It looks as if it will also make smoothies. But that's OK as in

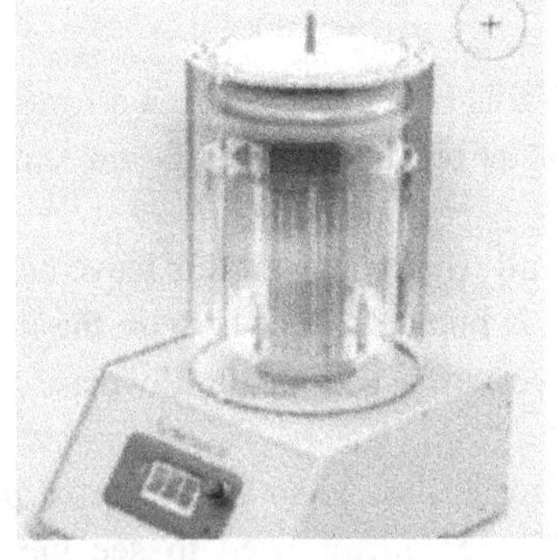

2015 he authored a paleo cookbook which featured a recipe for a breastmilk replacement for babies made from chicken livers and bone broth which the Public Health Association said could be fatal.

- Which one of the above will get the Nobel Prize for Medicine

There is obviously a great deal of money to be made in this Wellness World: According to Wikipedia: "Goop, and by extension Paltrow, have drawn criticism by showcasing expensive products and promoting medically and scientifically impossible treatments, many of which have harmful consequences. The controversies have included vaginal steaming, the use of jade eggs, a dangerous coffee enema device, and "Body Vibes", wearable stickers that were claimed to "rebalance the energy frequency in our bodies" and which Goop falsely claimed were made of a NASA-developed material. Goop settled a lawsuit regarding the health claims it made over the jade eggs. Jill Avery, a brand analyst, has noted how Goop's response to criticisms seems designed to "strengthen their brand and draw their customers closer", noting Goop's references to feminism, traditional Asian medicines and Eastern philosophies, and anti-establishment politics to do so.

On January 27, 2020, Truth in Advertising watchdog (TINA.org) filed a complaint with the district attorneys of California alleging that Goop has continued to engage in deceptive marketing alleging that Goop claims their products are "clinically-proven" to treat such symptoms as anxiety, depression, OCD and more".

"I know some people that, through that energetical (sic) transformation, through the power of prayer, through the power of gratitude, they manage to turn the most toxic food or the most polluted water, into the most healing water. Because water reacts and scientists have proven that, that molecules in the water react to our emotions, to what is being said". - Novak Djokovic

If this is the case, there's a fortune to be made turning these people into cholera water purifiers. Wow! Beam 'em up, Scotty! Let's go!

And where does all this leave us? There is a great demand for health advice, and it is human nature to seek the miracle cure. There is also a growing distrust of Western Medicine, until we are seriously ill, that is.

I remember when I first started practice and I was annoyed when one patient of another doctor used to see me when his usual doctor had gone home. But, unusually, this time he came and saw me in the middle of the day so, confused, I asked him why he had not gone and seen his usual doctor? He answered, "Aw gees, Doc, *I'm really sick this time!"*

And so, the Wellness Industry is arguably a diversion for such people and real doctors are reserved for when we are "really sick". Why even Novak had to get surgery when his Faith Healing failed.

For goodness sakes you should ensure your information and advice it is evidenced and the best available. To live longest healthiest, it is imperative we access the best information, but also, increasingly important, is to identify the silly, the dubious and the absurd which, due to our prosperity and the Internet, get more coverage while expert advice has been relegated to "if and only and when" we are seriously ill.

The latest short-term fad replaces the previous short-term fad. Religious loonies are cloning – they even look like us. And the various fad diets are just recycled after they have been forgotten. There is nothing new when it comes to fads. The Mediterranean Diet which forms the basis of this Newtrition Diet has been accredited by qualified experts as the best diet for the past number of years and is to be recommended above all.

CHAPTER 9

BIAS, MISINFORMATION, FAKE NEWS, RELIGIOUS ZEALOTS and VEGANMANIA

Introduction

This has nothing to do with Newtrition's dietary advice per se and not necessary if you just want to follow its nutritional recommendations.

And so, I will just outline the problems here, and if anyone wants to delve into the rather amazing details, I append the full chapter at the end. (It's really worth a read).

The problem is that there is a great deal of increasing nutritional bias, misinformation and manipulation as to nutritional advice and not just from the unqualified wellness industry but from formerly respected University or Nutrition Organizations, some of whom seem to have been infiltrated by the Vegan Lobby.

And this calls into question the validity of their findings let alone their recommendations. Cognitive bias in clinical medicine is increasingly recognized as an important source of medical error,[39] but it is not so easily recognized when applied to nutrition.

For every research paper there seems and immediate counter-claim: Milk good, milk bad; Plants good, meat bad; Eggs good, eggs bad; Saturated fat bad, saturated fat not bad; Carbs good, fat bad or Fat good, carbs bad; Breakfast important, breakfast not necessary, and so on, such that confusion reigns!

Where oh where is the truth, common sense and balance?

There are four major participations leading to bias in nutrition

1. Individual aggrandizement
2. Herd mentality
3. Religious dogma
4. Vested Interests

---

[39] J R Coll Physicians Edinb 2018; 48: 225-232

1. Individual aggrandizement

Researchers are under enormous pressure to churn out papers, "Publish or Perish".

Every year there are some two to three million papers / articles published with only about 1,400 retracted. This does not vouch well for the quality of the papers or the peer journal reviews. Thousands of scientists publish a paper every five days.

Researchers can't get a job if they don't have papers and a record of scholarship. This has led to data dredging, or p-hacking, the process of running exhaustive analyses on data sets to tease out small signals that might otherwise be unremarkable.

When such an interesting topic arises the derived article then creates a hypothesis to support whatever cherry-picked findings seem interesting.

This is the antithesis of what scientific method should be.

This reached its climax in 2018 when the "JAMA Network Retracts 6 Articles That Included Dr. Brian Wansink as Author" because of questions about their "scientific validity." Seven of his other papers had previously been retracted for similar reasons.

Wansink had been one of the most respected food researchers in America founding the Food and Brand Lab at Cornell University. On Sept. 20, the university announced that a yearlong investigation had found that he committed "academic misconduct in his research and scholarship, including misreporting of research data," and that he had tendered his resignation.

The more controversial or exaggerated the claims by an article or its title, the better as it will then attract media attention, the researcher gets press, funds and jobs follow. But many reporters inflame the headlines so as their articles get lots of clicks.

2. Herd Mentality

As reported in the BMJ (2nd May 2020) 'Lessons from the Covid-19 Pandemic':

"Inevitably perhaps, people are using aspects of the covid-19 pandemic to argue in support of something they already believed in. Vegetarians point to the origin of the virus to show the harms of eating meat. Libertarians fear that the pandemic is herding us towards a police state. Religious leaders see it as a timely reminder of eternal truths. Sometimes the evidence points both ways (*https://www.spectator.co.uk/article/we-re-all-guilty-of-recruiting-this-virus-to-our-cause*). Supporters of the NHS think the pandemic shows the value of socialised medicine. Detractors, on the other hand, say that it reveals a monolithic organization unable to react fast enough to avoid a population lock down".

People are attracted to those of like minds and so are researchers and if not, the Head of the Department soon makes it clear, "My way or the Highway", and so, one way or the other a unified approach is the result. Over the decades I have noticed how the Harvard T.H. Chan School of Public Health has become progressively vegetarian, anti-meat and then vegan. The end result (so far) was a ludicrous biased claim to "Save the Planet" at the Lancet-EAT Commission in 2019, which was later assessed in the light of cold day as "science fiction".

3. Religious Dogma

The Seventh Day Adventist Church insists it is their religious duty to spread the word about veganism. They have infiltrated nearly every nutritional organization and, by funding them, "persuaded" them to promote their message. They are incredibly aggressive, nearly ruining one surgeon's life, and take no prisoners while promoting their business interests.

4. Vested Interests

There are very, very many vested interests urging us what to eat. These include the Fast Food Industry, the Farmers Organizations, Nutrition Researchers, the Dietetics Organizations, Religious Zealots, Self-Appointed Gurus, Faddists, Loonies and the Frankly Strange.

There would also seem to be a very well organised ant-meat lobby such that when a pro-meat article, still under embargo, was about to be published in the prestigious Annals of Internal Medicine, the Editor received some 2,000 emails of complaint within 30 minutes. And this is not the only such case.

However, be reassured Newtrition has no Personal Aggrandisement, Herd Mentality, Religious Dogma or Vested Interests.

It is, so it would seem, one of the few sources of the best, unbiased information.

PART B

The EVIDENCE

How do we know what is the best food and diet

CHAPTER 10

BENEFITS: NEWTRITION MICRONUTRIENT DIET

1. **Improved All-Cause Mortality**
2. **Less Heart Attacks and Strokes**
3. **Prevention of Cardiovascular Disease**
4. **Reduced Deaths in Patients with CVD**
5. **Improved Post Heart Attack Survival**
6. **Lower Inflammatory & Coagulation Markers, raised HDL & lowered Triglycerides and BP**
7. **Lower Cholesterol & improved artery lining in men**
8. **Lipoprotein oxidation was reduced and lipid (LDL) fell**
9. **Metabolic Syndrome halved**
10. **Slower Aging**
11. **Long Lasting Benefits**
12. **Less Total Cancer**
13. **Less Uterine Cancer**
14. **Less Breast Cancer Risk**
15. **Less Colorectal Cancer**
16. **Less Prostate cancer**
17. **Less Diabetes**
18. **Less Age-Related Macular Degeneration (Blindness)**
19. **Brain Health and Protection**
20. **Less Alzheimer's**
21. **Less Depression**
22. **More Aged Physical Independence**
23. **Reduced Hip Fracture Risk in Women**
24. **Reduced Risk for Kidney Stones**
25. **Improved Survival of the elderly**
26. **Less Chronic Obstructive Pulmonary Disease**
27. **Reduced Apnoea-Hypopnoea Index**
28. **Improvement of erectile dysfunction.**
29. **Improved HDL**
30. **Further risk reduction: Cancer, CVD, Premature Death**
31. **Improved Memory**
32. **Bigger Brain**
33. **Less Gout**
34. **Less Asthma**
35. **Less Allergies**
36. **Improved Gut Microbiome**
37. **Promotes gut bacteria linked to 'healthy aging'**
38. **Improved bone density and less fractures in post-menopausal women**
39. **Improved IVF Results**
40. **More Long-Term Benefits**

1. Improved All-Cause Mortality

EPIC is the largest prospective cohort (similar people) study worldwide, with more than 521,000 research participants followed for almost 15 years. It found that closer adherence to this diet is associated with *reduced overall mortality as well as incidence of and mortality from cardiovascular diseases and cancer*. In a paper studying more than 70, 000 elderly men and women from nine European countries, it was shown that adherence to the Mediterranean diet can improve survival in this vulnerable group.[40] A 14-year follow-up study of almost 1000 adults aged 65 or over who participated in the British Diet and Nutrition Survey in 1994/95 concluded that the Mediterranean diet was inversely associated with All-Cause Mortality. The Moli-Sani study reported a 37% reduction in All-Cause Mortality.[41]

2. Less Heart Attacks and Strokes

A more recent PREDIMED study was stopped at 4.8 years because the benefits were so obvious and found persons at high cardiovascular risk, a Mediterranean Diet supplemented with extra-virgin olive oil and/or nuts reduced the incidence of major cardiovascular events.[42]

Analysis of 451,256 Europeans found the most pro-vegetarian style diets (70% of food coming from plant sources) had a 20% lower risk of dying from cardiovascular disease. Instead of drastic avoidance of animal foods, substituting some of the meat with plant sources may be a very simple way to lower cardiovascular mortality.[43]

Further. adults who closely followed the Mediterranean diet were 47% less likely to develop heart disease over a 10-year period compared to similar adults who did not closely follow the diet in a study of more than 2,500 Greek adults, ages 18 to 89 from 2001 to 2012. This difference was independent of other heart disease risk factors including age, gender, family history, education level, body mass index, smoking habits, hypertension, diabetes and high cholesterol.[44]

---

[40] Modified Mediterranean diet and survival: EPIC-elderly prospective cohort study. BMJ. 2005 Apr 30;330(7498):991.

[41] The observational Moli-sani study presented at ESC Congress 2016

[42] N Engl J Med 2013;368:1279-90 DOI: 10.1056/NEJMoa1200303

[43] American Heart Association. "Semi-veggie diet effectively lowers heart disease, stroke risk." ScienceDaily. ScienceDaily, 5 March 2015. <www.sciencedaily.com/releases/2015/03/150305110433.htm>.

[44] American College of Cardiology. "Mediterranean diet cuts heart disease risk by nearly half." ScienceDaily. ScienceDaily, 4 March 2015. <www.sciencedaily.com/releases/2015/03/150304190222.htm>.

3. Prevention of Cardiovascular Disease

Healthy individuals following this diet in a 12 year prospective UK study lowered their risk for both cardiovascular events and mortality, and the results were stronger in those who were more diligent. Almost 4% of all new cardiovascular cases and 12.5% of all cardiac-related deaths could be avoided if the population adhered to the Mediterranean diet.[45]

4. Reduced Deaths in Patients with Cardiovascular Disease and Lower All-Cause Mortality

21% reduced risk of death in patients with cardiovascular disease (CAD and stroke and all-cause mortality was 37% lower in those who had a higher adherence to the diet (score 6-9) compared to those who didn't (score 0-3) (taking a statin reduces mortality by around 25%).[46]

5. Improved Post Heart Attack Survival

The Lyon Heart Study (the Lancet in 1995) focused on patients who had sustained a heart attack. Those then adopting this Mediterranean Diet had a 76% less recurrence compared with those who didn't. This was a most influential trial.

6. Lower Inflammatory & Coagulation Markers, raised HDL and lowered Triglycerides and BP

Adherence lowers Inflammatory & Coagulation Markers, raised HDL and lowered Triglycerides and BP.[47]

7. Lower Cholesterol & improved artery (endothelial) lining function in high cholesterol men.[48]

8. Lipoprotein oxidation was reduced and lipid (LDL) fell29

---

[45] *BMC Med.* Published online September 29, 2016.
[46] The observational Moli-sani study presented at ESC Congress 2016
[47] J A Col Cardiol 2004;44:152-58
[48] Ann Int Med 2001;134:1115-19

9. Metabolic Syndrome halved

Metabolic Syndrome patients who had the Mediterranean Diet for 2 years had less than half its features compared to the control group.[49]

10. Slower Aging: Longer Telomeres

Greater adherence to the Mediterranean diet has been associated with greater telomere length, a biomarker of slower ageing. A pro-vegetarian diet with a higher proportion of plant-based compared to animal-based foods is linked to lower risks of dying from heart disease and stroke.[50]

11. Long Lasting Benefits

The health benefits of switching to a Mediterranean style diet for just eight weeks can still be seen a year after stopping the regime.[51] After one year, the prevalence of metabolic syndrome decreased 13.7% without changes in exercise, calorie expenditure, and weight.[52]

12. Less Total Cancer

4% reduction[53]

13. Less Uterine Cancer

Women who adhered to the Mediterranean diet most closely by eating between seven and nine of the beneficial food groups lowered their risk of womb cancer by more than half (57%). Those who stuck to six elements of the diet's components reduced their risk of womb cancer by 46% and those who stuck to five reduced their risk by a third (34%). But those women whose diet included fewer than five of the components did not lower their risk of womb cancer significantly.[54]

---

[49] JAMA 2004;292:1440-46

[50] American Heart Association EPI/Lifestyle 2015 meeting.

[51]. Long-term effects of an exercise and Mediterranean diet intervention in the vascular function of an older, healthy population. *Microvascular Research*, 2014; 95: 103 DOI: 10.1016/j.mvr.2014.07.015

[52] *Arch Intern Med.* 2008;168:2449-2458.

[53] *Ann Intern Med.* Published online July 18, 2016

[54]. Mediterranean diet and risk of endometrial cancer: a pooled analysis of three italian case-control studies. *British Journal of Cancer*, 2015; 112 (11): 1816 DOI: 10.1038/bjc.2015.153

14. Less Breast Cancer Risk

Women showed a 68 percent relatively lower risk of malignant breast cancer with the Mediterranean diet supplemented with extra virgin olive oil [EVOO] or nuts compared with a low-fat diet.[55]

Reduce risk by 40% for estrogen-receptor-negative breast cancer which has the highest risk of death.[56]

15. Less Colorectal Cancer[57]

By 9%.

16. Less Prostate cancer

Five servings a week of any type of nuts, including peanuts, cuts death from prostate cancer by 34%.[58]

17. Less Diabetes[59]

Less Age-Related Loss of Eyesight Macular Degeneration -

18. AMD (Blindness)[60]

People who closely follow the Mediterranean diet – especially by eating fruit – may be more than a third less likely to develop age-related macular degeneration.

19. Brain Health and Protection

The human brain needs key nutrients, such as polyunsaturated fatty acids Omega-3, essential amino acids, B-group vitamins (B12 and folate), vitamin D and minerals like zinc, magnesium and iron. A balanced and high-quality diet, such

---

[55] Mediterranean Diet and Invasive Breast Cancer Risk Among Women at High Cardiovascular Risk in the PREDIMED Trial. *JAMA Internal Medicine*, 2015; 1 DOI: 10.1001/jamainternmed.2015.4838
[56] Mediterranean diet adherence and risk of postmenopausal breast cancer: results of a cohort study and meta-analysis. International Journal of Cancer, First published: 5 March 2017, DOI: 10.1002/ijc.30654View/save citation
[57] *Ann Intern Med.* Published online July 18, 2016
[58] Harvard Medical School Study, British Journal of Cancer June 2016.
[59] *Ann Intern Med.* Published online July 18, 2016
[60] American Academy of Ophthalmology (AAO). "Fruit-rich Mediterranean diet with antioxidants may cut age-related macular degeneration risk by more than a third." Presented 17 October 2016.

as the Mediterranean, provides all of these.[61] Cognitively healthy old adults who stuck to a Mediterranean diet, the brain's aging process appeared to be slowed down by up to five years.[62]

Mediterranean dieters did not lose brain volume as fast as others.[63]

A Mayo Clinic Study of Aging suggests that eating a Mediterranean-style diet is linked not only to improved cognitive function but also to increased cortical thickness in certain brain lobes. Those with a higher consumption of fish or legumes also had larger cortical thickness. But those who consumed large amounts of carbohydrates and sugar had lower cortical thickness.[64]

Flavonols. Blueberries: In the Nurses' Health Study a half a cup of blueberries two to three times a week was shown to delay the onset of cognitive decline Dark cocoa powder may also be effective.[65]

By contrast a junk food diet is associated with cognitive impairment.

20. Less Alzheimer's

The evidence shows that fruits, vegetables, grains, low-fat dairy products, legumes, and fish are associated with reduced risk of Alzheimer's disease. Whereas meat, sweets and high-fat dairy products that characterize a Western Diet are associated with increased risk. Alzheimer's disease is the most common type of dementia and rates are rising worldwide. [66]

21. Less Depression

Studies have linked the Mediterranean diet with advantageous effects on neurologic and mental health. Adults who followed the Mediterranean dietary pattern the closest over 4.4 years had a significantly reduced risk of developing

---

[61] Nutritional medicine as mainstream in psychiatry. *The Lancet Psychiatry*, 2015; 2 (3): 271 DOI: 10.1016/S2215-0366(14)00051-0

[62] *Neurology* Source Reference: *Gu Y "Mediterranean diet and brain structure in a multiethnic elderly cohort" Neurology 2015; 85: 1-8.*

[63] *Neurology* 2015 Oct 21

[64] *Alzheimers Dement.* Published online July 25, 2016.

[65] Dietary intakes of berries and flavonoids in relation to cognitive decline. Ann Neurol. 2012;72:135-143. Abstract

[66]Using Multicountry Ecological and Observational Studies to Determine Dietary Risk Factors for Alzheimer's Disease.*Journal of the American College of Nutrition*, 2016; 35 (5): 476 DOI: 10.1080/07315724.2016.1161566

depression (40%-60%).[67] Also, a 2014 meta-analysis[68] found that 47% of the randomized controlled trials included reported improved depression outcomes with dietary interventions, levels comparable to those of drug trials.

22. More Aged Physical Independence

The Nurse's Health Study of 54,762 American Nurses studied for 30 years found those who ate lots of nuts, especially walnuts, vegetables and fruits especially oranges, apples, pears and leafy lettuce and avoided cakes, biscuits and take-outs were more physically independent as they aged.[69] (While not strictly the Mediterranean Diet the basics are there).

23. Reduced Hip Fracture Risk in Women[70]

In "The Women's Health Initiative" study over 90,000 postmenopausal women aged 50 to 79 years at 40 US clinical centers were enrolled. Women in the highest quintile for Mediterranean diet adherence had a lower risk for hip fractures over a follow-up period of about 16 years.[71]

24. Reduced risk for Kidney Stones[72]

This was a study based on the DASH Diet.[73]

25. Improved Survival of the elderly[74]

EPIC is the largest prospective cohort worldwide, with more than 521, 000 research participants followed for almost 15 years.

---

[67] Association of the Mediterranean dietary pattern with the incidence of depression: the Seguimiento Universidad de Navarra/University of Navarra follow-up (SUN) cohort. Arch Gen Psychiatry. 2009;66:1090-1098. Abstract

[68] The impact of whole-of-diet interventions on depression and anxiety: a systematic review of randomised controlled trials. Public Health Nutr. 2014 Dec 3:1-20.

[69] Nurse's Health Study, The Journal of Nutrition, 2016

[70] *JAMA Intern Med.* 2016;176(5):652-653. doi:10.1001/jamainternmed.2016.0494

[71] *JAMA Intern Med.* Published online March 28, 2016

[72] JAMA Intern Med. 2016;176(5):652-653. doi:10.1001/jamainternmed.2016.0494

[73] DASH-Style Diet Associates with Reduced Risk for Kidney Stones. doi: 10.1681/ASN.2009030276 JASN October 1, 2009 vol. 20 no. 10 2253-2259

[74] Modified Mediterranean diet and survival: EPIC-elderly prospective cohort study. BMJ. 2005 Apr 30;330(7498):991.

Less Chronic Obstructive Pulmonary Disease

26. Reduced Apnoea-Hypopnoea Index

27. Improvement of erectile dysfunction.75

28. Improved HDL76

A Mediterranean diet, particularly when enriched with virgin olive oil, appears to improve the function of high-density lipoprotein, the so-called good cholesterol, in patients at high risk for heart disease. A Mediterranean diet rich in virgin olive oil may help the body remove excess cholesterol from arteries, serve as an antioxidant and keep blood vessels open -- all of which are known to reduce cardiovascular risk.

29. Increased Consumption Fruit & Veg: Imperial College[77]

Reduced Risk by

4% cancer
15% premature death.
24% heart disease
33% stroke
28% cardiovascular disease
13% total cancer
31% in dying prematurely

30. Better Memory[78]

The Mediterranean Diet (MD) improved attention, memory, and language. Memory, in particular, was positively affected including improvements in delayed recognition, long-term, and working memory, executive function, and visual constructs. A study evaluated all the available papers between 2000-2015 that

---

[75] J Sex Med. 2010 Jul;7(7):2338-45. doi: 10.1111/j.1743-6109.2010.01842.x. Epub 2010 May 4.
[76] Mediterranean Diet Improves High-Density Lipoprotein Function in High-Cardiovascular-Risk IndividualsClinical Perspective. Circulation, 2017; 135 (7): 633 DOI: 10.1161/CIRCULATIONAHA.116.023712
[77] Int J Epidemiol dyw319. DOI: https://doi.org/10.1093/ije/dyw319
[78] Adherence to a Mediterranean-Style Diet and Effects on Cognition in Adults: A Qualitative Evaluation and Systematic Review of Longitudinal and Prospective Trials. Frontiers in Nutrition, 2016; 3 DOI: 10.3389/fnut.2016.00022

investigated if and how a MD may impact cognitive processes over time. Positive effects were found in countries around the whole world. The reason are thought because the MD changes some modifiable risk factors including reducing inflammatory responses, increasing micronutrients, improving vitamin and mineral imbalances, changing lipid profiles by using olive oils as the main source of dietary fats, maintaining weight and potentially reducing obesity, improving polyphenols in the blood, improving cellular energy metabolism and maybe changing the gut micro-biota.

31. "Bigger Brain"

Research suggests that a Mediterranean-style diet (MeDi) may be protective for the aging brain. Of more than 400 individuals from Scotland who were in their 70s, those who were low consumers of the MeDi had significantly lower total brain volume over a 3-year period than those who regularly adhered to this type of diet.[79]

32. Less Gout

The results of the study showed that both men and women of all ages adhering to Mediterranean diet reduced SUA levels. Approximately 44% (43.8%) of individuals managed to reduce serum uric acid SUA levels by following the Mediterranean diet. (A raised SUA causes gout).

33. Less Asthma

Greater adherence to a Mediterranean Diet by children is associated with decreased odds of having asthma.[80]

34. Less Allergies

The results of this study suggest a beneficial effect of commonly consumed fruits, vegetables and nuts, and of a high adherence to a traditional Mediterranean diet during childhood on symptoms of asthma and rhinitis. Diet may explain the relative lack of allergic symptoms in this population.[81]

---

[79] Neurology. published online January 4, 2017
[80] Evidenced Based Practice DOI.10 1097/EBP 000000000000466
[81] Thorax 2007 Aug 62(8): 677-683

35. Improved Gut Microbiome

Eating a Mediterranean diet (MedDiet) for just 1 year improved diversity in the gut microbiome of elderly participants and was associated with reduced frailty and better health, according to the results of a randomized multicenter study and adherence to the MedDiet modulates specific components of the gut microbiota that were associated with a reduction in risk of frailty, improved cognitive function, and reduced inflammatory status.[82]

37. Promotes gut bacteria linked to 'healthy aging'[83]

Ageing is associated with deteriorating bodily functions and increasing inflammation, both of which herald the onset of frailty. Sticking to the Mediterranean diet for 12 months was associated with beneficial changes to the gut microbiome. It was associated with stemming the loss of bacterial diversity; an increase in the types of bacteria previously associated with several indicators of reduced frailty, such as walking speed and hand grip strength, and improved brain function, such as memory; and with reduced production of potentially harmful inflammatory chemicals due to an increase in bacteria known to produce beneficial short chain fatty acids and a decrease in bacteria involved in producing particular bile acids, overproduction of which are linked to a heightened risk of bowel cancer, insulin resistance, fatty liver and cell damage. The changes were largely driven by an increase in dietary fiber and associated vitamins and minerals -- specifically, C, B6, B9, copper, potassium, iron, manganese, and magnesium. The findings were independent of the person's age or weight (body mass index), both of which influence the make-up of the microbiome.

36. Higher Bone Density and Muscle Mass in Post Menopausals[84]

A higher Mediterranean diet score (MDS), meaning better adherence to the Mediterranean diet, was significantly associated with higher bone mineral density measured at the lumbar spine and with greater muscle mass, and this association was independent of whether the women used hormone therapy previously, their

---

[82] published online February 17 in the journal *Gut.*

[83] Mediterranean diet intervention alters the gut microbiome in older people reducing frailty and improving health status: the NU-AGE 1-year dietary intervention across five European countries. ***Gut,*** 2020; gutjnl-2019-319654 DOI: 10.1136/gutjnl-2019-319654

[84] The Endocrine Society. "Mediterranean diet is linked to higher muscle mass, bone density after menopause." ScienceDaily. ScienceDaily, 18 March 2018. <www.sciencedaily.com/releases/2018/03/180318144826.htm>

prior smoking behaviour or their current level of physical activity, as measured by wearing a pedometer for six days.

37. Improved IVF Results[85]

A Mediterranean diet may help improve success of in vitro fertilization (IVF). Lower rates of pregnancy (29.1% versus 50.0%) were seen among with the lowest compliance to the Mediterranean diet when compared with women with the highest compliance.

38. More Long-Term Benefits[86]

An analysis of 121 diet studies of over 21,000 people found the Mediterranean Diet provided the only long-term reductions in LDL, and hence CVD risk.

"Estimated effects at the 12 month follow-up for weight loss and cardiovascular risk factor improvements diminished for all popular named diets, except for the Mediterranean diet."

The other diets studied included: Atkins, Zone, DASH, Paleo, Low Fat, Jenny Craig, Volumetrics, Weight Watchers, Rosemary Conley, Ornish, Portfolio, Biggest Loser, Slimming World, South Beach, Dietary Advice

Mediterranean Diet World's Best Diet of 2020

Experts gathered by *U.S. News* this year ranked 35 diet plans and for the third year in a row, the Mediterranean diet has been named the best diet overall. The expert panel included nationally recognized experts in diet, nutrition, obesity, food psychology, diabetes, and heart disease.

Winner for 2020:

- Best Overall
- Best for Healthy Eating
- Easiest Diet to Follow
- Best Diets for Diabetes
- Best Plant-Based Diet

This Newtrition Micronutrient Revolution Diet offers the latest benefits and information.

---

[85] "Adherence to the Mediterranean diet and IVF success rate among non-obese women attempting fertility" Hum Reprod 2018; DOI 10.1093/humrep/dey003

[86] BMJ 2020;369:m696

CHAPTER 11

HOW DO WE KNOW: THE EVIDENCE

"OBSERVATION MY DEAR Dr WATSON"
- ***Sherlock Holmes***

All nutrition studies are *observational*, meaning the researchers can't prove a cause-and-effect relationship between diet and health outcomes but only show that there *may be a link* between the two.

As stated previously, the Gold Standard for evidence are Random Controlled Trials (RCT) where a statistical number of participants are randomly divided into two groups unknown to the trial organisers who then administer the ingredient or drug and a placebo or fake substitute, which they also don't know which is which. Then after a due time, preferably many years, independent analysts assess the result(s).

RCTs are therefore impossible to do with nutrition: It would take half of 100,000 participants, eating only the one fixed diet or food item with the other half eating only a placebo for seven years.

So, all that can be done is observe and try to conclude a link. This is not all bad as in 1949, from observation, smoking was linked, associated with, lung cancer (but it took until 1991 to prove it) and much nutrition observational studies are compelling, but some are also biased.

In addition, nutrition science has burgeoned. We now know the macro-nutrients, Protein, Carbohydrates/carbs and Fat (PCF), the 13 Vitamins, the Amino Acids – which are essential for life, and now, as you will read, we are just discovering the world of Micro-nutrients. These are not essential for life, but many seem to confer health benefits.

All are available from a variety of fresh foods. Supplements and vitamins are not necessary. Foods contain micronutrients which allow their vitamins and essentials to not only be absorbed better (than a synthetic pill) but then allow them to work better. Vitamins, after all, come from foods not pills and in a better form and in the correct dose. An orange, as well as its vitamin C, contains at least 70 other micronutrients to ensure the essential vit C works best.

As an indulgent aside, when I specialised in Edinburgh, I was attached to the Doyen of Scottish Medicine, Sir Hugh Munro, who used to pause me at the door and instruct me "to diagnose the ward". (I think I averaged around 19 out of 30, but once got 29).

This I had to do by pure observation which I still practise. It was the proud Edinburgh school of medicine that Conan Doyle, the author of Sherlock Holmes, was subjected to when he was a medical student there.

Credit was given to Dr Joseph Bell (of Bell's Palsy fame) who used to stagger and impress his students and patients by "knowing" much about his patients without having previously met, talked to, or examined them – all by observation.

Conan Doyle was bright enough to adapt this, 'School of Observation', to create "the Great Detective" and I have always thought of Medicine as an exercise in being a great detective.

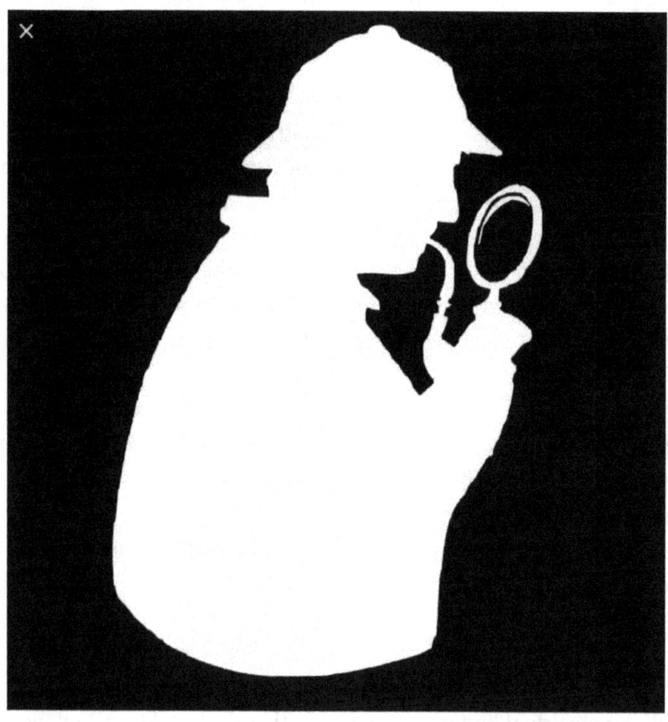

CHAPTER 12:

THE OUTSTANDING STUDIES

The studies and evidence on which Newtrition is based:

1. THE SEVEN COUNTRIES STUDY
2. THE NORTH KARALIA PROJECT
3. THE LYON HEART STUDY
4. THE PREDIMED STUDY
5. EPIC
6. FRESH FRUIT
7. IMPERIAL COLLEGE Increased Fruit & Veg
8. WHOLE GRAIN
9. NUTS
10. HYPO- CALORIC / LO-CAL DIETS
11. FIBER
12. SPICY FOOD
13. NURSES and HEALTH PROFESSIONALS STUDIES
14. PROTEIN
15. LANCET: EAT
16. ULTRAPROCESSED FOODAND MORTALITY - FRANCE
17. VITAMINS ONLY FROM FOOD
18. AUTISM
19. PURE, WHITE and DEADLY
20. COMPARISON OF MACRONUTRIENT PATTERNS OF 14 POPULAR NAMED DIETS

1. THE SEVEN COUNTRIES STUDY (SCS)

In the early 50s Ancel Keys, a Minnesotan physiologist, observed how Italians had far fewer heart attacks than most Western nations and he studied their diets comparing it with the Mediterranean Diet.

In what would become known as the Seven Countries Study, Keys recruited groups of middle-aged men for a long-term project in Finland, the United States, Japan, Italy, the Netherlands, Greece, and Yugoslavia for their diet history and a battery of tests every five years.

A pattern soon emerged: The farther north the men lived, the more animal products they consumed and the more heart attacks they suffered. In Greece and Italy, where people ate mostly a plant-based diet, men were largely free of heart disease—an observation that eventually informed our understanding of the value of the traditional Mediterranean diet.

Keys was criticized for omitting government data on diet and heart disease from certain countries that he compared early on but there were good reasons: Death certificates were undependable, and World War II had disrupted the food supply in those countries.) In places like North Karelia (the study's northern extreme), conversely, men were 30 times more likely to die of heart attacks than in places like Crete. In fact, North Karelian men on average were dying 10 years earlier than their counterparts in the south.

He published this as the "Seven Countries Study" and it formerly laid down and popularised the basis for what we now call the Mediterranean Diet.

There is a U-Tube of Keys proposing all this, but I also noted he was lean and rode a bicycle. He lived to be 100.

2. THE NORTH KARALIA PROJECT[87]

In 1970 Finnish men had the world's highest death rate from heart disease.

The Finnish Minster of Health at the time recognized the novelty of the problem and appointed a 27-year old physician with a master's degree in social sciences, named Puska, to lead a pilot project in the region to tackle the problem. Not because he was good, but because he was young, and the problem was going to

[87] *Adapted from Dan Buettner's book* The Blue Zones Solution: Eating and Living Like the World's Healthiest People.

take a long time to solve. He made the right choice. In the ensuing decades, Puska pioneered a strategy that lowered male cardiovascular mortality in a population of 170,000 Finns by some 80 percent—an unparalleled accomplishment. And he achieved it by breaking established rules of public health.

Dr Puska persuaded the province of North Karalia to adopt, in effect, the Mediterranean Diet with the result heart attacks plunged by 75% - probably also a world record. It was an amazing achievement with the whole province on side.

I am particularly impressed with this community program as it shows what can be done and what could be done if we had politicians of the same calibre and not those in the pockets of the fast food industry.

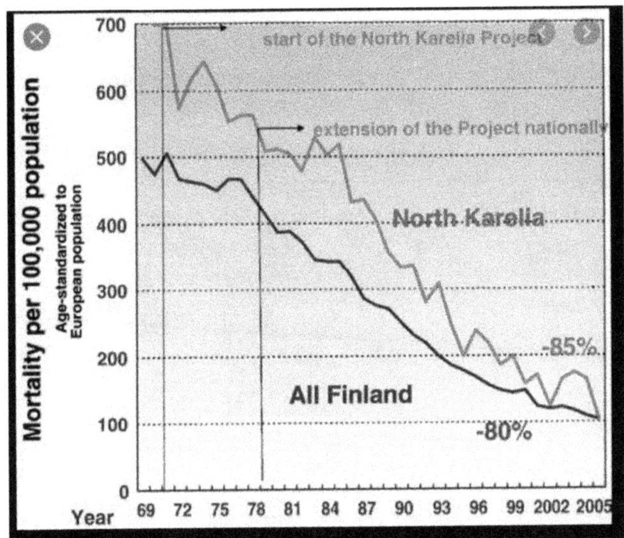

3. THE LYON HEART STUDY[88]

In the mid 90s, Prof Michelle De Logeril of Lyon, home of Paul Bocouse and great French cuisine, carried out a randomized secondary prevention trial aimed at testing whether a Mediterranean-type diet may reduce the rate of recurrence after a first myocardial infarction. An intermediate analysis showed a striking protective effect after 27 months of follow-up. An extended follow-up (with a mean of 46 months per patient) found the rate of cardiac death and nonfatal infarction in the experimental group after 46 months (1.24 per hundred patients

[88] Mediterranean Diet, Traditional Risk Factors, and the Rate of Cardiovascular Complications After Myocardial Infarction Final Report of the Lyon Diet Heart Study
Originally published16 Feb 1999https://doi.org/10.1161/01.CIR.99.6.779Circulation. 1999;99:779–785

per year) is similar to that observed after 27 months (1.32). The rate in control subjects was 4.07 after 46 months, whereas it was 5.55 after 27 months. Hence, the data confirm the impressive protective effect of the Mediterranean diet.

The result was that those who did not have the Mediterranean Diet suffered three to five times more subsequent heart attacks than those on the Mediterranean diet.

4. THE PREDIMED STUDY[89]

This came in for some early criticisms which were nit-picking

The study specified that participants were to be randomly assigned, in a 1:1:1 ratio, to one of three dietary intervention groups: 1) a Mediterranean diet supplemented with extra-virgin olive oil, 2) a Mediterranean diet supplemented with nuts, or 3) a control diet. The primary composite endpoint (myocardial infarction, stroke, or cardiovascular death) was reduced by 30% and 28% respectively, as compared with the control group. And later reviews concluded "Other potential doubts related to data should not be causes of concern.

The points are that EVOO and Nuts reduced CVD events by some 30%.

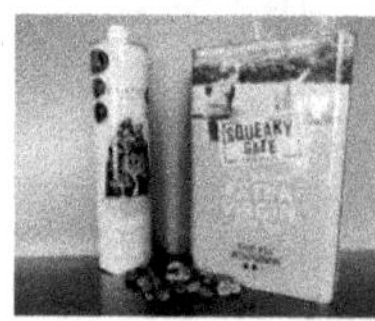

5. EPIC

The European Prospective Investigation into Cancer and Nutrition (EPIC) study is one of the largest cohort studies in the world, with more than half a million (521,000) participants recruited across 10 European countries and followed for almost 15 years. It was designed to investigate the relationships between diet, nutritional status, lifestyle and environmental factors, and the incidence of cancer and other chronic diseases.

89 June 21, 2018 N Engl J Med 2018; 378:e34 DOI: 10.1056/NEJMoa1800389

6. FRUIT: 500,000 Chinese Can't Be Wrong
Fresh Fruit Consumption and Major Cardiovascular Disease in China.

A seven-year study of half a million adults in China found that people who ate fresh fruit on most days are at lower risk of heart attack and stroke than people who rarely eat fresh fruit. Fruit is a rich source of active compounds and contains little sodium or fat and relatively few calories. The study found that fruit consumption (which was mainly apples or oranges) was strongly associated with many other factors, such as education, lower blood pressure, lower blood glucose, and not smoking. But, after allowing for what was known of these and other factors, a 100g portion of fruit per day was associated with about one-third less cardiovascular mortality and the association was similar across different study areas and in both men and women.[90] This was supported by the Copenhagen General Population Study (CGPS) and Copenhagen City Heart Study which showed that those who ate the most fruit and vegetables had a 13% lower risk of CVD and a 20% lower risk of all-cause mortality compared with the subgroup that ate these foods only rarely.[91]

Resume

Daily fruit consumption cuts the risk of cardiovascular disease (CVD) by

- 40% (0.5 million Chinese Kadoorie Biobank)
- 13% (Copenhagen General Population Study (CGPS) and Copenhagen City Heart Study)
- And 20% lower risk of all-cause mortality

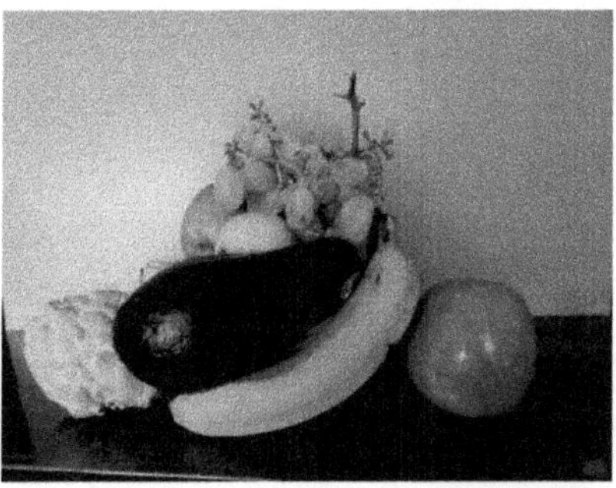

[90] Fresh Fruit Consumption and Major Cardiovascular Disease in China. New England Journal of Medicine, 2016; 374 (14): 1332 DOI: 10.1056/NEJMoa1501451

[91] Genetically high plasma vitamin C, intake of fruit and vegetables, and risk of ischemic heart disease and all-cause mortality: a Mendelian randomization study. Am J Clin Nutr 2015; 101:1135-1143

7. IMPERIAL COLLEGE Increased Intake Fruit and Veg[92]

It has been found that the greatest benefit came from eating more than previously recommended (which is why I increased each to 20% for Newtrition). The study was a meta-analysis of all available research in populations worldwide, included up to 2 million people, and assessed up to 43,000 cases of heart disease, 47,000 cases of stroke, 81,000 cases of cardiovascular disease, 112,000 cancer cases and 94,000 deaths. Risk comparison to not eating any fruit and vegetables concluded that eating up to 800g fruit and vegetables a day – or 10 portions – was associated with a:

- 4 per cent reduced risk in cancer risk
- 15 per cent reduction in the risk of premature death.
- 24 per cent reduced risk of heart disease
- 33 per cent reduced risk of stroke
- 28 per cent reduced risk of cardiovascular disease
- 13 per cent reduced risk of total cancer
- 31 per cent reduction in dying prematurely

FRUITS	CAD	Stroke:	Ischemic	Hen'rage	CD	All Cause Mortality	Cancer
Apples, pears	10	6			7	5	
Bananas	3					2	
Berries	6	5	3	3	2	3	
Citrus fruits	14	8	7	3	6	6	5
Dried fruits	2	2			3		2
Fruit juices	2	2 (citrus)	2		2	1	1
Grapes	4	2			3		
Strawberries	2	2			3		
Tinned fruits					3	3	3
VEGETABLES							
Watermalon	2						
Allium vegetables	3	2	2				
Broccoli					3		2
Carrots					2		
Cuciferous vegetables	7	4	5	2		6	5
Non Cuciferous Veg						2	2
Green Leafy vegetables	10	4	4				3
Green Yellow Veg							5
Mushrooms						2	1
Pickled vegetablea		2					2
Onions	3					3	2
Potatoes	5	4	5	3	3	4	2
Root veg		2	3	2		2	
Salads						7	4
Tomatoes	3	3			4		3
Beta-carotene rich F&V	3				2		
Lutin rich F&V	3						
Viitamin C rich F&V	3		2		1		
Raw V	2				2		2
Cooked veg							5
Yellow veg							3

[92] Fruit and vegetable intake and the risk of cardiovascular disease, total cancer and all-cause mortality–a systematic review and dose-response meta-analysis of prospective studiesInt J Epidemiol dyw319. DOI: https://doi.org/10.1093/ije/dyw319
Published: 22 February 2017 Article history

8. WHOLE GRAIN

Consumption and risk of cardiovascular disease, cancer, and All-Cause and Cause-specific mortality: Two Major Studies Confirm Reduced Risks (despite the Paleos).

One report, in BMJ[93], found that whole grain consumption was associated with a reduction in the risk for death from cancer, coronary heart disease, respiratory disease, infectious disease and diabetes. Calculations from 45 studies of 90 grams of whole grains a day compared with eating none, reduced risk for all-cause mortality by 17%.

The other analysis, in Circulation[94], used data from 14 prospective studies with 786,076 participants and found that compared with those who ate the least whole grain foods, those who ate the most had a 16% reduced risk for all-cause mortality and an 18% reduced risk for cardiovascular mortality. Each 16-gram increase in whole grain intake reduced mortality risk by 7%.

Resume
Reduce All-Cause Mortality by 9%
Reduce CVS mortality by 15 - 20%
Less CAC
Protect against Diabetes 2 by 21%
Risk Ratio (the lower the better)
CHD, stroke, CVD = 0.81
total cancer = 0.85
all causes = 0.83
respiratory diseases = 0.78
diabetes = 0.49
infectious diseases = 0.74
CNS diseases = 1.15
all non-cardiovascular, non-cancer causes = 0.78

[93] Whole grain consumption and risk of cardiovascular disease, cancer, and all cause and cause specific mortality: systematic review and dose-response meta-analysis of prospective studies *BMJ* 2016; 353 doi: https://doi.org/10.1136/bmj.i2716 (Published 14 June 2016) Cite this as: *BMJ* 2016;353:i2716
[94] Whole Grain Intake and Mortality From All Causes, Cardiovascular Disease, and Cancer A Meta-Analysis of Prospective Cohort Studies Circulation. 2016;133:2370-2380

9. NUT consumption and risk of cardiovascular disease, total cancer, all-cause and cause-specific mortality: a systematic review and dose-response meta-analysis of prospective studies.

Analysis of 29 published world studies of 819,000 participants, including more than 12,000 cases of coronary heart disease, 9,000 cases of stroke, 18,000 cases of cardiovascular disease and cancer, and more than 85,000 deaths found that 20g of nuts a day reduced the risk of CAD by 29%, CVD (strokes) by 21%, Cancer by 15%, Respiratory Disease by 52%, Diabetes by 39%, Infectious Diseases by 75% and Premature death by 22 %.[95]

Resume

20g nuts / day	% Risk Reduction
All-Cause Mortality	**20**
CAD	29
CVD	21
Cancer	15
Respiratory Disease	52
Diabetes	39
Infectious Disease	75
Premature death	22

Anti-cancer Effects

Walnuts, pecan, peanuts especially

10. HYPO-CALORIC / LO-CAL DIETS

The 1934 discovery that calorie restriction extended lifespan by 50% in rats motivated research into the delaying and prevention of ageing.

There is historical, and recent evidence as well as on-going research that hypo or low calorie diets increase longevity.

In the USA Dustbowl Depression of the 30s people starved but then lived six years longer. In World War 2 when food in the UK was severely rationed people were never healthier. With the USA embargo against Castro's Cuba again severe rationing saw improved health across all parameters. I had some friends who survived the starvation of the WW2 Japanese Prisoner of War Camps. One became a Minister in the Australian Government and one was my Accountant.

---

[95] Nut consumption and risk of cardiovascular disease, total cancer, all-cause and cause-specific mortality: a systematic review and dose-response meta-analysis of prospective studies. *BMC Medicine*, 2016; 14 (1) DOI: 10.1186/s12916-016-0730-3

While they were obvious "survivors", mentally, I wondered, as they lived well past 90 years of age, if enforced starvation had not primed their immune system.

The Okinawans, one of the longest living peoples advise "never feel full".

When I was a medical student one of my teachers advised "leave a third of your meal on the plate". Before you think this is wasteful, he was really pointing out to cut our food by a third. He was ahead of his time as animal experiments now have shown reducing consumption by 35% prolongs life and increases health.

Animal research finds hypo-caloric diets increase health and lifespans.

With restricted calorie consumption, there was almost a linear increase in lifespan in mice experiments. It was found that calorie restriction allows for ribosome repair. Ribosomes are the cell's protein makers and use 10-20% of the cell's total energy. This energy production slow down and causes the aging process to slow.

In two groups of mice one group had unlimited access to food while the other was restricted to consume 35% fewer calories but all the necessary nutrients.

Hypo-caloric diets have long been proposed as prolonging life, but this study was the first to show that general protein synthesis slows down and to recognize the ribosome's role in facilitating those youth-extending biochemical changes. The calorie-restricted mice were more energetic and suffered fewer diseases and it was not just that they're lived longer, but because they were better at maintaining their bodies, they were younger for longer as well.[96]

When I started Preventive Medicine, more than 50 years ago, I observed "the lean live longest". An adult heart pumps about 6,000-7,500 liters (1,500-2,000 gallons) of blood daily. And, wait for it, there are seven miles (11.2 km) of new blood vessels for every pound or 2.2 kg of fat gained. When you gain a pound or kilogram of fat, your body makes seven new miles or 11.2 km of blood vessels that the heart has to try and pump through. This is an incredible daily impost, which eventually leads to high blood pressure and heart failure. In contrast, in the lean person there is no such burden on the heart.

---

[96] Mechanisms of In Vivo Ribosome Maintenance Change in Response to Nutrient Signals. *Molecular & Cellular Proteomics*, 2017; 16 (2): 243 DOI: 10.1074/mcp.M116.063255

11. FIBER

Reduces

- heart disease,
- diabetes,
- diverticulitis,
- constipation,
- metabolic syndrome
- total & LDL cholesterol
- CAC: a 10% reduction for each 10 g/day intake but right gut microbiome necessary

"The evidence from prospective studies is remarkably consistent that a higher intake of fiber is related to lower risk of type 2 diabetes, cardiovascular disease and weight gain."

12. SPICY FOOD[97]

The habitual consumption of spicy foods was inversely associated with total and certain Cause-specific mortality, independent of other risk factors of death.

This was a Chinese study of 199 293 men and 288 082 women aged 30 to 79 years between 2004 and 2013 who had no cancer, heart disease, and stroke.

Compared with those who ate spicy foods less than once a week, those who consumed spicy foods 6 or 7 days a week showed a 14% relative risk reduction in total mortality. The inverse association between spicy food consumption and total mortality was stronger in those who did not consume alcohol than those who did. Inverse associations were also observed for deaths due to cancer, ischemic heart diseases, and respiratory diseases.

---

[97] BMJ 2015; 351 doi: https://doi.org/10.1136/bmj.h3942 (Published 04 August 2015) Cite this as: BMJ 2015;351:h3942

13. THE NURSES HEALTH AND HEALTH PROFESSIONALS FOLLOW UP STUDIES 131,342 participants from 1980 to 2012.

Increased risk of protein

All Cause		%	H.R. Worse
Processed red meat	=	34	0.66
Unprocessed red meat	=	12	0.88
Poultry	=	06	0.94
Fish	=	06	0.94
Egg	=	19	0.81
Dairy	=	08	0.92
CVD			
Processed red meat	=	39	0.61
Unprocessed red meat	=	17	0.83
Poultry	=	09	0.91
Fish	=	12	0.88
Egg	=	12	0.88
Dairy	=	11	0.89
Cancer			
Processed red meat	=	14	0.86
Unprocessed red meat	=	04	0.96
Poultry	=	01	0.99
Fish	=	02	0.98
Egg	=	17	0.83
Dairy	=	00	1.00
Other			
Processed red meat	=	45	0.55
Unprocessed red meat	=	16	0.84
Poultry	=	07	0.93
Fish	=	06	0.94
Egg	=	24	0.76
Dairy	=	14	0.86

14. ANIMAL PROTEIN: A NOTE: Further Risks and Benefits[98]

There are many studies and the reader who wants greater detail is referred to "Protein" from the Harvard T.H.Chan, The Nutrition Source.

But in resume: There is growing evidence that *high-protein food choices* do play a role in health—and that eating healthy protein sources like fish, chicken, beans, or nuts *in place of red meat* (especially processed red meat) can lower the risk of several diseases and premature death.

This Harvard Nutrition Source details the increased risks from additional red meat especially processed meats for *Cardiovascular disease, Diabetes, Cancer and Osteoporosis.*

According to their studies there is overwhelming evidence that a plant-based diet is best and animal protein, especially as red and processed meat, is bad.

However, the fact remains that the human race would have self-destructed and been exterminated unless it ate meat and offal as it was the only source of essential micronutrients, especially Vitamin B12, and no population willingly adopted a vegetarian diet until recently when supplements became available.

Given the evangelical zeal of the Seventh Day Adventist Church to convert us all to be vegans, I now wonder if the T,H,Chan School is not populated and funded by the SDA. It certainly receives fund from one of their businesses.

Below are the results from the Nurses Health Study of 131,342 participants from 1980 to 2012, which certainly present meat in a bad light. It is very long but so important I feel it had to be included for you to view- even if just to skim the tabled results.

However, the even larger EPIC study of 448,568 people from ten different European countries, followed for a median of 12.7 years, found that red meat posed *no detectable risk, as judged by all-cause mortality.*

It did conclude that, "analysis supports a moderate positive association between processed meat consumption and mortality, in particular due to cardiovascular diseases, but also to cancer".

---

[98] Harvard T.H.Chan,The Nutrition Source, Protein

- This supports my contention that, as the human race could not have survived if we were vegetarians and, as we had canine teeth evolved for tearing and eating meat, it is obvious humans were meant to eat meat
- And I contend that it is the amount, quality, cooking and preserving of "modern" meat that is the problem. We are eating too much. It is altered from its previous natural state in that it can be full of growth promoters (steroids), antibiotics and feeds the cattle normally don't eat and often with unknown supplements. Finally, it is then overcooked at too high a temperature and charred
- The people with the lowest reported levels of vascular aging and the lowest prevalence of coronary atherosclerosis of any population yet studied (the Tsimane of the Bolivian Amazon)99 eat meat; albeit wild game.
- Grass-fed, organic beef has a fatty acid profile different from these new lot-fed, growth-boosted animals
- I feel we can eat small amounts of grass fed, lean organic beef
- But we cannot eat processed-preserved meats. If it is preserved it would seem carcinogenic chemicals have been added.

But we should all have access to the correct information as presented here: Neither extremely vegetarian nor carnivore but based on the best independent and unbiased studies. Again, there is little doubt we should cut down our ingestion of red meat and eat just a little say two times a week, and totally avoid processed meat. We should seek organic, lean beef (pork and poultry) and learn to cook it gently and marinate it.

15. EAT: The Lancet Commission on Healthy Diets[100]

This was promoted as a vegetarian diet to save the planet but was flawed methodologically, with wrong conclusions, strange impositions ignoring traditional diets and finally labelled "science fiction". What was even more ridiculous was that their proposed diet was both more expensive and culturally incompatible, than those of the people they claimed to save.

[99] Coronary atherosclerosis in indigenous South American Tsimane: a cross-sectional cohort study. *The Lancet*, 2017; DOI: 10.1016/S0140-6736(17)30752-3

[100]Food in the Anthropocene: the EAT–*Lancet* Commission on healthy diets from sustainable food systems. *Lancet.* 2019; 393: 447-492

16. ASSOCIATION BETWEEN ULTRAPROCESSED FOOD and RISK OF MORTALITY AMONG MIDDLE-AGED ADULTS IN FRANCE[101]

In this cohort study of 44 551 French adults 45 years or older, a 10% increase in the proportion of ultra-processed food consumption was statistically significantly associated with a 14% higher risk of all-cause mortality.

The same study observed more cancers among heavy consumers of these foods. The question remains, what is it about these foods that causes negative impacts on health? One popular hypothesis is the presence of additives.

17. VITAMINS ONLY FROM FOOD[102]

A decade long study of more than 30,000 people, published in April, 2019, in the respected Annals of Internal Medicine, found that certain vitamins and minerals may help extend your life and keep you from dying of cardiovascular disease – but only if you get those beneficial nutrients from foods, not supplements or pills.

Vitamin or Supplement	**Patients number tested**	**Benefit(s): Harm**
Anti-oxidants	992,129	Nothing, zilch, blot
Beta carotene		Nil
Calcium		Nil
Calcium +Vitamin D		Increased stroke risk
Folic acid		Nil
Iron		Nil
Multivitamins		Nil
Omega-3 fatty acids		Nil
Selenium		Nil
Vitamin A		Nil
Vitamin B complex		Nil
Vitamin B6		Nil
Vitamin B3 - niacin		Nil
Vitamin C		Nil
Vitamin D		Nil

[101] JAMA Intern Med. 2019 Apr 1;179(4):490-498. doi: 10.1001/jamainternmed.2018.7289.
[102] *Ann Intern Med.* 2019;170(9):604-613. DOI: 10.7326/M18-2478

And while this analysis didn't record vitamin E other studies have shown Vitamin E is potentially unsafe if taken by mouth in high doses. If you have a condition such as heart disease or diabetes, do not take doses of 400 IU/ day or more. Some research suggests that high doses might increase the chance of death and possibly cause other serious side effects.

After analysing nearly 300 trials and one million participants, the conclusions are that there is no high-quality evidence that any vitamin pill or supplement has a beneficial effect on overall mortality.

18. AUTISM[103]

Molecular changes that happen when neural stem cells are exposed to high levels of an acid commonly found in processed foods have been identified. Propionic Acid (PPA), used to increase the shelf life of packaged foods and inhibit mould in commercially processed cheese and bread, reduce the development of neurons in foetal brains. The combination of reduced neurons and damaged pathways impede the brain's ability to communicate, resulting in behaviours that are often found in children with autism.

19. PURE, WHITE and DEADLY

John Yudkin was a Professor of Nutrition in London and felt sugar was more to blame than saturated fat, as proposed by Ancel Keys, for the epidemic of CVD.

The chapter "The Diet Pioneers", details the history of their dispute. Yudkin wrote this for the public in 1972 how sugar is hidden inside everyday foods, and how it is damaging health. It has been updated by childhood obesity specialist Dr Robert Lustig M.D. Readers are also directed to the Chapter on Sugar.

---

[103] Scientific Reports June 19, 2019

20. COMPARISON OF DIETARY MACRONUTRIENT PATTERNS OF 14 POPULAR NAMED DIETARY PROGRAMMES FOR WEIGHT AND CARDIOVASCULAR RISK FACTOR REDUCTION IN ADULTS:[104]

Diet v usual diet	Weight loss (kilograms)	Systolic blood pressure reduction (mm Hg)	Diastolic blood pressure reduction (mm Hg)	Low density lipoprotein reduction (mg/dL)	High density lipoprotein reduction (mg/dL)	C-reactive protein reduction (mg/dL)
Atkins	5.46	5.14	3.30	-2.75	3.41	0.64
Zone	4.07	3.46	2.33	-2.89	-0.33	0.27
DASH	3.63	4.68	2.84	3.93	-1.90	NA
Mediterranean	2.87	2.94	1.03	4.59	-0.61	0.25
Paleolithic	5.31	14.56	3.85	7.27	-2.52	0.52
Low fat	4.87	3.95	2.22	1.92	-2.13	0.33
Jenny Craig	7.77	7.86	7.81	0.21	-2.85	0.19
Volumetrics	5.95	2.93	1.95	7.13	-0.13	NA
Weight Watchers	3.90	2.80	1.03	7.13	-0.88	0.87
Rosemary Conley	3.76	2.39	1.44	7.15	-2.04	NA
Ornish	3.64	0.69	0.20	4.71	-4.87	1.11
Portfolio	3.64	5.97	3.98	21.29	-3.26	-0.37
Biggest Loser	2.88	3.17	2.20	3.90	-0.01	NA
Slimming World	2.15	NA	NA	NA	NA	NA
South Beach	9.86	NA	NA	-0.64	0.36	NA
Dietary advice	0.31	0.58	0.40	-2.01	-1.71	-1.15

"Among the most effective" with moderate to high certainty
"Inferior to the most effective/superior to the least effective" with moderate to high certainty
"Among the least effective" with moderate to high certainty
"Maybe among the most effective" with very low to low certainty
"Inferior to the most effective/superior to the least effective" with very low to low certainty
"Maybe among the least effective" with very low to low certainty
"Maybe worse than usual diet"

Only the Mediterranean diet showed a statistically significant difference compared with usual diet in LDL cholesterol reduction. Estimated effects at the 12-month follow-up for weight loss and cardiovascular risk factor improvements diminished for all popular named diets, except for the Mediterranean diet.

[104] BMJ 2020;369:m696

21. ASSOCIATIONS OF PROCESSED MEAT, UNPROCESSED RED MEAT, POULTRY, OR FISH INTAKE WITH INCIDENT CARDIOVASCULAR DISEASE AND ALL-CAUSE MORTALITY[105]

These findings suggest that, among US adults, higher intake of processed meat, unprocessed red meat, or poultry, but not fish, was significantly associated with a small increased risk of incident CVD, whereas higher intake of processed meat or unprocessed red meat, but not poultry or fish, was significantly associated with a small increased risk of all-cause mortality.

As noted elsewhere: This large 6-cohort study found that a higher intake of processed meat and unprocessed red meat, but not poultry or fish, significantly correlates with a small increase in the risk for all-cause mortality and increased relative risks for these associations, ranging from approximately 3% to 7% and increased absolute risks for less than 2% during a follow-up period that lasted up to 30 years.

This is the longest study so far (30 years and ~30,000 participants) and based on a larger and more diverse sample and longer follow-up than most published studies. An absolute risk of just 2% over 30 years with it not being clear if this included processed meat, but eating meat four times a week, I would regard as 'acceptable', and certainly modifiable by reducing all meat and cutting out processed meats, as Newtrition recommends. And it certainly does not warrant further hysterical outbursts of the Veggie Loonies, as above.

---

[105] *JAMA Intern Med.* 2020;180(4):503-512. doi:10.1001/jamainternmed.2019.6969

CHAPTER 13

MEDICALLY BENEFICIAL DIETS: GENERAL

1. **NEWTRITION MICRONUTRIENT DIET**
2. **THE MEDITERRANEAN DIET**
3. **THE MEDITERR*ASIAN* DIET**
4. **THE ANTI-INFLAMMATORY DIET**
5. **LYON HEART DIET**
6. **PREDIMED**
7. **DASH - HYPERTENSION -DIET**
8. **MIND**
9. **NORDIC DIET**
10. **POLYPHENOL: BERRY-CHOCOLATE**
11. **POLYMEAL**
12. **PLANT BASED**
13. **VEGETARIAN**
14. **WORLD'S BEST CORONARY ARTERIES**
15. **PORTFOLIO**
16. **PRUDENT**
17. **PALEO**
18. **DETOX and CLEANSING**
19. **CHOLESTEROL**
20. **INFLAMMATORY BOWEL DISEASE (IBD)**
21. **INUIT**

MEDICALLY BENEFICIAL DIETS: GENERAL

It is of interest that some diets favoured specific ingredients but, as more studies were done, the conclusion is that it would seem no one ingredient could be isolated to donate exclusive benefits. The MIND Diet emphasized blueberries and refuted other fruits but then found the Traditional Mediterranean Diet, which embraced all fruits, had equal brain healthy results in patients not at risk. Next it was thought one fat was superior, but this was confused by the fact that the Lyon Diet had trans-fats from margarine and less poly-unsaturates than the normal French diet and so on. And so, it has slowly emerged that there are good and bad fats with the latest PREDIMED Trial recording benefits from Extra Virgin Olive Oil and nuts.

It would seem benefit is gained from ***the mixture, variety and amalgam of the ingredients*** **in the Mediterranean Diets** (they differ slightly from country to country)

The corollary is that processed foods and altered (trans) fats are bad.

Not all of the following diets are beneficial.

1. NEWTRITION MICRONUTRIENT REVOLUTION DIET

Newtrition is the combination of all these other best diets *with* the added benefit of the latest studies, discoveries and beneficial micronutrients. It is the easiest to do and everyone can do it vegans to meat eaters.

Ratios of ingredients such as fruit and vegetables are increased due to the latest research, Superfoods identified, EVOO recommended but in addition what *not* to eat is emphasised making it the most complete, up-to-date and beneficial of all diets.

2. THE TRADITIONAL MEDITERRANEAN DIET

This has been well and truly covered but in resume:

Adopting the Traditional Mediterranean Diet was the most significant advance in modern nutrition. It varied between those countries around the Mediterranean but with ingredients common to all.

It was 'legitimized' by Ancel Keys' research of the 50s to become popular after publication in the 70s and then augmented by Professor De Logeril's Lyon Heart

Study published in the Lancet in 1995 and then latest the PREDIMED study of 2013.

Constituents: High intake of vegetables, legumes, fruits, nut, unrefined cereals, olive oil but low intake of saturated lipids, moderately high intake of fish, low to moderate intake of dairy products (& then in the form of cheese or yoghurt), low intake of meat & poultry, regular moderate intake of ethanol, usually as wine with meals.

3. THE MEDITERRASIAN DIET

Traditional Mediterranean and Asian diets have many similarities. They are rich in vegetables, with a primary focus on legumes, fruits, and fresh foods. Both are moderately rich in fish and associated omega-3 fatty acids. They include some lean meats and eggs but avoid processed foods, artificial flavoring, high-fructose corn syrup, saturated fat, and trans-fat. They're high in antioxidants that protect the body from many chronic diseases.

The rise of Asian cooking has broadened our tastes and many Asian ingredients and techniques can now be incorporated into the traditional Mediterranean diet to enhance and give it more variety without any loss of benefits. This is mainly due to herbs such as coriander, lemon grass and chillies whereas coconut oil (saturated fat) and fish sauce (high salt) should be minimized. There was also some concern about certain fermented Soy sauces and the high rate of stomach cancer in Japan. It is also difficult to recommend the deep frying.

Chillies seem beneficial:[106] Consumption of hot red chili peppers is associated with a 13% reduction in total mortality -- primarily in deaths due to heart disease or stroke. Capsaicin is believed to play a role in cellular and molecular mechanisms that prevent obesity and modulate coronary blood flow, and also possesses antimicrobial properties that may indirectly affect the host by altering the gut microbiota. Bok Choi has been shown to have cancer suppressing qualities in laboratory experiments so other Asian vegetables may also have qualities yet to be determined. It may be of interest that most Asian societies eat little and often and not three big meals a day. (This is not to be confused with Western "grazing" which is eating lots and often).

---

[106] The Association of Hot Red Chili Pepper Consumption and Mortality: A Large Population-Based Cohort Study. *PLOS ONE*, 2017; 12 (1): e0169876 DOI: 10.1371/journal.pone.0169876

The traditional Asian diet focuses on oily fish; miso soup; and fermented foods such as kimchi, pickles, and natto (fermented soybeans) that encourage and stimulate a favorable microbiome. This is associated with a lower incidence of irritable bowel disease. The mushrooms consumed in the Asian diet (shiitake, enoki, and oyster) are actually now being studied in cancer centers in the United States because they've been linked to improvement in cancer risk and recurrence. The inclusion of herbs, medicinal garnishes, spices, turmeric, phenol, and green seaweed, just to name a few aspects of this diet, offer important antioxidants.

4. THE ANTI-INFLAMMATORY DIET

Inflammation is the natural body protective reaction and initiate healing. If, however, it continues to become chronic, cycles of cytokines and anti-inflammatory mediators continue and can increase. The body's immune response then produces mediators that allow inflammation to occur in an ongoing and out-of-control manner. This chronic inflammation can increase our lifetime risk for obesity, type 2 diabetes, heart disease, and some forms of cancer as well as other autoimmune diseases.

The Basics of the Anti-inflammatory Diet: Phytochemicals have anticarcinogenic and anti-cardiovascular disease properties. It includes beneficial antioxidants (eg, polyphenols, flavonoids), oleic acid (olives) and polyunsaturated fatty acids and, especially, monounsaturated fatty acids. These combine to produce an anti-inflammatory, antithrombotic prostaglandin pathway.

Arguably the best anti-inflammatory diet is based on the “Mediterranasian” Diet combining the Asian diet and the Mediterranean diet. The combination of the two is thought to be one of the healthiest ways of eating on a daily basis.

The essential ingredients are fresh foods with the emphasis is on fruits and vegetables that have important antioxidants as well as herbs, nuts, seeds, and green tea, while avoiding processed foods, artificial flavors, high-fructose corn syrup, and trans-fats. Instead, it incorporates healthy monounsaturated and polyunsaturated fats, which have a higher omega-3 to omega-6 fatty acid ratio. It includes a variety of sources of plant proteins that are high in fiber with a low glycemic index, such as beans and other legumes. It is lower in saturated animal fat and thus includes healthier fats.

Because this diet is high in fiber and has a low glycemic index, there is a decreased risk for diabetes. The higher magnesium content reduces inflammation and improves cognitive ability. Spices that are rich in phytochemicals such as ginger, garlic, cayenne, black pepper, rosemary, and turmeric, are associated with maintaining a favorable microbiome. Other phytochemicals in these diets (e.g. alpha linolenic acid, beta-carotene) offer important anti-inflammatory mediators.

The Asian diet is relatively less studied than the Mediterranean diet. However, an ongoing China Project from Cornell University demonstrated an association that the consumption of the Asian diet in rural China protected against many of the cancers we see in Western civilization. There was also a decrease in the incidence of cardiovascular disease and significantly greater longevity. However, as soon as the rural Chinese moved into cities and acquired the Western diet, a much higher incidence of diabetes, breast cancer, colon cancer, and cardiovascular disease was reported.

Given the latest studies on chilies the Mediterrasian Diet may well be the healthiest.

5. THE LYON HEART STUDY DIET (LHS)

The Lyon Diet Heart Study has been accredited as "the cornerstone of modern Cardiovascular Health".

The LHS was for secondary prevention i.e. for people who had suffered a heart attack (and was incredibly successful)

It was the first randomized trial for secondary prevention of heart disease, testing whether a Mediterranean-type diet may reduce the rate of recurrence after a first myocardial infarction. An intermediate analysis showed a striking protective effect after 27 months of follow-up. The protective effect of the Mediterranean dietary pattern was maintained up to 4 years after the first infarction, confirming previous interim analyses.

The secondary prevention Lyon Diet Heart Study showed a large reduction in rates of coronary heart disease events with a modified Mediterranean diet enriched with alpha-linolenic acid (a constituent of walnuts, canola, soybean, flaxseed oil and fish)

This alerted the medical world as to potential benefits and now attention moved to primary prevention

Recommendations

1. Multigrain bread every day
2. No day without fruit
3. No day without vegetables
4. Eat more fish, less meat
5. Use Extra Virgin Olive Oil
6. Handful of nuts every day
7. More fresh herbs & garlic
8. A glass of red wine with food daily
9. No butter, no cream
10. Eat in a pleasant environment

This diet reduces death from heart disease by 76% & minor coronary events by 30% in post infarct patients.

6. PREDIMED (Primary Prevention of Cardiovascular Disease with a Mediterranean Diet)[107]

PREDIMED (2013) now addressed primary prevention of cardiovascular disease i.e. among high-risk persons who were initially free of cardiovascular disease. In this trial, *an energy-unrestricted Mediterranean diet supplemented with either* ***extra-virgin olive oil or nuts*** *resulted in a relative risk reduction of approximately 30%.*

Favorable trends were seen for both stroke and myocardial infarction. Extra-virgin olive oil and nuts were considered probably responsible for most of the observed benefits of the Mediterranean diets. Differences were also observed for fish and legumes but not for other food groups.

But a paper on medical statistics discovered some potential problems with PREDIMED's randomization methodology and the authors retracted the original paper, and published a new report in 2018 and Steven Nissen, MD, head of cardiovascular medicine for the Cleveland Clinic, credited the updating of their work, "But it didn't really change the findings," he said. "The Mediterranean diet still has the best evidence of any diet."

There is considerable evidence as to the benefits of both EVOO and all Nuts[108].

---

[107] N Engl J Med 2013; 368:1279-1290April 4, 2013DOI: 10.1056/NEJMoa1200303

[108] Health Benefits of Nuts and Dried Fruits edited by Cesarettin Alasalvar, Jordi Salas-Salvado, Emilio Ros, Joan Sabat

7. DASH DIET

The DASH (Dietary Approaches to Stop Hypertension) was trialed in the USA from 1994 – 96. It concentrated on reducing sodium (salt), advising high amounts of fruit and vegetables, low saturated fat and cholesterol, low-fat or non-fat dairy, with whole grains. Its unique recommendations were for dairy and low salt. It is a high fiber, low to moderate fat diet, rich in potassium, calcium, and magnesium and moderately increased protein. BP was slightly reduced (max 5.5 mm Hg). It was developed to lower blood pressure without medication in research sponsored by the US National Institutes of Health. The first DASH diet research showed that it could lower blood pressure as well as the first line blood pressure medications, even with a sodium intake of 3,300 mg/day. Since then, numerous studies have shown that the DASH diet reduces the risk of many diseases, including some kinds of cancer, stroke, heart disease, heart failure, kidney stones, and diabetes. Despite its proven benefits and media awards new research has found it has been largely ignored. In reality it is just the Mediterranean Diet with emphasis on lowering sodium.

8. MIND DIET

The MIND (Mediterranean-DASH Intervention for Neurodegenerative Delay) diet was developed by researchers at Chicago's Rush University Medical Center whose study suggested that certain foods could help prevent the onset of Alzheimer's disease The MIND diet combines elements of the heart-healthy Mediterranean diet and the DASH diet but also includes 'brain-healthy' foods: A person would need to eat at least three servings of whole grains, a green leafy vegetable, and one other vegetable each day, along with having a glass of wine. They would also need to snack most days on nuts, have beans every other day or so, and eat poultry and berries at least two times a week (berries are the only fruits allowed in the MIND diet) and fish at least once a week. It has 15 dietary components, including 10 "brain-healthy" food groups and five unhealthy groups (i.e. red meat, butter and stick margarine, cheese, pastries and sweets, and fried or fast food). To adhere to the MIND diet, a person has to limit intake of the designated unhealthy foods, especially butter (<1 tablespoon/day), sweets and pastries, whole fat cheese, and fried or fast food (<1 serving a week for any of the three).

No difference wrt Cognition[109]

---

[109] Alzheimer's Association International Conference (AAIC) 2017. Abstracts P2-546, P2-555, and P2-599, presented Monday, July 17, 2017.

After adjusting for factors that might affect cognition, including age, sex, race, low education, obesity, hypertension, diabetes, depression, smoking, physical activity, and energy intake, the analysis showed that adherence to either the Mediterranean or DASH diet appeared to protect cognition.

9. THE NORDIC DIET[110]

People who ate more of the Nordic Diet Foods - essentially the same as the Mediterranean Diet - were 14% less likely to experience a stroke during the following decade or so than those who didn't follow the diet as closely. The Nordic Diet features fruits, vegetables, and whole grains which are good sources of potassium, fiber, and other substances that appear to improve high blood pressure and other risk factors associated with stroke and popular in Scandinavian countries, uses the Healthy Nordic Food Index, which includes six food categories: fish, apples and pears, root vegetables (such as carrots and celery root), cabbages (which also include broccoli, cauliflower, kale, and Brussels sprouts), rye bread and oatmeal, reduced

10. THE POLYPHENOL ("CHOCOLATE- BERRY") DIET

A 2016 published study has shown that increasing the polyphenol content of the diet via consumption of fruit and vegetables (F&V) which included one portion of berries/day and 50g of Lindt 70% cocoa dark chocolate, resulted in a significant improvement in cardiovascular risk in hypertensive participants. Participants in the study were allowed to make their own choices of type of F&V to be consumed. They also had hypertension and other cardiovascular risk factors. The results, therefore, are more relevant to 'real-life' than studies involving inpatient admission or supervised meals. A well-tolerated polyphenol-rich diet through the simple addition of berries and dark chocolate could have a positive effect on microvascular function and cardiovascular risk.[111]

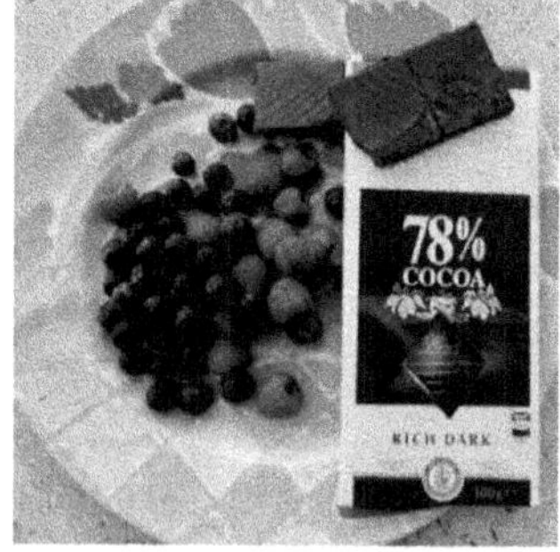

[110] *Stroke*, February 2017.

111 Beneficial Effect of a Polyphenol-Rich Diet on Cardiovascular Risk A Randomised Control Trial Heart. 2016;102(17):1371-1379.

11. THE POLYMEAL[112]

2003: The 'POLYPILL' promised great Cardiovascular risk benefits but it is still unproven.

2004: data taken from published research & the Framingham heart study evolved a 'Polymeal' Diet which would theoretically reduce Cardiovascular events by 76% Increase total life expectancy by 6.6 years

The Polymeal Diet:

Wine	150ml
Dark chocolate	100 g
Fruit & vegetables	400 g
Garlic	2.7 g
Almonds	68 g
Fish	114g x4 weekly

12. PLANT BASED

Plant-Based infers that meat is also used but has become a euphuism to promote vegetarianism. The claimed benefits of vegetarian diet are usually accompanied by criticising meat but this is confused by the

- increased high-risk behaviour of meat eaters (smoking, drinking, overweight, sedentary)
- dubious quality of the meat eaten (supplements, growth hormones)
- poor quality of cooking high temperature charred steaks & poultry.

We are eating too much fatty, artificially fed and preserved meats. Organic, grass-fed, "fresh" meats, eaten sparingly (twice a week) would seem OK.

13. VEGETARIAN

A vegetarian diet is one of the healthiest. However, it would seem impossible for most populations in the history of the world to have ever willingly adopted a vegan diet because, before the era of supplements, such a diet would have resulted in the illness and extermination of that tribe or society.

---

[112] BMJ 2004;329:1447-50

There are some traditional vegetarian, but not vegan societies: Jains and Buddhists traditionally are vegetarians and not vegans. Jains are lacto-vegetarians, which means they consume dairy products. Most Buddhists including the monks follow a vegetarian diet but ate meat that died naturally, not slaughtered. The only food Jains avoid are meat and root vegetables (onion, garlic etc.). The same goes for Buddhist diet, which is heavily influenced by Hindu and Jain vegetarian diet. Dairy products can be a good source of vitamin B12.

It has been pointed out that B12 deficiency is a slowly progressing disease. Symptoms mimic those of aging. It may be that many died with severe B12 deficiency.

Vegetarians abstain from the consumption of any meat and may also include abstention from by-products of animal slaughter.

Vegans have no intake of animal products. They are total vegetarians in that they don't eat food that comes from animals in any way, including milk products, eggs, honey and gelatin (which comes from bones)

Lacto-ovo vegetarians consume dairy products and/or eggs 1 or more times per month but no fish or meat.

Pesco-vegetarians consume fish once or more per month but no meat.

Semi-vegetarians consumed meat or poultry less than once a week and 1 or more times per month.

Non-vegetarians consumed animal products 1 or more times a week.

- Vegetarian diets are associated with an overall lower incidence of colorectal cancers. Pesco-vegetarians in particular have a much lower risk compared with nonvegetarians[113]
- Every 3% increase in calories from plant protein reduces the risk of death by 10% and 12% for risk dying from heart disease
- Vegetarian Californian Seventh Day Adventists are non-smoking, non-drinking and live 7 years longer than the general population
- All Vegetarians have less CAD, less cancer (mostly lung/smoking) and are thinner with less Diabetes 2
- The issue is clouded because meat eaters more often smoke, eat processed junk food & drink to excess

---

[113] *JAMA Intern Med.* 2015;175(5):767-776. doi:10.1001/jamainternmed.2015.59.

- There would seem evidence that a plant-based diet not only prevents heart disease but can reverse it
- The number of people in Britain who follow a vegan diet has increased 360% over the last decade
- The European Prospective Investigation found that BMI [body mass index] was highest in meat eaters, lowest in vegans, and intermediate in fish eaters. The foods in vegetarian diets may also help in the prevention of type 2 diabetes.[114]
- Other research suggests vegetarianism lowers the risk of diabetes, stroke and obesity[115]
- Another study found[116]
- Both vegetarians and non-vegetarians consumed the same amount of eggs and fruit. The researchers defined vegetarians as people who did not eat any meat or fish.
- Compared with non-vegetarians, vegetarians consumed more dietary fibers and plant protein, but less protein, fat, and vitamin B_{12}. More vegetarians than non-vegetarians had an inadequate intake of vitamin B_{12} (64% vs 33%).
- Homocysteine increases with either folate or vitamin B_{12} deficiency, because folate and vitamin B_{12} are intertwined with the metabolism of methionine and homocysteine. In addition to thinking of this vitamin as necessary to the proper functioning of metabolic pathways, there is also the view that vitamin B_{12} may be a **general nerve-protecting and nerve-regenerating compound**.
- Overall, vegetarians in cohort 2 had a 48% lower risk of overall stroke than non-vegetarians, a 60% lower risk of ischemic stroke, and a 65% lower risk of hemorrhagic stroke, following adjustments for other factors.

Vegan, Vegetarian Diet Risks

Vegans need supplements especially vitamin B12 and D and calcium-fortified drinks[117] Zinc intake should be monitored. Many vegetarians also struggle to get enough protein, iron, vitamin D, vitamin B12 and calcium which are essential for health. One study found that vegetarians had approximately 5% lower bone-mineral density (BMD) than non-vegetarians.

---

[114] *Diabetes Care*. 2009;32:791-796

[115] Journal Molecular Biology and Evolution, March 2016

[116] *Neurology* 2020; DOI: 10.1212/WNL.0000000000009093

[117] Food and Nutrient Intake and Nutritional Status of Finnish Vegans and Non-Vegetarians. PLOS ONE, 2016; 11 (2): e0148235 DOI: 10.1371/journal.pone.0148235

A study that examined vegan populations showed that 52% of individuals were "frankly deficient" in vitamin B12 and that 23% had "insufficient" levels. A case report of 30 vegan mothers found that 60% of their offspring had developmental delays and that 37% had cerebral atrophy. There is a strong correlation between eating no meat and higher rates of depression and anxiety and worse quality of life. Although in some ways the vegan diet makes sense, in that the North American diet is heavily laden with animal products, that doesn't mean the solution is to eat no seafood.[118]

100% vegan, but may contain lots of Additives and be Highly-Processed[119]

The additives in some plant-based food cast doubt on health claims

Some of the most popular vegan meals, contain more chemical additives than conventional meat and fish products and are ultra-processed relying on a cocktail of chemical food additives to replicate the taste, appearance and texture of meat and fish.

According to Joanna Blythman, an investigative food journalist and author of *Swallow This: Serving Up the Food Industry's Darkest Secrets*, said: "Vegan products are often just high-protein flours with gums, glues, water and a range of additives. A lot contain a rogues' gallery of additives and dodgy ingredients that I wouldn't touch with a bargepole."

The imitation meat products with chemical additives include: titanium dioxide, yellow gelling agent polysorbate 80 (E433), also used in soaps and cosmetics, propylene glycol, a non-toxic chemical used in antifreeze and e-cigarette fluid, butylated hydroxyanisole "reasonably anticipated to be a human carcinogen. Many processed vegan products use phosphate to mimic the texture of meat and fish, but a 2012 review warned of a link between phosphate consumption and heart and kidney problems.

Male vegetarians are at greater risk for depression than their meat-eating counterparts.[120]

---

[118] American Psychiatric Association (APA) 2016 Annual Meeting: Presented May 17, 2016.
[119] January 26 2020, The Sunday Times
[120] *J Affect Disord.* 2017;225:13-17.

14. WORLD'S BEST CORONARY ARTERIES[121]

The Tsimane people (pronounced chee-MAH-nay) - a forager-horticulturalist population of the Bolivian Amazon - have the lowest reported levels of vascular aging and the lowest prevalence of coronary atherosclerosis of any population yet studied (done by CT Scans). Tsimane spend only 10% of their daytime being inactive: Men spend an average of 6-7 hours of their day being physically active and women spend 4-6 hours in a subsistence lifestyle of hunting, gathering, fishing and farming

Their diet is 72% carbohydrate-based and includes non-processed carbohydrates, which are high in fiber such as rice, plantain, manioc, corn, nuts and fruits. Protein constitutes 14% of their diet and comes from animal meat. The diet is very low in fat with fat compromising only 14% of the diet -- equivalent to an estimated 38 grams of fat each day, including 11g saturated fat and no trans fats.

Av LDL was 2.35 mmol/L (91 mg/dL), HDL 1.0 mmol/L (39.5 mg/dL).

Authors note: Surely it is the LDL that would be the lower reading?

In addition, smoking was rare.

85% had no risk of heart disease, 13% had low risk and only 3% had moderate or high risk. These findings also continued into old age, where almost two-thirds of those aged over 75 years old had almost no risk and 8% had moderate or high risk and suggest that coronary atherosclerosis can be avoided by most people by achieving a lifetime with very low LDL, low blood pressure, low glucose, normal body-mass index, no smoking and plenty of physical activity.

Summary:

Non-processed, high-fiber (complex) carbohydrates 72%
Protein 14% from (wild) animal meat
Fat 14%
Exercise - some 17,000 steps a day
No smoking

---

[121] Coronary atherosclerosis in indigenous South American Tsimane: a cross-sectional cohort study. *The Lancet*, 2017; DOI: 10.1016/S0140-6736(17)30752-3

15. THE PORTFOLIO DIET

The Portfolio Eating plan is a recognized dietary approach to lowering cholesterol. It involves a combination of plant sterols/stanols, almonds, plant fibers and soya protein alongside regular physical activity and a largely vegetarian diet. It uses commercial foods (spreads / margarine, yoghurt, milk) fortified with plant sterols plus soya, oats and almonds.

It was made popular by Dr David Jenkins, a researcher in Toronto Canada. In short term studies the portfolio diet lowered cholesterol about as much as a low dose statin In longer studies the portfolio diet lowered cholesterol on average by 20%.

16. THE PRUDENT DIET

The term "prudent diet" has been in use to describe the fat and cholesterol-controlled diet followed by subjects participating in the anticoronary program of the New York City Department of Health since 1957. This diet curtailed the intake of eggs, whole milk, and whole milk-based dairy products, liver, shellfish, and commercial pastry products. Lean meats are permitted but preference is given to fish which is recommended for use at least four or five times a week.

17. THE PALEO DIET

The Paleo Diet advocates fresh fruits and veggies, nuts, grass-fed meat and the like (*but no grains*) -- gained traction with the idea that people's bodies didn't evolve to handle all the industrial foods now available. While such diets certainly have their benefits, paleoanthropologist Peter Ungar (*Scientific American*) points out fad paleo is not what real paleo-humans ate. *"From the standpoint of paleoecology, the Paleolithic diet is a myth. Food choice is as much about what is available to be eaten as it is about what a species evolved to eat. And just as fruits ripen, leaves flush and flowers bloom predictably at different times of the year, foods available to our ancestors varied over deep time as the world changed around them from warm and wet to cool and dry and back again. Those changes are what drove our evolution".*

And that Dietary Flexibility is the hallmark of humanity.

Cereal grains were staples for some cultures long before domestication and, at any given time, diets varied dramatically across the globe. One culture ate nothing but marine animals while another got 70% of its calories from grains.

The Paleos argue that the harvesting and processing of grains effectually prevented ancient humans from eating much grains, that they didn't use fires so couldn't cook grains and finally that the introduction of cereal grains into the human diet adversely affected human health (e.g., oral health, bone density). However, humans did develop salivary amylase, more than any other animal, and this allowed us to eat starches which gave us more energy to fuel the most energy-demanding organ in the human body, our brain and why humans have bigger, more complex, brains.

The Paleos claim benefits because adherents:

- Only consume carbohydrates from fruits and vegetables (not grains and sugar)
- Have never been exposed to industrial seed oils and other oxidizing agents.
- Haven't been overmedicated with antibiotics & other gut-disrupters
- Eat plenty of anti-inflammatory foods (fish, coconut oil, etc)
- Walk every day and have plenty of leisure time
- Their circadian rhythm is in-check (plenty of sleep)
- They don't sit at a desk for 40+ hours per week
- They're not exposed to environmental toxins
- Well, nice work if you can get it and all good stuff, except this odd set against grains, and who said the Paleos "walked every day"?
- As studies show, unrefined grains donate significant benefits. The rest is just common sense – except the fad coconut oil – and recommended by all good nutritional advice.

18. DETOX and CLEANSE DIETS – see separate chapter end of book

19. CHOLESTEROL LOWERING FOODS

By all means try these but there are those, who despite such efforts and controlling their weight, still have high cholesterol. At this stage of medicine, statins would then seem the best option. I am not sure where they get these claimed % reductions.

1. Monosaturated and Polyunsaturates Oils 18%
2. Bran (oats, rice) 7-14%
3. Flax seeds 8-14%
4. Garlic 9-12%
5. Almonds 7-10%
6. Lycopene Foods 0-17%
7. Walnuts and Pistachios 10%
8. Whole Barley 7-10%
9. Dark Chocolate 2-5%
10. Green Tea 2-5%

20. IBD

Foods typically labelled as junk food showed an association with inflammatory bowel disease (IBD) among U.S. adults in a secondary analysis of the National Health Interview Survey 2015. French fries in particular were consumed by more people with IBD, who also drank less 100% fruit juice and ate more cookies and cheese than the non-IBD population. The odds ratios of having had a diagnosis of IBD rose significantly with the intake of fries and sports, energy drinks and soda/soft drinks. In contrast, the odds fell with the intake of popcorn and milk.

21. INUIT

A landmark 1970s study connected the low incidence of coronary artery disease (CAD) among the Inuit of Greenland to their diet, rich in whale and seal blubber but later researchers have found that the Inuit actually suffered from CAD at the same rate as their Caucasian counterparts. Fish oil capsules have no effect on CAD, but the Inuit suffer more strokes and when Dr Hugh Sinclair did the Inuit diet for 100 days his bleeding time went from 3 to 50 minutes, making hemorrhagic strokes more likely.

CHAPTER 14

INDIVIDUAL SPECIFIC PROTECTIVE DIETS

1. **BRAIN and ALZHEIMER'S**
2. **CVD**
3. **CANCER**
   a. **GUT**
   b. **LIVER**
   c. **PROSTATE**
   d. **BREAST**
   e. **UTERUS**
   f. **PANCREAS**
4. **PREGNANCY**
5. **OSTEOPOROSIS**
6. **DEPRESSION**
7. **ARTHRITIS**
8. **CROHN'S AND ULCERATIVE COLITIS**
9. **EYES**
10. **ELDERLY**
11. **RESPIRATORY**
12. **INFECTIOUS**

The Newtrition Diet covers all needs and recommendations. Minor tweaking may be noted. References can be found in Part C Notes.

Percentages (%) are the *reduction* in risk unless otherwise indicated (as in increased risk)

DIETARY REDUCTION OF ALL-CAUSE MORTALITY

1. Newtrition / Mediterranean Diet 25%
2. Grains 9 - 17%
   (each 16g increase reduced mortality risk by 7%)
3. Fruit and Vegetables (20%)
4. Nuts 22%
5. Coffee 10 -16%
6. Tea 24%

1. BRAIN PROTECTION and ALZHEIMER'S DISEASE (AD)

Brain Protection

The human brain can make new brain cells (neurogenesis) such that by age 50 years all he cells we were born with have been replaced. When I was a medical student, we were told brain cells could not regenerate so this is relatively recent research. The importance of this is that there are foods and lifestyles that stimulate this production of new brain cells and there are foods and behaviors that inhibit this neurogenesis.

Obviously getting our old worn-out brain cells replaced is good for us, preserving, protecting and even promoting our brain and to that end maybe staving off Dementia and Alzheimer's Disease.

Neurogenesis

Stimulation	**Inhibition**
Hypo-caloric diet 20 - 30% less cals	Over-eating
Blueberries (probably all berries)	Lack of
Omega-3 oils (fish)	Saturated fats
Dark Chocolate	Sweets / sugar
Exercise (including sex)	Sedentary
Calm	Stress

Resveratrol, the flavonoid in red wine, also seems to preserve new brain cells

Older adults who scored high on cardiorespiratory fitness (CRF) tests performed better on memory tasks than those who had low CRF. Further, the more fit older adults were, the more active their brain was during learning. Difficulty remembering new information represents one of the most common complaints in aging and decreased memory performance is one of the hallmark impairments in Alzheimer's disease.[122]

Best Advice: Strict adherence to the Mediterranean Diet

Consistently, individuals who adhered the closest to the Mediterranean diet enjoyed the highest cognitive function throughout the observational study's 10-year window. Strict adherence to the Mediterranean diet was specifically defined as habitual consumption of whole fruits, vegetables, whole grains, nuts, legumes, fish and olive oil, as well as reduced amounts of red meat and alcohol. Fish and

---

[122] FMRI activity during associative encoding is correlated with cardiorespiratory fitness and source memory performance in older adults. *Cortex*, 2017; DOI: 10.1016/j.cortex.2017.01.002

vegetables appeared to have the biggest impact on outcomes. Routine fish intake was concurrently associated with higher rates of cognitive functioning and the lowest rate of decline over time.[123]

And

Individuals whose diets consisted mainly of highly processed and starchy foods were significantly more likely to develop dementia than those whose diets also included processed foods and incorporated a wider variety of healthy foods.[124]

Alzheimer's Disease

People who did not have dementia were more likely to have a lot of diversity in their diet, that usually included healthier foods, such as fruit and vegetables, seafood, poultry or meats. The more diversity in diet, and greater inclusion of a variety of healthy foods, is related to less dementia.[125]

Protein Pump Inhibitors (PPI) – Cease / reduce

PPIs affect the synthesis of the neurotransmitter acetylcholine, which plays a significant part in conditions such as Alzheimer's disease.[126]

A large study in *JAMA Neurology* showed that people who use PPIs also ran a higher risk of dementia. https://www.ncbi.nlm.nih.gov/pubmed/26882076

A study in *Alzheimers Research & Therapy* showed healthy young individuals who took PPIs for ten days had worse memory tests than previously, compared with a placebo group. https://www.ncbi.nlm.nih.gov/pubmed/26714488

According to a study published in *PLOS ONE* the use of PPIs in the population more than doubled from 4 to 9.2 percent between 2002 and 2009. https://www.ncbi.nlm.nih.gov/pubmed/23418510

Given the underlying pathology it is difficult to imagine any diet reversing this. While the illness destroys brain connections, mental exercises may open alternate pathways as much as possible.

---

[123] Alzheimer's & Demenita 13 April 2020 **https://doi.org/10.1002/alz.1207**
[124] *Neurology*. Published online April 22, 2020.
[125] American Academy of Neurology.
[126] Department of Neurobiology, Care Sciences and Society, Karolinska Institutet

Diet and Cognitive Decline: Untangling the Evidence

1. *Whole Diets*
   a. The Mediterranean-style diet: There's a lot of evidence that this diet may reduce a person's risk of developing Alzheimer's and cognitive impairment over time.
   b. Caloric restriction and even, most recently,
   c. The MIND diet (Mediterranean-DASH Intervention for Neurodegenerative Delay): Suggests a reduction in the likelihood of developing cognitive impairment significantly over several years.[127, 128] The MIND and Mediterranean diets had comparable protective relations to AD suggesting that the MIND diet is not specific to the underlying pathology of Alzheimer disease.[129]
   d. The Polyphenol-Chocolate Diet incorporates the noted benefits of blueberries/ polyphenols.
   e. Consumption of one can of diet soda or more each day was associated with a three times increased risk for stroke and dementia over a 10-year follow-up period compared with individuals who drank no artificially sweetened beverages.

A link between consumption of both sugar-sweetened and artificially sweetened beverages and reduction in brain volume in a middle-aged cohort has been shown.[130]

Consumption of one can of diet soda or more each day was associated with a three times increased risk for stroke and dementia over a 10-year follow-up period compared with individuals who drank no artificially sweetened beverages.[131]

2. *Single or multiple nutrients*

Flavonols. Blueberries: In the Nurses' Health Study[132], a half cup of blueberries two to three times a week delayed the onset of cognitive decline. Dark cocoa powder may be effective for boosting memory.

---

[127] MIND diet slows cognitive decline with aging. Alzheimers Dement. 2015;11:1015-1022.
[128] diet associated with reduced incidence of Alzheimer's disease. Alzheimers Dement. 2015;11:1007-1014.
[129] Alzheimers Dement. MIND Diet Associated with Reduced Incidence of Alzheimer's Disease, 2015 Sep; 11(9): 1007–1014. Published online 2015 Feb 11. doi: 10.1016/j.jalz.2014.11.009
[130] Alzheimer's and Dementia March 5, 2017
[131] *Stroke* April 20, 2017
[132] Dietary intakes of berries and flavonoids in relation to cognitive decline. Ann Neurol. 2012;72:135-143. Abstract

Omega-3 fatty acids DHA and EPA have the most evidence for reducing a person's risk of developing cognitive decline. People with an *ApoE4* gene may respond more favorably.

E vitamins, curcumin, vitamin D, and caffeinated foods: Are all different dietary components that may or may not play a role.

With high homocysteine levels, then B complex vitamins—folic acid, B12, and B6 slow overall brain atrophy as well as increase memory function but only work in patients who have high homocysteine levels and those who have an adequate level of omega-3's in the blood.

Regular consumption of any tea (green, black or oolong) lowers the risk of cognitive decline in the elderly by 50% while impairment risk by as much as 86 per cent. This study was on Chinese elderly but the results could apply to other races.[133]

Eight nutrients to protect the aging brain[134]

Brain health is the second most important component in maintaining a healthy lifestyle according to a 2014 AARP study. Food Technology published eight nutrients that may help keep your brain in good shape.

1. Cocoa Flavanols: A study showed cocoa flavanols may improve the function of a specific part of the brain which is associated with age-related memory (Brickman, 2014).

2. Omega-3 Fatty Acids: A study on mice found that omega-3 polyunsaturated fatty acid supplementation appeared to result in better object recognition memory, spatial and localizatory memory (facts and knowledge), and adverse response retention (Cutuli, 2014). Foods rich in omega-3s include salmon, flaxseed oil, and chia seeds.

3. Phosphatidylserine and Phosphatidic Acid: Studies showed that phosphatidylserine with phosphatidic acid can help benefit memory, mood, and cognitive function in the elderly (Lonza, 2014).

---

[133] Tea consumption reduces the incidence of neurocognitive disorders: Findings from the Singapore longitudinal aging study. *The journal of nutrition, health & aging*, 2016; 20 (10): 1002 DOI: 10.1007/s12603-016-0687-0

[134]Institute of Food Technologists (IFT). "Eight nutrients to protect the aging brain." ScienceDaily. ScienceDaily, 15 April 2015. <www.sciencedaily.com/releases/2015/04/150415203340.htm>.

4. Walnuts: A diet supplemented with walnuts may have a beneficial effect in reducing the risk, delaying the onset, or slowing the progression of Alzheimer's disease in mice (Muthaiyah, 2014).

5. Citicoline: Citicoline is a natural substance found in the body's cells and helps in the development of brain tissue, which helps regulate memory and cognitive function, enhances communication between neurons, and protects neural structures from free radical damage. Clinical trials have shown citicoline supplements may help maintain normal cognitive function with aging and protect the brain from free radical damage. (Kyowa Hakko USA).

6. Choline: Choline, which is associated with liver health and women's health, also helps with the communication systems for cells within the brain and the rest of the body. Choline may also support the brain during aging and help prevent changes in brain chemistry that result in cognitive decline and failure. A major source of choline in the diet is eggs.

7. Magnesium: Magnesium supplements are often recommended for those who experienced serious concussions. Magnesium-rich foods include avocado, soybeans, bananas and dark chocolate.

8. Blueberries: Blueberries are known to have antioxidant and anti-inflammatory activity because they boast a high concentration of anthocyanin, a flavonoid that enhances the health-promoting quality of foods. Moderate blueberry consumption could offer neurocognitive benefits such as increased neural signaling in the brain centers.

9. Vitamin K Rich Foods may help

There is evidence that eating green leafy vegetables and other foods rich in vitamin K, lutein, folate and beta-carotene include brightly colored fruits and vegetables can help to keep the brain healthy to preserve functioning. Of more than 950 older adults over 5 years, those who ate one to two servings per day had the cognitive ability of a person 11 years younger than those who consumed none.[135]

---

[135] Federation of American Societies for Experimental Biology (FASEB). "Eating green leafy vegetables keeps mental abilities sharp." ScienceDaily. ScienceDaily, 30 March 2015. <www.sciencedaily.com/releases/2015/03/150330112227.htm>.

Summary

1. Mediterranean Diet may reduce risk by 15% to 40%
2. No sodas, soft drinks, artificial sweeteners or SSBs
3. Hypo-caloric Intermittent Fasting
4. Blueberries: All berries
5. Dark chocolate / Cocoa
6. Green leafy vegetables
7. Omega 3 oils: Fish
8. Tea
9. Coffee
10. Mental activity
11. Physical activity
12. Vit C: citrus, kiwi
13. Vit E: grains, nuts, milk, egg yolk
14. Folate: if low
15. B complex only if homocysteine high and good omega 3 levels
16. Rosemary seems to enhance memory
17. NSAIDS – no convincing evidence

2. CARDIOVASCULAR - Heart and Strokes

The Traditional Mediterranean Diet reduced Cardiovascular Disease. Secondary prevention (i.e. for those people who had suffered a heart attack) was demonstrated by the Lyon Heart Study. The DASH diet lowered sodium and improved blood pressure and stroke rates. The PREDIMED diet demonstrated primary prevention. All in **Newtrition PHYTO.**

Summary

1. Fruit & Veg 13% (Copenhagen) to 40% (China)
2. Grains 15-18%. Every 28g /day lowered CVS risk by 9%
3. Nuts 29%
4. Olive Oil
5. Fish, not fried, 50% reduction in fatal IHD 58% reduction arrhythmias
6. Tea 27%:
7. Coffee 16 -26%
8. Chocolate 11 - 29%

Worse

1. Processed Meats: Each 1.5oz = 20% increase in CVS deaths
2. Red Meat 3oz / day increased risk of CVS death by 13%

STROKES - risk reduction %

1. Coffee 22-25%
2. Nuts 21%
3. Apples, pears, white fruits
4. Orange 20%
5. Tea 18%
6. Chocolate (dark - cocoa) 22%
7. Consumption of one can of diet soda or more each day was associated with a three times increased risk for stroke
8. Homocysteine (see)
9. Reduced salt intake, omega-3 LC-PUFA use, and folate supplementation could reduce risk for some cardiovascular outcomes in adults. Combined calcium plus vitamin D might increase risk for stroke.[136]

3. CANCER (Ca OR CA)

Cancer is a disease resulting from dysregulated cell growth & is caused by an interaction of dietary, genetic & environmental risk factors and, as such, is largely preventable.

A direct association between intake of ultra-processed food and incidence of total cancer and breast cancer.[137]

Malignant cancer cells seem to feed on sugar, and diets high in refined carbohydrates may lead to a range of adverse health effects primarily due to their impacts on body fatness and on the dysregulation of insulin and glucose, both of which are factors that may increase cancer risk. It would appear that healthy carbohydrate sources, such as legumes, tend to protect us from cancer, but non-healthy ones, such as fast foods and sugary beverages, seem to increase the risk of these cancers.[138]

- Conservative estimates are that 40% of cancers are preventable Diet and exercise may contribute up to 35%. Smoking is the worst provocateur. Alcohol accounts for 4% (usually upper GIT).
- Excess weight is directly associated with increase in Ca colon CAC), breast (post menopause), endometrium, esophagus, kidney[139]

---

[136] *Ann Intern Med.* 2019;171:190-198. doi:10.7326/M19-0341
[137] The BMJ (doi:10.1136/bmj.k322),
[138] Federation of American Societies for Experimental Biology (FASEB). "Cancer link offers another reason to avoid highly processed carbs." ScienceDaily. ScienceDaily, 5 April 2016.
[139] Lancet Oncology 2002;3:565-74

- Vitamin D 1,000 IU / day (to maintain serum 25-OH vitamin D concentrations > 30ng/ml) is associated with reduction in colon, breast, prostate & ovarian Cancer.[140]
- No pesticide residual foods i.e. organic. Results indicate that higher organic food consumption is associated with a reduction in the risk of overall cancer. [141]

Vegetables

Phytates: are the main storage of phosphorus in the body and found in nuts, edible seeds, beans/legumes, bran (grains) and *in the laboratory* has have been found to inhibit all cancer cell growth and even cause cancer cells to become normal.

1. Omega 3 from Fish
2. Orange capsicums - prostate
3. Cruciferous / Brassicas: Bok Choy (best), Cabbages, Cauliflower, and Kale. Cuciferous vegetables (cabbage, cauliflower, broccoli, brussel sprouts, kale) reduce Ca by 50%.
4. Alliums: Garlic, spring onions, Leeks. Garlic most effective against Ca of prostate, breast, stomach. 2nd to leeks for renal Ca
5. Legumes such as beans, lentils and peas were associated with 32% lower risk of all overweight- and obesity-related cancers, including breast, prostate and colorectal cancers.[142] Beans, lentils, peas, nuts & cereals contain inostol pentakisphosphate which inhibits an enzyme that promotes Ca growth[143]
6. Chillies
7. Nuts: Walnuts, Pecan, Peanuts (Not tomatoes, lettuce, carrot)
8. *Ca Experimental:* Turmeric - curcumin has anti-Ca properties[144]

Omega 3 Anti-Cancer[145]

Marine-based omega-3s are eight times more effective at inhibiting tumor development and growth when comparing the cancer-fighting potency of plant- versus marine-derived omega-3s on breast tumor development.

---

140 BMJ 2006;3332:70

141 *JAMA Intern Med.* 2018;178(12):1597-1606. doi:10.1001/jamainternmed.2018.4357

142 Federation of American Societies for Experimental Biology (FASEB). "Cancer link offers another reason to avoid highly processed carbs." ScienceDaily. ScienceDaily, 5 April 2016.

143 Uni Col Lon Sep 2005

144 U Texas 2005

145 Marine fish oil is more potent than plant based n-3 polyunsaturated fatty acids in the prevention of mammary tumors. *The Journal of Nutritional Biochemistry*, 2017; DOI: 10.1016/j.jnutbio.2017.12.011

There are three types of omega-3 fatty acids: a-linolenic acid (ALA), eicosapentaenoic acid (EPA) and docosahexaenoic acid (DHA). ALA is plant-based and found in such edible seeds as flaxseed and in oils, such as soy, canola and hemp oil. EPA and DHA are found in marine life, such as fish, algae and phytoplankton.

Omega-3s prevent and fight cancer by turning on genes associated with the immune system and blocking tumor growth pathways Exposure to marine-based omega-3s reduced the size of the tumors by 60 to 70 per cent and the number of tumors by 30 per cent.

Based on the doses given in the study, humans should consume two to three servings of fish a week to have the same effect.

Summary

A diet low in fat and sugars, together with a healthy lifestyle, regular exercise, weight reduction and not smoking, may contribute to prevent many cancer types.

1. Diet and exercise. No excess weight. (35%)
2. Fish x3 / week – reduction in tumors 30% and up to 70% in size.
3. Vitamin D 1000 i.u./day
4. Green leafy vegetables (50%) - cabbage family Bok Choy
5. Allums - onion family - garlic
6. Legumes - beans, peas, lentils (32%)
7. Chillis
8. Nuts (walnuts, pecans, peanuts) 15-21%
9. Curcumin - Tumeric
10. Vegetarian
11. Grains

CANCER.

a) GUT: COLORECTAL CANCER (CAC) PREVENTION

1. Restrict Calories to < 2500 M & 2000 F (less is sedentary)
2. Reduce dietary fat to <25% of total Calorie intake and saturated fat to <10%

Gut - Dairy & Calcium (Ca++)

Dietary calcium 1000 to 1200 mg/day. No benefit > 1400mg /day[146]

Milk / dairy

Both dairy and calcium consumption have an inverse relationship for Colorectal Ca

- Milk is the most effective dairy product but is limited to distal colon and rectum
- 1.5 glasses / day had a 33% lower risk than < 2 glasses / wk

Vitamin D

1. Higher blood vitamin D concentration showed a strong dose—response inverse association for colorectal cancer risk. Subjects in the highest fifth of blood vitamin D levels showed a 40% reduced risk. Subjects with very low levels showed a significantly higher risk of colorectal cancer development[147]
2. Vitamin D 650 IU / day (fish, fortified milk). Later recommendations are for 1,000 i.u. / day D3)

Red Meat

- Absolute risk of developing colorectal Ca within 10 years after age 50: = 1.71% for highest intake cf 1.28% for lowest.
- Long-term red meat or pork increases Colorectal Ca risk as does heavy drinking
- Diet rich in red & processed meats, fat, sweets and refined grains (Western Diet) seems to increase risk of recurrence.
- Avoid processed meats. Processed meats had a 50% higher rate compared with fresh meats

---

[146] Am J Clin Nutr. 2006;83:527-8, 667-73

[147] Association between pre-diagnostic circulating vitamin D concentration and risk of colorectal cancer in European populations: a nested case-control study. BMJ. 2010 Jan 21;340:b5500. PMID: 20093284

Prediagnostic 25-hydroxyvitamin D, VDR and CASR polymorphisms, and survival in patients with colorectal cancer in western European populations. Cancer Epidemiol Biomarkers Prev. 2012 Apr;21(4):582-93. PMID: 22278364

- Prudent diet (fish, poultry, fruit, veg, whole grains) was not protective[148]
- Reduce red meat & pork. Don't char. Not smoked
- Red and processed meat increases the risk of colorectal cancer:35% higher rate of CAC if eating > 160 g/day cf those eating <20 g/day
- Eating more red meat doubled development of Ca distal colon: Distal Colon Ca risk increases by 70% for every additional 100 g of red meat eaten / day[149]
- Eating meat > 10 times a week x 1.8 chances of bowel Ca. Processed meat x 5 /wk = 1.5 times[150]

Fish

- Risk inversely related to eating fish. Increase consumption
- 31% risk reduction who consume 1 portion fish 2nd daily (>80g/day) cf <10g/day (once a week)[151]

Fruit and Vegetables

- Fruit and Vegetables (FV) & (250 g / day)
- Garlic protects against colorectal cancer[152]
- FV Low intake associated with increased colorectal cancer. < 1.5 serves a day had a 65% increased risk of colorectal cancer cf with those who had > 2.5 serves a day[153]
- Citrus reduce Ca of mouth and stomach (and strokes)
- Gut and Insoluble vegetable fiber (Bran) > 25 g / day
- Eating > 25g fiber a day is 40% less likely to develop bowel cancer than eating less than 10g[154]

Miscellaneous

- Avoid salty foods (pickles, fish)[155]
- Green tea – no real evidence

---

[148] JAMA 2007;298:754
[149] Int J Ca 20 Feb 2005
[150] BMJ 2002;324;1544
[151] J Nat Ca Inst 2005;97:906-916. BMJ2005;330:1406
[152] J Nut 2007;137:2264
[153] J National Car Institute 2001; 93; 525 - 33
[154] Lancet 2003;361
[155] NEMJ 2001;344:675-6

- Reduce beer consumption & heavy drinking (don't exceed 2 –3 glasses red wine a day). 2 units (pint beer) increase risk by 10%. >30g of alcohol by 25%[156]
- High magnesium intake[157] - maybe.
- Selenium (200 mcg / day) only if low. Test.
- Folate 400 mcg/day Anti-oxidant supplements not advised
- NSAIDS & Aspirin maybe protect after 10 years
- No smoking

Summary

1. Calorie restriction
2. Fat < 10%
3. Calcium Ca++ 1200 to 1400 mg / day
4. Milk 1.5 glasses / day 33% lower risk
5. Vitamin D 40% less with highest levels (1,000I.U./day D3)
6. Fish: 31% risk reduction eating fish 2nd daily
7. Fruit and Vegetables low intake = 65% increased risk
8. Fiber > 25g/day = 40% less
9. Reduce alcohol 10 - 30% increase risk
10. Magnesium - maybe
11. Green tea - no use
12. Processed red meat: 35% increase CAC if eating > 160g/day
13. Unprocessed red meat: risk increases 70% every additional 100g

b). Ca MOUTH, LARYNX and STOMACH

1. Citrus esp. oranges
2. Coffee

c). Ca LIVER

Molluscs, crustaceans and coffee reduce risk by 14%

d). PROSTATE (PCA)

PCA occurs in 50% of men older than 80 years but not too many die from it. Rates differ from country to country but if a man migrates to a Western country and eats

---

[156] Int J Cancer 2007 Jul19

[157] JAMA 2005;293:86-9 & 2599

a Western diet their rate of PCA goes up. Chinese men have a rate 120 times less than African Americans. This is thought to be the Chinese diet being higher in soya (isoflavone phytoestrogens) while the American diet is high in fat and animal protein. No nutritional intervention has been shown to have an effect once cancer established.

Regular consumption of processed lunch foods such as pizza, burgers and meat sandwiches, doubled prostate cancer risk or sugary beverages, such as sugar-sweetened soft drinks in addition to fruit juices, which can be naturally high in sugar and often contain added sugars. (Americans consume almost half of their added sugars in beverages and sugar-sweetened beverages have been shown to increase the risk of obesity and diabetes and may also have a detrimental impact on cancer risk).

Men with prostate cancer could reduce their risk of premature death by more than a third if they eat nuts regularly. Five servings a week of any type of nuts could cut the chances of death by 34%. There was no evidence nuts prevented getting prostate cancer in the first place. Nuts are rich in tocopherol a type of vitamin E. Nuts also protect against heart disease and type 2 diabetes and reduce cholesterol and increase insulin sensitivity to prevent diabetes.[158]

Summary

1. No preventive nutrition - only slowing of Ca
2. Processed foods implicated
3. Highest in those eating meat, poultry, dairy, alcohol, fats (processed foods). Reduce animal protein. Reduce fat intake.
4. Lowest with diet of: cereals, nuts, soybeans, fatty fish
5. Nuts- 34% less
6. Orange peppers/capsicums = 75% suppression
7. Garlic
8. Coffee
9. Flax - ground
10. Almond milk - 30% suppression
11. Quercetin found in apples, onions, tea & red wine blocks androgen activity in lab tests (Mayo Clinic) & hence the growth of prostate cancer cells may be prevented or stopped
12. Boron (grapes, red wine, nuts,) seems specifically protective
13. Cranberries raw

---

[158] British Journal of Cancer, 50,000 men aged over 26 examined at Harvard Medical School

14. Vit E 250 I.U. / day (?33% reduction, ?the benefit from nuts)
15. Vit D
16. Coffee 4 cups a day
17. Selenium (check levels first ?49% reduction)[159]
18. Increase intake of lentils
19. Drugs – Finasteride and Dutasteride – a 50% reduction.
20. Aspirin /NSAIDS
21. Pumpkin seeds
22. Green tea catechins (GTC)
23. Lycopene (tomatoes, strawberries) of no proven benefit
24. Soy - maybe
25. African Tree Bark (Pygeum africanum) not confirmed
26. Saw Palmetto - of no use
27. Trinoven / red clover / phytoestrogen supplements not proven
28. *Bad*
29. Eggs (>2.5 a week = 81% increased risk of death
30. Chicken and Turkey x4 risk of worsening progression
31. ? cows milk

e). BREAST CANCER

A direct association between intake of ultra-processed food and incidence of total cancer and breast cancer.[160]

Women with the highest consumption of fiber had an eight percent lower risk of breast cancer. Soluble fiber was associated with lower risks of breast cancer, and higher total fiber intake was associated with a lower risk in both premenopausal and postmenopausal women.[161]

Hypo-Caloric diet (53% less)

Weight gain after 18 (10-15 kg = 40% more)

Preschool diet of French fries linked to later breast Ca risk while milk slightly reduced[162]

Exercise -- at least 30 minutes of moderate exercise a day, five days a week, or 75 minutes of vigorous exercise per week. Two to three sessions of strength training for large muscle groups.

---

[159] Cancer 24 Sep 2007
[160] The BMJ (doi:10.1136/bmj.k322),
[161] Maryam Farvid, PhD, of the Harvard T.H. Chan School of Public Health,July 2019.
[162] Int J Cancer 2006;118:74

Less than one drink (any alcohol type)

No alcohol if Family History (70% increase risk).

Calcium and Vit D may have a lower risk in premenopausal

Healthy carbs (legumes, non-starchy vegetables, whole grains) associated with a 67% lower risk.[163]

Statins & lipid lowering drugs (70-60% less)

NSAIDs may help

HRT - debatable

Minimise red meat

Fruit: Maybe an association between higher fruit intake and lower risk of breast cancer. Especially adolescence[164]*Fats:* inconsistent results: SFAs may increase and w-3 PUFA maybe associated with reduced risk.[165] Whereas post-menopausal woman seem to be at greater risk from w-3 PUFA. Fat from fermented milk products was negatively associated with breast cancer risk The highest ingestion of vegetable oil-based dietary fats and dried soup powders showed positive associations. Dietary fiber did not influence associations[166] Other studies are contradictory or poor quality data from diet studies may dilute better quality evidence[167] Current dietary guidelines concerning fat intake are thus generally not supported by our observational results.[168]Postmenopausal breast cancer is associated with high intakes of omega6 fatty acids (Sweden).[169]

Sugar intake of the average "Western diet" directly promotes breast cancer development and metastasis to the lungs.[170]

---

[163] Federation of American Societies for Experimental Biology (FASEB). "Cancer link offers another reason to avoid highly processed carbs." ScienceDaily. ScienceDaily, 5 April 2016.
[164] Fruit and vegetable consumption in adolescence and early adulthood and risk of breast cancer: population based cohort study
BMJ 2016;353:i2343
[165] Int J Prev Med. 2014 Jan; 5(1): 6–15.
[166] Journal Nutrition and Cancer Volume 53, 2005 - Issue 2 Fat From Different Foods Show Diverging Relations With Breast Cancer Risk in Postmenopausal Women Published online: 18 Nov 2009 Download citation http://dx.doi.org/10.1207/s15327914nc5302_2
[167] BMJ 2016; 354 doi: http://dx.doi.org/10.1136/bmj.i4219 (Published 15 August 2016) Cite this as: BMJ 2016;354:i4219
[168] Journal of Internal Medicine Dietary fat intake and early mortality patterns – data from The Malmö Diet and Cancer Study, Volume 258, Issue 2 August 2005 Pages 153–165
[169] Cancer Causes Control2002;13:883-93.
[170] published online January 1, 2016 in the journal Cancer Research.

For patients with breast cancer, physical activity and avoiding weight gain are the most important lifestyle choices that can reduce the risk of cancer recurrence and death.

Vit C reduced mortality by 25% on breast cancer patients in Japan.

Diet -- Data from more than 6,000 women with breast cancer found that post-diagnosis consumption of natural foods (supplements not studied) containing isoflavones (mostly soy) was associated with a 21 percent decrease in all-cause mortality (but only in women with hormone-receptor-negative tumors, and in women who were not treated with endocrine therapy). No specific type of diet has been shown to reduce the risk of breast cancer recurrence. Evidence indicates that patients do not need to avoid soy, and it may help with weight management if used to replace higher-calorie meat protein.

Vitamin D supplements may be taken to maintain adequate levels for bone strength, since chemotherapy and hormonal treatments can reduce bone density.

Smoking: While it is unclear if stopping smoking after a breast cancer diagnosis affects recurrence, the risk of death from smoking-related health issues is a strong reason to quit.

Summary

Less Risk

1. Omega 3 from fish x 3 /week
2. Hypo-Caloric diet (53% less)
3. No alcohol if Family History (70% increase risk).
4. Calcium and Vit D may be associated with a lower risk in premenopausal
5. Exercise
6. Healthy carbs (legumes, non-starchy vegetables, whole grains) associated with a 67% lower risk
7. Fruit: Maybe an association between higher fruit intake and lower risk of breast cancer. Especially adolescence
8. Soy
9. Statins & lipid lowering drugs (70-60% less)
10. Coffee 4 (+) cups a day

11. Fat from fermented milk products was negatively associated with breast cancer risk
12. NSAIDs may help
13. Minimise red meat
14. Low GI after menopause
15. Luteolin, thyme and parsley, celery and broccoli,

Increased risk

1. Weight gain after 18 (10-15 kg = 40% more)
2. Red meat
3. Preschool diet of French fries linked to later breast Ca risk while milk slightly reduced
4. HRT
5. Fats: inconsistent results: SFAs may increase and w-3 PUFA maybe associated with reduced risk. Whereas post-menopausal woman seem to be at greater risk from w-3 PUFA
6. The highest ingestion of vegetable oil-based dietary fats and dried soup powders showed positive associations. Dietary fiber did not influence associations. Fat from fermented milk products was negatively associated with breast cancer risk
7. Dietary restrictions concerning fat intake are generally not supported by observational results. Other studies are contradictory or have been challenged alleging poor quality data
8. Postmenopausal breast cancer is associated with high intakes of omega6 fatty acids (Sweden)
9. The sugar intake of the average "Western diet" directly promotes breast cancer development and metastasis to the lungs

f). UTERINE CA

Coffee > 4 cups a day beneficial.

g). PANCREATIC CA

Some circumstances, such as smoking habits, being overweight and diabetes, have been identified as potentially predisposing factors to pancreatic cancer, suggesting that diet might play a role. A diet low in fat and sugars, together with a healthy lifestyle, regular exercise, weight reduction and not smoking, may contribute to prevent pancreatic cancer and many other cancer types. In addition, increasing evidence suggests that some food may have chemo preventive properties. Indeed, a high intake of fresh fruit and vegetables has been shown to reduce the risk of developing pancreatic cancer, and recent epidemiological studies have associated nut consumption with a protective effect against it.[171]

High CHO in sedentary & overweight women implicated in greater risk.

Smoking[172]

Epidemiological studies have associated nut consumption with a protective effect against Pancreatic Cancer.[173]

High triglycerides are a documented risk

Processed meats increases the risk of pancreatic Ca by 67%

Summary

1. Fruit and Veg
2. Nuts
3. Risks: High Triglycerides
4. No processed meats (sausages and hot dogs)

4. PREGNANCY

- Omega 3 – Fish – increase (good for brain development; may reduce eczema)
- Folate: 400 micrograms of folic acid each day before conceiving and until the 12th week of pregnancy
- Vitamin D: 10 micrograms of vitamin D each day throughout pregnancy and continue taking this supplement while breastfeeding
- Increase fruit & veg or supplement especially apples (may prevent asthma)
- There is benefit and little risk associated with Fish Oil (n–3 LCPUFA) supplementation.

Drinking

Four in 10 British women drink when pregnant. Some binge-drink in the first few months because they don't know they are pregnant. Only Ireland, Denmark and

---

[171] Diet and Pancreatic Cancer Prevention: Cancers (Basel). 2015 Dec; 7(4): 2309–2317. Published online 2015 Nov 23. doi: 10.3390/cancers7040892

[172] BMJ 2002;325;566

[173] Diet and Pancreatic Cancer Prevention: Cancers (Basel). 2015 Dec; 7(4): 2309–2317. Published online 2015 Nov 23. doi: 10.3390/cancers7040892

Belarus have worse rates. Britain has the highest rates of Fetal Alcohol Syndrome in the world.

Caffeine Drinks

A woman is more likely to miscarry if she and her partner drink more than two caffeinated beverages a day during the weeks leading up to conception. Women who drank more than two daily caffeinated beverages during the first seven weeks of pregnancy were also more likely to miscarry.[174]

Fish Oil Supplementation in Pregnancy175

There is benefit and little risk associated with n−3 LCPUFA supplementation. Offspring of women who received 2.4 g per day of n−3 LCPUFAs from 24 weeks of gestation until 1 week after delivery had a lower risk of asthmatic symptoms and fewer respiratory infections than the offspring of women who were assigned to placebo.

Multivitamins in Pregnancy "Are a Waste of Money"

A review of available evidence, published in the Drug and Therapeutics Bulletin, says pregnant women who want to help ensure their baby has the best start in life by taking multivitamin and mineral supplements are wasting their money because they are unlikely to need them and should focus on improving their overall diet instead. They should also follow official advice to take folic acid and vitamin D supplements, the researchers say.

Folic Acid and Vitamin D

The NHS recommends that pregnant women should eat a healthy, varied diet. Additionally, they should take:

10 micrograms of vitamin D each day throughout pregnancy and continue taking this supplement while breastfeeding

A study confirmed vitamin D at this level is not only safe for you, but for your baby, and the researchers from this study now recommend this daily dosage of

---

[174] Lifestyle and pregnancy loss in a contemporary cohort of women recruited before conception: The LIFE Study. Fertility and Sterility, 2016; DOI: 10.1016/j.fertnstert.2016.03.009

[175] N Engl J Med 2016; 375:2599-2601December 29, 2016DOI: 10.1056/NEJMclde1614333

vitamin D for all pregnant women. The average prenatal vitamin only contains 400 IU of vitamin D, so additional supplementation should be taken daily[176]

400 micrograms of folic acid each day before conceiving and until the 12th week of pregnancy to help prevent neural tube defects

5 milligrams of folic acid a day where there is a family history of neural tube defects or where they have diabetes or have had a previous baby with a neural tube defect

They also caution against taking vitamin A supplements, or any multivitamin containing vitamin A (retinol), because too much could harm the baby.

There is no need for pregnant women to 'eat for two'. This is a myth and all that is required is a normal, balanced amount of food.

USA: New FDA, EPA Fish Consumption Guidance for Pregnant Women and Young Kids 2017

The FDA and Environmental Protection Agency have broken down which fish are safest to eat — based on mercury levels — for young children and women of childbearing age.

The agencies recommend that women of childbearing age eat two to three servings of fish every week. Children should eat one to two servings weekly. "Fish to avoid" because of their high mercury content include king mackerel, marlin, orange roughly, shark, swordfish, Gulf of Mexico tilefish, and bigeye tuna. The chart linked below categorizes 62 types of fish based on their average mercury levels.

FDA chart categorizing 62 types of fish (Free)

Summary

1. Omega 3 - Fish oil – Fish – increase (good for baby brain development; may reduce eczema)
2. Folate: 400 micrograms of folic acid each day before conceiving and until the 12th week of pregnancy
3. Vitamin D: 10 micrograms of vitamin D each day throughout pregnancy and continue taking this supplement while breastfeeding

---

[176] Vitamin D and Pregnancy - American Pregnancy Association americanpregnancy.org/pregnancy-health/vitamin-d-and-pregnancy/

4. Increase fruit & veg or supplement especially apples (may prevent asthma in baby)
5. There is benefit and little risk associated with Fish Oil (n−3 LCPUFA) supplementation. But see Part D, Notes
6. Restrict coffee
7. Cease alcohol
8. Cease caffeine
9. Restrict salt
10. Restrict Soy
11. No smoking

5. DIABETES 2

Diabetes 2 is now an epidemic in Western civilisations. Common sense would seem to implicate our changed diet from natural to processed foods, inactivity and obesity.

Type 2 diabetes is the most common form of diabetes, occurring mostly in people aged 50 years and over. Although uncommon in childhood, it is becoming increasingly recognized in that group. People with Type 2 diabetes produce insulin but may not produce enough or cannot use it effectively. Type 2 diabetes may be managed with changes to diet and exercise, oral glucose-lowering drugs, insulin injections, or a combination of these. Another strong factor is a genetic predisposition shown by family history and ethnic background. Several modifiable risk factors also play a role in Type 2 diabetes—notably obesity, physical inactivity and an unhealthy diet. The metabolic syndrome substantially increases the risk of Type 2 diabetes.

Most T2D can be cured or controlled by weigh loss.

The Diabetes Remission Clinical Trial (DIRECT)[177] first year findings, announced in December 2017, showed that 46% of participants were in remission after twelve months. A year later, 70% of those participants are still in remission.

Remission is closely linked to weight loss, 64% of participants who lost more than 10 kilos were in remission at two years. Participants regained some weight, as expected, between the first and second years of the trial. However, those who were in remission after one year, and who had stayed in remission, had lost a greater

[177] The LANCET, VOLUME 391, ISSUE 10120, P541-551, FEBRUARY 10, 2018

amount of weight on average (15.5 kilos) than those who didn't stay in remission (12 kilos).

As well as resulting in remission for some people, there appear to be additional benefits to taking part in a weight management programme overall. These include a reported better quality of life, improved blood glucose levels and a reduced need for diabetes medications.

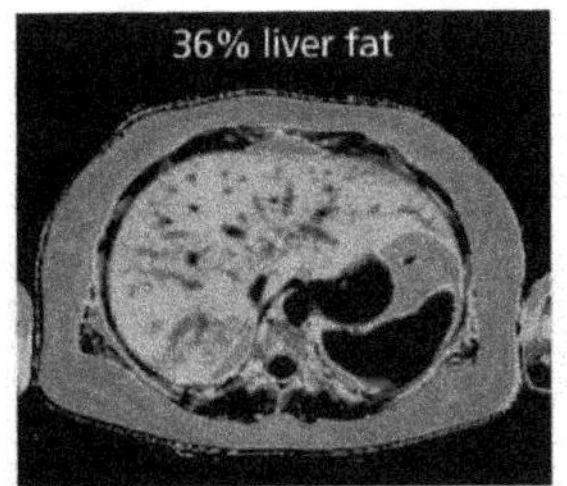

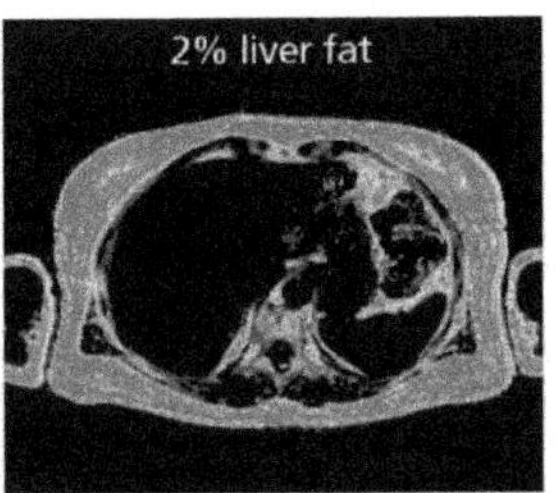

An MRI liver scan: Great amounts of (green) fat left with much less after a low-calorie diet (right) *Simple vs Complex Carbs and Diabetes 2*

Repeatedly eating foods that cause surges in blood sugar makes the pancreas work harder. Over time, that can lead to insulin resistance and an increased risk of Type 2 diabetes. Refined grain products Simple carbs) like white bread, crackers, and cookies, which tend to be low in fiber, deliver large amounts of carbohydrates per serving and are digested very quickly, raising blood sugar and insulin levels. Sugars enter into the bloodstream especially rapidly when you consume carbohydrates in liquid form, such as in sugary sodas.

Reduced Risk
Nuts (39%) less risk
Plant based 20% less risk
Strict adherence to a Mediterranean diet yielded an 83% relative reduction in the risk of developing type 2 diabetes.
Prudent: veg, fruit, fish, poultry, whole grains, less red meat results in 34% less
At ten years, higher diet quality was associated with 25% lower risk
BMI < 25
Exercise
Low Glycaemic Index Diet
Nuts
Coffee 6 cups a day
Fiber = 40% less
Alcohol: One drink a day

Increased Risk;

Western Diet: red & processed meats, dairy, refined grains, sweets, sugar-sweetened beverages: 16 % increase

Eggs: a modest elevated risk of DM with ≥3 eggs/wk was suggested

Sugary drinks

- Women who drink two (+) sugar-sweetened soft drinks per day have a 24% higher risk
- Each extra 250 mL serving of sugar sweetened beverages each day, was associated with an 18% increased risk
- Children and young adults— higher exposures and risks.
- The consumption of sugary drinks in 2016 was two to four times higher than it was in the 1980s
- Two or more daily fruit drinks (which contain little, if any, real fruit juice) lead to a 31% higher risk.

Meat.

- Women who eat the most red meat (about one serving per day) have about a 20% higher risk
- Men who eat processed meats like hot dogs, bacon, and lunch meats five times a week are twice at risk
- Trans fats. Trans fats have been a 30% increased risk of diabetes among women

Of Interest

Not restricting calories but concentrating on the nutritional value of carbohydrates, a randomized pilot study of a *calorie unrestricted* very low carbohydrate/high fat diet in overweight patients with type 2 diabetes or prediabetes resulted in a significant improvement in glycaemic control and even discontinuation of diabetes medications within 3 months in comparison to a moderate carbohydrate, low-fat calorie-restricted diet (consistent with guidelines from the American Diabetes Association), with no adverse effect on blood lipids.[178] A critical review in Nutrition also concluded that dietary carbohydrate restriction is the "single most effective intervention for reducing all of the features of the metabolic syndrome" and should be the first approach in diabetes

---

[178] A randomized pilot trial of a moderate carbohydrate diet compared to a very low carbohydrate diet in overweight or obese individuals with type 2 diabetes mellitus or prediabetes. *PLoS ONE* 2014;9:e91027. doi:10.1371/journal.pone.0091027

management with the very low carbohydrate ketogenic diet (<10% carbs) revealing the greatest falls in glycated hemoglobin.

A short course of intensive lifestyle and drug therapy achieved on-treatment normoglycemia and promoted sustained weight loss. It may also achieve prolonged, drug-free diabetes 2 remission and strongly supports ongoing studies of novel medical regimens targeting remission. Type 2 diabetes was reversed in just four months in 40% of patients by cutting calories, exercising and keeping glucose under control, a Canadian trial has shown. The treatment plan involved creating a personalized exercise regime for each trial participant and reducing their calories by between 500 and 750 a day. The participants also met regularly with a nurse and dietician to track progress and continued to take medication and insulin to manage their blood sugar levels.[179]

Summary

1. Get fit
2. Exercise
3. BMI < 25 (but see above "Of Interest" Trial)
4. Mediterranean (Newtrition) Diet
5. Low Glycaemic Index Diet
6. Nuts
7. Coffee 4 cups a day
8. Fiber = 40% less
9. Alcohol: One drink a day
10. Use good fats - Olive Oil
11. Cut out sugary drinks (colas, sodas, soft drinks, fruit juice)
12. Cut out simple carbs
13. Reduce eggs
14. You may wish to discuss the above Canadian Trial with your Doctor

6. DEPRESSION

During the past decade there has been a great deal of evidence that food and diets are strongly correlated with risk and relief of depression.

The first-ever randomized controlled clinical trial[180] to test a dietary intervention as a treatment for clinical depression found that in the treatment group, about 32% of patients achieved remission, compared with 8% in the control group. In terms

---

[179] Piloting a Remission Strategy in Type 2 Diabetes: Results of a Randomized Controlled Trial J Clin Endocrinol Metab jc.2016-3373. DOI: https://doi.org/10.1210/jc.2016-3373 Published: 15 March 2017

[180] A randomized controlled trial of dietary improvement for adults with major depression (the 'SMILES' Trial). BMC Medicine. 2017;15:23.

of risk-benefit profiles, a dietary intervention is emerging as very safe and effective.

The Newtrition Diet recommends all the foods in this trial (plus more as documented). The trial diet was called the Modified Mediterranean Diet, or the Modi-Medi Diet, by combining recommendations from the Australian government and the Greek government recommending an increase consumption of *foods in 12 food categories: Whole grains, fruits, vegetables, nuts and legumes, and lean meats, chicken, and seafood, and a decrease consumption of foods that are correlated with a higher risk for depression: empty carbohydrates, refined starches, and highly processed foods.*

(Research found a significant 7.1-point difference on the Montgomery-Asberg Depression Rating Scale) in favor of the treatment group and extrapolated that there was a 2.2-point reduction in the MADRS for every 10% adherence to the healthier dietary pattern).

Neurogenesis

There is some research that suggests those foods or lifestyles that inhibit neurogenesis (see MIND Diet) both block anti-depressants and may contribute to depression.

New 'Brain Food' Scale Flags Best Nutrients for Depression[181]

A new evidence-based scale rates animal and plant-based foods that improve depressive symptoms. There is increasing evidence regarding the crucial role that diet plays in brain health, particularly in the areas of depression and dementia. Plant foods are high on the brain food scale of brain essential nutrients (BEN) that affect the treatment and prevention of depression. Key nutrients include long-chain omega 3 fatty acids, magnesium, calcium, fiber, and vitamins B1, B9, B12, D, and E. In addition to plant sources of these nutrients some nutrients, such as vitamin B12, are predominantly found in meat and other animal products and are absolutely critical for brain health. Possible mechanisms by which these foods may boost brain function include neuronal membrane stabilization and anti-inflammatory effects.

These nutrients are key to brain function, but 2009 statistics from the U.S. Department of Agriculture show that most Americans are not getting enough of them. For example, the percentages of the US population that do not meet the recommended daily allowances for these key nutrients are as follows:

---

[181] American Psychiatric Association (APA) 2016 Annual Meeting: Presented May 17, 2016.

1. Vitamin E: 86%
2. Folate: 75%
3. Calcium: 73%
4. Magnesium: 68%
5. Zinc: 42%
6. Vitamin B6: 35%
7. Iron: 34%
8. Vitamin B12: 30%

Summary

In addition to leafy green vegetables, organ meats, game meats, nuts (pecans, walnuts, and peanuts), bivalves (mussels, clams, oysters), mollusks (octopus, squid, snail), and fish (salmon and sardines). 8 to 12 ounces of fish a week, grass-fed and pastured animals.

Increase consumption of foods in 12 food categories: Whole grains, fruits, vegetables, nuts and legumes, and lean meats, chicken, and seafood, and to decrease consumption of foods that are correlated with a higher risk for depression: empty carbohydrates, refined starches, and highly processed foods. Ensure adequate of the above vitamins and minerals

Male vegetarians are at greater risk for depression than their meat-eating counterparts.[182]

7. OSTEOPOROSIS

- Calcium, Vitamins B, C, D, K also zinc, magnesium, phytoestrogens. Calcium: 800 - 1400 mg / day.
- Dairy (not butter & cream), green leafy veg, soybean, canned fish with bones
- Less: Salt), protein, caffeine, phosphates (soft drinks)
- Early Postmenopausal: Calcium ineffective. Vit D good
- Vit D: Elderly less exposed to sun, less precursor in skin, absorbed less & eat less. Increase Vit D in diet or 1,000 i.u. D3 / day
- *Vit K:* Increased intake needed with age
- *Protein:* High Protein diets increase Calcium loss
- *Oxalates:* (e.g. spinach) binds Calcium; as does fiber
- *Boron:* Fruit & veg
- *Soy:* May increase BMC
- *Onions (GPCS):* reduced bone loss[183]

---

[182] J Affect Disord. 2017;225:13-17.
[183] J Ag & Food Chem, 4May 2005

8. ARTHRITIS RHEUMATOID

- 'Greek Diet': Olive and Canola oils, fish (any), legumes, cereals, poultry. It's probably the Oleic A & Vit E which are anti-inflammatory. Can give x3 times relief after 6 weeks.
- BMI has a paradoxical effect (The higher the BMI the lower the mortality)
- Certain antioxidants (carotenoids: beta-cryptoxanthin & zeaxanthin) found in yellow/orange fruit & vegetables were associated with a lower chance of developing inflammatory arthritis.
- These diets are not a miracle but are worth trying and sticking to even if somewhat disappointing.

9. CROHN'S and ULCERATIVE COLITIS

New Diet Helps Children with Crohn's Disease, Ulcerative Colitis Reach Remission

No grains, dairy, processed foods, and sugars, except for honey. The diet promotes only natural, nutrient-rich foods, which includes vegetables, fruits, meats and nuts.

10. EYES:

AMD (age-related macular degeneration)

The Age-Related Eye Disease Studies (AREDS) found a high dose of antioxidants (vitamin C, vitamin E, beta-carotene) and zinc reduced progression of AMD by 25% and the same reduction when beta carotene was replaced with lutin/zexanthin (presumably because of the dangers of beta carotene - lung cancer increase)

Fruit-rich Mediterranean diet may cut risk by 35% (higher diet adherence scores meant lower AMD risk)

Those who consumed 150 grams (five ounces) or more of fruit a day: 54.5% did not have AMD and 45.5% had AMD. People who ate that much fruit or more each day were almost 15% less likely to have AMD

Broccoli

Caffeine and antioxidants also were protective

Higher consumption of antioxidants such as caffeine, beta-carotene and vitamins C and E were protective against AMD. Those who consumed high levels of caffeine (about 78mg a day, or the equivalent of one shot of espresso): 54.4% did not have AMD and 45.1% had AMD

Zeaxanthin: Helpful against age-related macular degeneration and impaired eyesight. It is found in pumpkins but a newly deliberately University developed strain of Sweet Corn "SuperGold" (not GM) has ten times the zeaxanthin content as normal corn

Cataracts

Fruit and vegetables two servings each a day (Vitamin C) had a 20% lower risk

Ten years later those who took twice the recommended daily allowance of Vitamin C 150 instead of 75 mg for women and 180 instead of 90 mg for men, had 33% lower risk of their cataracts progressing

Oranges, cantaloupe, kiwi, broccoli and green leafy vegetables are recommended

Carnosine showed a success rate of 80% in advanced senile cataracts, and 100% in patients with mild to moderate cataracts, over the 6 months trial period

Summary
Vitamin C
Vitamin E
Lutin
Zexanthin
Zinc
Caffeine (coffee)
Carnosine
Fruit & Veg as above

11. ELDERLY

The Elderly need less food but the highest quality must be maintained and emphasized. Some Nutritionists suggest 800 calories less per day. But old age can lead to reduced absorption of such nutrients as Vitamin B12. Any unexplained weight loss or poor hydration are major bell ringers.

There are a number of nutritional plans that can be used:

- Malnutrition Universal Screening Tool (MUST)
- Malnutrition Screening Tool (MST)
- Nutritional Risk Screening 2002 (NRS 2002)
- Geriatric Nutritional Risk Index (GNRI)
- Simplified Nutritional Assessment Questionnaire (SNAQ)
- Nutritional Assessments
- Mini-Nutritional Assessment (MNA) and Mini-Nutritional Assessment Short Form (MNA-SF)
- Subjective Global Assessment

But, again, the key is regular monitoring, even if this means watching just what they eat plus ensuring a wide variety of foods while ensuring adequate protein. If they are eating like little birds then a multivitamin may be warranted. Those living alone or in Nursing Homes are especially at risk.

Memory[184]

High consumption of fruit and vegetables was linked to lowered odds of memory loss and its comorbid heart disease. High consumption of protein-rich foods was associated with a better memory.

People aged 80 years and over with a low consumption of cereals are at the highest risk of memory loss and its comorbid heart disease, her research showed.

12. RESIRATORY DISEASES

Nuts 52% reduction in risk

13. INFECTIOUS DISEASES

Nuts 75% reduction in risk

---

[184] ScienceDaily. ScienceDaily, 18 February 2020. <www.sciencedaily.com/releases/2020/02/200218124351.htm>

PART C

NOTES

ON

INDIVIDUAL FOODS

AND

NUTRIENTS

The following NOTES may have confusing and contradictory studies. That is how medicine and science often work and while it can be perplexing and annoying, as we all want an absolute simple answer, the truth or the best recommendations eventually reveals themselves by such on-going studies. In addition, some foods have been studied more than others and while this does not detract from any benefits they may bestow, there are many others yet to be so exhaustively investigated. Variety would seem to be the key at this stage of our knowledge as no one food can make claim to contributing unique total benefits. Superfoods, so called, are those which may contain high amounts of micronutrients but again a variety of foods may contribute other micronutrients which make the "super" food ingredients work better.

I have often included the chemical and study details for your interest or rejection, but they do show the considerable detailed research which forms the basis for **Newtrition**.

We have been immersed in "The Age of Kale" where organic, biodynamic smoothies have become an almost religious ritual as the disciples queue like Lemmings to get their fix. Well it's certainly better than colas and sugar drinks but it's all a fad that each year or so sees some amazing new "superfood" discovered which somehow seems to have escaped the best research and studies. There is nothing wrong with Kale by the way it's just that it doesn't have any advantages over most other cruciferous vegetables with Bok Choy having the most anti-cancer properties. Maybe we are entering the "Age of Bok"?

However, the media and glossy mags tell us the new "super-super foods for 2017 are NotMilk, made with almonds, peas, rice, nuts, linseed, coconut and vanilla. Beetroot too has been superseded by anthocyanin-rich blackcurrants. Inulin is being used as a sweetener while Himalayan or South African rock salt is hailed as they have 35% less sodium and more micronutrient minerals. But wait! The Super-super foods continue with Maqui berries, Watermelon seeds replacing chia and pumpkin seeds which are now pushed to the back cupboard with the kale. Chaga mushroom tea, it would seem will allow you win an Olympic Gold Medal without even training while nut oils are to be "used sparingly" (just in case you fail the drug tests before the Medal Ceremony). But the final essential Super-super food, we are assured, will be Algae fats. Meanwhile, however, on the other side of the world we are assured, just as enthusiastically that the "superfoods" for 2017 will be Raw Cacao Nibs, Red Algae, Kakadu Plum (also known as Gubinge), Turmeric, Goji Berries, Bone Broth, Coconut Sugar, Insects, Pea Protein, Black Bean Pasta, Avocado oil, Goat Meat, Tilapia, Maca Powder, Buckwheat noodles and Macadamia Nuts.

Fast forward to 2020 and we now must have Watermelon seeds, Tahini, Tempeh, Moringa, Casava, Golden Berries, Broccoli Sprouts, Tiger Nuts (?).

But how sad! The guru who advocates these obviously hasn't heard of her rival guru's Nervines, Chlorella, Raw cacao and Digestive bitters.

Like the Touchstone that turns lead into gold we humans love to hope and believe in magic. To that end we eagerly seek these self-appointed gurus' anointed superfoods and may ascribe properties to foods that they don't have. On one hand we have people who seek any new fad while on the other hand when patients are ill, especially with cancer, they are extremely vulnerable and will try anything from macrobiotic diets to cabbage soup let alone the Charlatan Mix of chemicals that don't work.

But after all is said and done it comes down to the results of exhaustive medical studies and trials and the amalgam of beneficial micronutrients from the variety the Newtrition Micronutrient Revolution Diet provides.

All these 'new discoveries' may well be nutritious but the Newtrition Foods provide all the macro and micro-nutrients humans need. By all means try these new additions but, again:

It is the variety of foods and the 20/20 split between the various food groups that provide the full spectrum of foods that then combine in an amalgam to provide these beneficial nutrients.
No one food does it.

NEWTRITION does not promote, endorse or recommend anything that is not proven as much as can be and the nutritional advice has evolved from first rate evidenced trials and can be endorsed and recommended. However, before evidence can be gathered there is a long period of observation and suspicion as to possible benefits.

The following NOTES are research extracts, which either further supports the evidence or highlights research of interest, which may (or may not) later be proven. But if they do no harm in the interim, I can't object to incorporating them while awaiting evidence. Of course, there is nothing anyone can do about conflicting studies except keep an open mind and see what develops.

Alcohol

One unit translates to approximately 2 deciliters (dl) or 200 ml or 6.8 fluid ounces of beer, 1 dl or 3.4 ounces of wine, or 4 centiliters (cl) or 1.35 ounces of hard liquor.

Level of alcohol consumption:

Low = up to seven drinks a week
Moderate: Women = seven to 14; men = seven to 21 drinks/wk
High = women =14 (+); men = 21 (+) /wk
Heavy episodic (Binge) drinking = five or more drinks in one sitting at least once per month

- The World Health Organization defines a standard drink as 10 g of pure ethanol, with both men and women advised not to exceed 2 standard drinks per day. Although the WHO's definition of a standard drink is the one most often used, 50% of countries with drinking guidelines don't use it
- In the most conservative countries, low-risk consumption means drinking no more than 10 g of pure ethanol per day for women, 20 g for men
- Research, which was presented at the American Association for the Advancement of Science's annual conference, has found that moderate drinking is linked to a longer life. Drinking about two glasses of wine or beer a day was linked to an 18% drop in a person's risk of early death—an even stronger effect than the life-preserving practice of exercise,
- Compared with moderate drinkers (Moderate alcohol consumption seems associated with lower cardiovascular risks, but the relationship is highly nuanced, as follows:
    - Nondrinkers had increased risks for unheralded cardiac death (hazard ratio, 1.56), unstable angina, myocardial infarction, abdominal aortic aneurysm, heart failure, peripheral arterial disease, and ischemic stroke (HR, 1.12).
    - Heavy drinkers showed increased risks for cardiac arrest/sudden death (HR, 1.50), intracerebral hemorrhage, peripheral arterial disease, ischemic stroke, heart failure, unheralded coronary death, and transient ischemic attack (HR, 1.11).
    - Occasional drinkers had higher risks for heart failure (HR, 1.19), myocardial infarction, unheralded coronary death, and peripheral arterial disease (HR, 1.11).
    - Former drinkers showed some increased risks, but the authors say the findings align with the "sick quitter" hypothesis — that is, many people stop drinking when they become ill.
    - From 87 previously published studies on drinking and death from all

causes it was found all but 13 of these experiments had a critical flaw. Recommendations: Never binge drink and drinking small amounts when drinking - with meals - is a good rule of thumb. People should not drink for health reasons. If they choose to drink - usually for reasons other than health - they should not exceed two drinks on any given day to minimize their health risks[185]

  * A random sample of the Finnish population found that consumption of wine with meals was associated with high socioeconomic status and high subjective well-being[186]

- The more you earn the more you drink: Official UK figures relate that those who earn $80,000 a year or more are more than twice as likely to drink every day as those earning $20,000 a year or less and increasing with income. 45% consume more than a third of the weekly limit in a single day[187]
- Drinking alcohol does not result in a net health benefit and, in fact, increases the risk for alcohol-related cancers by 51%, according to a study of almost 115,000 people from 12 countries. Heavy drinking increases the risk for death by 31% to 54%.

Over a follow-up of about 4 years, current drinking was linked to:

24% lower risk for heart attack
51% increased risk for alcohol-related cancers (mouth, liver, esophagus, stomach, colorectal, breast, ovary, head and neck)
29% increased risk for injury

There was no reduction in the risk for death or stroke among current drinkers.

The risk for cardiovascular disease was lower in wine drinkers than in never drinkers, and the risk for heart attack was significantly lower. However, the risk for cancer was 38% higher in wine drinkers than in never drinkers, 69% higher in spirit drinkers, and 20% higher in beer drinkers.

The reduction in risk of heart attack is consistent with previous literature. However, this may be offset by increases in risk for other outcomes.

---

[185] J Stud Alcohol Drugs 2016.
[186] Alcohol and Alcoholism (doi:10.1093/alcalc/agw016)
[187] Office of National Statistics UK 2016

People with high alcohol intake had a 31% increased risk for death. Those with heavy episodic drinking had a 54% increased risk for mortality and a 71% increased risk for injury.[188]

- Women who drink beer at most once or twice per week run a 30% lower risk of heart attack, compared with both heavy drinkers and women who never drink beer. These are the findings of a Swedish study, which has followed 1,500 women over a period of almost 50 years.[189]In male smokers and women, even light-to-moderate drinking is associated with increased risk for alcohol-related cancers. Women who consumed up to one standard drink daily had a 13% increased risk for all alcohol-related cancers combined (cancers of the colon-rectum, breast, oral cavity, pharynx, larynx, liver, and esophagus), relative to abstainers. The association was due mainly to an increase in breast cancer risk. Among men, consuming up to two drinks daily was associated with increased risk for alcohol-related cancers — but only among men who'd ever smoked. Using data from recent two large cohort studies in the United States, when All-Cause Mortality attributable to alcohol is considered, drinking more than 10 g of pure alcohol per day for women or 20 g for men over a lifetime can lead to a magnitude of risk not considered acceptable for voluntary behavior in modern societies. Light to moderate drinking should be limited to no more than 10 g of pure alcohol a day for women and 20 g for men (roughly one standard drink a day for women and two standard drinks for men, as defined in most countries).

In women, light to moderate drinking was associated with an increased risk of cancers with an established link to alcohol consumption—that is, cancer of the colon-rectum, female breast, oral cavity, pharynx, larynx, liver, and esophagus. The increased risk was driven mainly by breast cancer. Similar findings emerged for light to moderate male drinkers who had ever smoked. No significant association was found in men who never smoked, or in women outside the relation with breast cancer[190]

- Long-term moderate ingestion of alcohol, especially wine, is associated with a smaller risk of death from CVS diseases and other causes but also a greater life expectation. (A 40 year Dutch study)[191]
- Wine drinkers in Denmark buy healthier food such as olives, fruits, vegetables, fish, lean meats and dairy compared with beer drinkers who were

[188] Published online the Lancet.September 17, 2015

[189] A 32-year longitudinal study of alcohol consumption in Swedish women: Reduced risk of myocardial infarction but increased risk of cancer. Scandinavian Journal of Primary Health Care, 2015 DOI: 10.3109/02813432.2015.1067515

[190] BMJ 2015;351:h4400

[191] Science/Health 1 march 2007

more likely to buy frozen dinners, cold cuts, pork, mutton, sugary foods, butter, margarine and soft drinks. Wine drinkers also tended to have higher education levels, higher earnings and be in better psychological health[192]

- A glass of wine per day can cut risk of heart failure by a fifth, and with better outcomes than abstaining but heavy drinkers (>21 drinks per week) were more likely to die from any cause[193]
- Wine reduces the risk of death from all causes. Red wine has been found superior to white wine, rose, beer, spirits and grape juice. Red wine contains polyphenols, which block the peptides, which constrict (coronary) arteries and thus make it more beneficial
- Resveratrol in grapes has been found to inhibit initiation, promotion & progression of cancer. It is an endogenous fungicide and killed if the grapes have been sprayed (with a fungicide)
- A moderate amount (8 to 21 glasses a week, 2/day) confers maximum benefit and is slightly better than a light amount. More than a daily intake of 4 glasses for men and 2 for women, however, increases mortality. Women with a family history of breast cancer should limit their intake. No alcohol should be taken when pregnant. Alcohol is also empty calories and it is hard to lose weight if drinking a lot
- Red wine reduces death from all causes
- 8 - 21 glasses (5 oz.) / week confers max benefit
- Even in men at low risk on the basis of BMI, physical activity, smoking and diet moderate alcohol intake is associated with lower risk of a heart attack[194]

-

- Drinking red grape juice or wine -- in moderation -- could improve the health of overweight people by helping them burn fat better, Four natural chemicals are found in Muscadine grapes, a dark-red variety native to the south-eastern United States. One of the chemicals, ellagic acid, proved particularly potent: It dramatically slowed the growth of existing fat cells and formation of new ones, and it boosted metabolism of fatty acids in liver cells. The findings suggest that consuming dark-colored grapes whether eating them or drinking juice or wine, might help people better manage obesity and related metabolic disorders such as fatty liver but are not a weight-loss miracle[195]
- Wine only protects against cardiovascular disease (CVD) in people who exercise, according to results from the In Vino Veritas (IVV) study The only

[192] Ugeskrift for Laeger Feb 2007
[193] Eur Heart J 2015; online 20 Jan
[194] Arch Int Med 2006;166:2145
[195] Ellagic acid modulates lipid accumulation in primary human adipocytes and human hepatoma Huh7 cells via discrete mechanisms. The Journal of Nutritional Biochemistry, 2015; 26 (1): 82 DOI: 10.1016/j.jnutbio.2014.09.010

positive and continuous result was in the subgroup of patients who took more exercise, which means regular exercise at least twice a week, plus the wine consumption. In this group HDL cholesterol increased and LDL and total cholesterol decreased in the red and white wine groups. There may be some synergy between the low dose of ethyl alcohol in wine and exercise, which is protective against CVD[196].

- The mortality benefits of light-to-moderate drinking appear to be much narrower than previously reported. In fully adjusted analyses, only men aged 50 to 64 and women 65 and older saw significant mortality benefits from drinking relative to never-drinkers. Among these men, benefits were seen only at 15-to 20-alcohol units/week or 0.1 to 1.5 units on the heaviest drinking day. Among these women, benefits were seen at 10 or fewer units/week and all levels of heaviest-day drinking[197]
- Moderate drinking in later years may damage heart
- Moderate to heavy alcohol intake, drinking two or more alcoholic beverages daily may damage the heart of elderly people with subtle changes in the structure and efficiency of the heart. Women may be particularly vulnerable to negative cardiac effects of alcohol at moderate to higher levels of consumption.
- The more people drank, the greater the subtle changes to the heart's structure and function.
- Among men, drinking more than 14 alcoholic beverages weekly (heavy drinking) was linked with enlargement of the wall of the heart's main pumping chamber (left ventricular mass).
- Among women, moderate drinkers had small reductions in heart function
- "Women appear more susceptible than men to the cardiotoxic effects of alcohol, which might potentially contribute to a higher risk of alcoholic cardiomyopathy[198]
- A 2015 survey commissioned by the Alcohol Health Alliance found that 47% of Britons — much more than previously thought — were at risk from the amount they drank. Until now, it was believed that 34% of men and 28% of women drank more than recommended, based on official figures from the General Lifestyle Survey 2011

---

[196] European Society of Cardiology. "Wine only protects against CVD in people who exercise." ScienceDaily. ScienceDaily, 31 August 2014
. www.sciencedaily.com/releases/2014/08/140831125255.htm

[197] BMJ 2015

[198] Relationship Between Alcohol Consumption and Cardiac Structure and Function in the Elderly The Atherosclerosis Risk in Communities Study. Circulation: Cardiovascular Imaging, May 2015
DOI: 10.1161/CIRCIMAGING.114.002846

- increasing the size of wine glasses led to an almost 10% increase in wine sales by encouraging people to drink more,[199]
- *Light-to-moderate drinking good for your heart*
- The greater the drinking frequency, the lower the risk
- A study, which looked at the relationship between heart failure and alcohol, followed 60,665 participants who had no incidence of heart failure at that time
- The more often participants consumed alcohol within normal amounts, the lower their risk of heart failure turned out to be. Those who drank five or more times a month had a 21% lower risk compared to non-drinkers and those who drank little, while those who drank between one and five times a month had a 2% lower risk
- *Drinking isn't necessary for a healthy heart*
- Adjusted analyses showed that each additional one-drink increment decreased the risk of Acute Myocardial Infarction (AMI) - heart attack - by 28 %
- Coronary computed tomography angiography (CCTA) found no association between light to moderate alcohol consumption and coronary artery disease (CAD) whereas some previous studies suggested that light alcohol consumption may actually reduce the risk for CAD. However, data regarding regular alcohol consumption and its association with the presence of CAD remains controversial [200]
- *Alcohol may increase other problems*
- The risk of a number of other diseases and social problems can increase as a result of higher alcohol consumption. For example, the risk of dying from various types of cardiovascular disease increased with about five drinks a week and up, while those who drank more moderate amounts had the lowest risk. High alcohol consumption was also strongly associated with an increased risk of death from liver disease[201]
- For the association between alcohol intake and myocardial infarction (MI), ischemic stroke (IS) and hemorrhagic stroke (HS) there appears to be a consistent finding of an immediately higher cardiovascular risk following any

---

[199] Does wine glass size influence sales for on-site consumption? A multiple treatment reversal design. BMC Public Health, 2016; 16 (1) DOI: 10.1186/s12889-016-3068-z

[200] Radiological Society of North America. "Alcohol consumption shows no effect on coronary arteries." ScienceDaily. ScienceDaily, 29 November 2016.

[201] Light-to-moderate drinking and incident heart failure — the Norwegian HUNT study. International Journal of Cardiology, 2016; 203: 553 DOI: 10.1016/j.ijcard.2015.10.179
Alcohol consumption is associated with a lower incidence of acute myocardial infarction: results from a large prospective population-based study in Norway. Journal of Internal Medicine, 2015; DOI: 10.1111/joim.12428

alcohol consumption but by 24 hours, only heavy alcohol intake conferred continued risk. Alcohol may have markedly different effects on immediate and long-term risk

- Moderate alcohol consumption was associated with an immediate higher cardiovascular risk, attenuated after 24 hours, and even protective for MI and HS (≈2-4 drinks: = 30% lower risk), and protective against IS within one week (≈ 6 drinks: 19% lower risk). Heavy alcohol drinking was associated with higher cardiovascular risk the following day (≈ 6-9 drinks) and week (19-30 drinks)
- Even moderate alcohol consumption -- one drink a day for women and up to two drinks a day for men -- may raise a person's risk of a heart attack or stroke approximately two-fold within the hour following consumption compared to other times. However, heavy alcohol use was associated with higher heart attack and stroke risks at all times studied. Six to nine drinks in a day nearly doubled the risk, and 19 to 30 drinks weekly elevated the risk by up to six times more[202]
- Beer consumption may protect against Aβ aggregation in the brain which is one of the pathological signs of Alzheimer's disease.[203]
- Grenache, has two to three times the amount of flavonoids as compared to other red wines. Small doses of this antioxidant-rich beverage throughout the day could explain fewer heart attacks and lower levels of stress among men in Sardinia. Grenache is also grown in the Rhone and Australia.
- 34% of the women and 16% of the men survived to their 60s, those who drank 5–15 g/d of alcohol had 'the highest probability of reaching 90[204].

A Supplement That May Block the Toxic Effects of Alcohol[205]

Ethyl alcohol is metabolized to acetaldehyde by alcohol dehydrogenase in the liver. Acetaldehyde is metabolized to acetate by aldehyde dehydrogenase and then to carbon dioxide and water. Depending on the alcohol dose, some of the acetaldehyde may escape hepatic metabolism and enter the general blood circulation.

---

[202] Alcohol and Immediate Risk of Cardiovascular Events: A Systematic Review and Dose-Response Meta-Analysis Circulation. 2016; published online before print March 2 2016, doi:10.1161/CIRCULATIONAHA.115.019743

[203] Beer Drinking Associates with Lower Burden of Amyloid Beta Aggregation in the Brain: Helsinki Sudden Death Series. Alcoholism: Clinical and Experimental Research, 2016; DOI: 10.1111/acer.13102

[204] Age and Ageing, afaa003, https://doi.org/10.1093/ageing/afaa003
Published: 09 February 2020

[205] George D. Lundberg, MD At Large at Medscape September 26, 2017

Some people, mostly East Asian and (I think) the Mongol genetics in Russia, are genetically deficient in aldehyde dehydrogenase and can't metabolize booze well (the classic "two-pot screamer"). The drug disulfiram also inhibits this detoxification.

For most, certainly European, people they metabolize roughly one standard drink per hour. If you drink more than that, depending on body weight, gastric contents, and the efficiency of your metabolic alcohol breakdown, acetaldehyde will build up because aldehyde dehydrogenase capability can be overwhelmed.

Acetaldehyde is a close cousin to formaldehyde. Both are known carcinogens. Our body's defence mechanism against excess acetaldehyde is the amino acid l-cysteine and glutathione. These molecules, similarly to thiamine, contain a sulfhydryl group that is chemically active against aldehydes.

If you quit drinking at 11:00 PM, then around about 1:00 AM, your acetaldehyde level may be elevated and you may feel symptoms of acetaldehyde toxicity, including skin flushing, tachycardia, palpitations, anxiety, nausea, thirst, chest pain, and vertigo. Of course, you are trying to "sleep it off," so you may not feel toxic until the next morning when that dreaded hangover appears.

Metabolizing Alcohol

To repeat the above, you can enhance the metabolism of blood alcohol to acetate, carbon dioxide, and water and minimize the acetaldehyde molecular logjam by taking oral supplements. *L-cysteine, vitamin C, and vitamin* B_1 are purported to help. At supplement doses, they are cheap and harmless at worst. At best: Goodbye, acetaldehyde toxicity; hello, restful sleep. About 200 mg of L-cysteine per ounce of alcohol consumed is sufficient to block a major portion of the toxic effect of acetaldehyde. But because alcohol is absorbed and metabolized rapidly, it may be necessary to take L-cysteine before and concurrently with consumption to maintain protection. Also, an excess of vitamin C (perhaps 600 mg) can help keep the L-cysteine in its reduced state and "on the job" against acetaldehyde. Experts recommend these doses (with or without extra B_1): one round before drinking, one with each additional drink, and one when finished.

Unfortunately, this concoction may have little effect on next-day hangovers, the causes of which are complex and resistant to prevention—except, obviously, by not drinking too much, which is, of course, the best answer to alcohol anyway.

Anthocyanins

Anthocyanins are regarded as the most versatile compound in terms of human health. Others, like carotenoids or glucosinolates, are recognized for benefits against one chronic disease, or a narrow spectrum of conditions. But anthocyanins have demonstrated efficacy against an extremely broad range of health impediments.

Anthocyanins, members of the flavonoid family of polyphenols, are among the most abundant flavonoids and may play important roles in helping reduce the risk of CVD, cognitive decline, and cancer[206] and possibly type 2 diabetes, metabolic syndrome, hypertension and gastrointestinal issues.

They are found some types of pigmented grains (e.g. black rice, purple corn); in certain varieties of root and leafy vegetables such as aubergine (egg plant), red cabbage, red onions, radishes, beans; but especially in red and purple fruits, vegetables and red wine. Content in vegetables and fruits is generally proportional to their color: it increases during maturation.

Anthocyanin rich foods foodstuff	Anthocyanin in mg per 100 g
aubergine (egg plant)	750
black currant	130-400
blackberry	83-326
blueberry	25-497
cherry	350-400
chokeberry	200-1000
cranberry	60-200
elderberry	450
orange	~200
plum - Queen Garnet	150 - 280
radish	11-60
raspberry	10-60
red currant	80-420
red grape	30-750
red onions	7-21
red wine	24-35
strawberry	15-35

One of the "secrets" of the Okinawans, among the world's longest living people is their high ingestion of purple sweet potato.

206 Dietary anthocyanin-rich plants: biochemical basis and recent progress in health benefits studies. *Mol Nutr Food Res.* 2012;56(1):159-170

Antibiotics

While not nutrients antibiotics are freely administered to the livestock we eat. Only about a fifth is to treat human illness. Most of the rest is given to livestock -- and not because the animals are sick. Instead -- despite increasing antibiotic resistance among pathogens -- the drugs are used for what the FDA calls "production purposes": to help animals gain weight more rapidly or to improve feed efficiency. In 2012 the FDA asked farmers voluntarily to agree only to use antibiotics to promote animal health and only then if the use is approved by a veterinarian. The FDA guidance "politely requests in an absolutely nonbinding manner that pharmaceutical companies change their drug labeling to suggest antibiotics shouldn't be used to promote growth in farm animals."

Yeah – sure.

The European countries and Australia are far ahead of the USA - they've already banned antibiotics in animal feed.

Evidence is mounting that nonhuman use of antibiotics is a risk factor for human health. In November, researchers in Pennsylvania found that proximity to high-density swine production operations was associated with greater risk of acquiring methicillin-resistant *Staphylococcus aureus* (MRSA). And in 2012, other researchers made a similar finding, this time looking at farms in the Netherlands.[207]

Antioxidants

People who get a lot of antioxidants in their diets, or who take them in supplement form, don't live any longer than those who just eat well overall, according to a long-term study of retirees in California. High doses of beta-carotene may increase the risk of lung cancer in smokers, high doses of vitamin E may increase risks of prostate cancer and one type of stroke, and antioxidant supplements may also interact with some medicines. Antioxidant supplements should not be used to replace a nutritionally adequate diet[208]

---

207 MedPage Dec 29, 2013

208 December 29, 2014, American Journal of Epidemiology. http://bit.ly/1Fgx3a8. Extra Antioxidants May Make Little Difference in Lifespan.

Daily intake = 17 mmom/dL
Coffee = *11*
Fruit = *1.8*
Tea = *1.4*
Wine = *0.8*
Grains = *0.8*
Veg = *0.4*[209]

The consumption of fruit & vegetables reduces the risk of major chronic degenerative diseases. The active compounds & mechanisms in this protective effect have not been well defined. Leutin, zeaxanthin & lycopene seem to contribute most. Beta-carotene Alpha-tocopherol (VitE) & VitC contribute <10%[210]

Treatment with beta-carotene, vitamin A and vitamin E may increase mortality. The potential roles of vitamin C and selenium need further study[211]

Supplements are not effective and may interfere with statins.

Eating foods rich in antioxidants, as well as taking antioxidant supplements, can actually promote cancer, rather than fight or prevent it[212]

Apples

Skin contains more antioxidants and micronutrients than the flesh.

Estimates are that the skin contains over 90% of nutrients and the rest is high in sugar and calories

Red Delicious have the highest concentration of antioxidants (up to 27% more than lowest variety)

Apple seems to have a protective effect on the gastric mucosa

Apples during pregnancy may protect child against wheeze and asthma[213]

An apple a day can reduce All-Cause Mortality by 35%. Women who ate more than 100 grams or one small apple a day had a longer life expectancy than those

---

209 J Nutrit 2004;134:562-67
210 J Nutrit 2004;134:
211 JAMA 2007;297:842-57
212 The Promise and Perils of Antioxidants for Cancer Patients. *New England Journal of Medicine*, 2014; 371 (2): 177 DOI: 10.1056/NEJMcibr1405701
213 Thorax 2007 doi;10.1136/thx.2006.074187

who only ate 5 g a day. Other fruit reduced the risk of mortality from cardiovascular disease (banana or total fruit intake) or cancer. Apples have high soluble fiber with magnesium, potassium, vitamin C and flavenoids in their skin[214]

An Apple (or white fruit) a day keeps the Strokes Away

During 10 years of follow-up, 233 strokes were documented. Green, orange/yellow and red/purple fruits and vegetables weren't related to stroke. However, the risk of stroke incidence was 52 percent lower for people with a high intake of white fruits and vegetables compared to people with a low intake

Each 25-gram per day increase in white fruits and vegetable consumption was associated with a 9% lower risk of stroke[215]

Granny Smith Apples

The non-digestible compounds in apples including dietary fiber and polyphenols, and low content of available carbohydrates which, despite being subjected to chewing, stomach acid and digestive enzymes, remain intact when they reach the colon. Once there, they are fermented by bacteria in the colon and benefits growth of friendly bacteria in the gut[216]

May help prevent disorders associated with obesity. The balance of bacterial communities in the colon of obese people is disturbed. Re-establishing a healthy balance of bacteria in the colon stabilizes metabolic processes that influence inflammation and the sensation of feeling satisfied, or satiety

The nondigestible compounds in the Granny Smith apples actually changed the proportions of fecal bacteria from obese mice to be similar to that of lean mice. The study showed that Granny Smith apples surpass Braeburn, Fuji, Gala, Golden Delicious, McIntosh and Red Delicious in the amount of nondigestible compounds they contain[217]

---

[214] University of Western Australia March 2016 (some 1500 Women aged 70 t0 85 years followed for 16 years).

[215] American Heart Association (2011, September 16). An apple or pear a day may keep strokes away. *ScienceDaily*. Retrieved September 30, 2011, from http://www.sciencedaily.com-/releases/2011/09/110915163523.htm

[216] Food Chemistry, 2014; 161: 208 DOI: 10.1016/j.foodchem.2014.03.122

[217] Assessing non-digestible compounds in apple cultivars and their potential as modulators of obese faecal microbiota in vitro. Food Chemistry, 2014; 161: 208 DOI: 10.1016/j.foodchem.2014.03.122

Aphrodisiacs

Any product that bears labeling claims that it will arouse or increase sexual desire, or that it will improve sexual performance, is an aphrodisiac drug product. But there is a lack of adequate data to establish general recognition of the safety and effectiveness of any of these ingredients, or any other ingredient, for OTC use as an aphrodisiac:

Advertised products (that don't work): Anise, cantharides, don qual, estrogens, fennel, ginseng, golden seal, gotu kola, Korean ginseng, licorice, mandrake, minerals, methyltestosterone, nux vomica, Pega Palo, sarsaparilla, strychnine, testosterone, vitamins, yohimbine, yohimbine hydrochloride, and yohimbinum have been present as ingredients in such drug products.

Foods: These, too, are products of hope and imagination not to mention the placebo effect. Most have gained their reputation from their appearance. Oysters, avocados, pistachios, bananas; or hope, chai tea, or an euphoric effect, red wine and chocolate.

Artificial Sweeteners

Artificial sweeteners can possibly increase risk of developing diabetes or exacerbation of glycemic control in patients with diabetes, and the same for obesity with increased body weight and waist-to-hip ratios i.e. a central obesity pattern seen in metabolic syndrome. These changes were all related to this exposure to non-caloric artificial sweeteners, and there seemed to be a dose-related effect: Those people who used more of these non-caloric artificial sweeteners had even more pronounced effects[218] Saccharine and aspartame elevated blood glucose more than sugar. However, opinions are that they are better than sugar laden soda-colas.

A link between consumption of both sugar-sweetened and artificially sweetened beverages and reduction in brain volume in a middle-aged cohort has been shown.[219]

Consumption of one can of diet soda or more each day was associated with a three times increased risk for stroke and dementia over a 10-year follow-up period compared with individuals who drank no artificially sweetened beverages.[220]

---

[218] sweeteners induce glucose intolerance by altering the gut microbiota. Nature. 2014;514:181-186.
[219] Alzheimer's and Dementia March 5, 2017
[220] Stroke April 20, 2017

Update

While more research is warranted, preliminary studies have shown artificial sweetener consumption may disrupt the gut microbiome, Aspartame in particular has been under fire in recent years as human research has suggested the popular sweetener in diet beverages may disrupt antioxidant function, induce oxidative stress, and damage cell membrane integrity, which could lead to inflammation and pose a health risk. Some human data suggests aspartame increases cortisol levels and impairs insulin function.[221]

Sucralose may predispose people to metabolic syndrome.[222]

Atherosclerosis

Is actually an immune disease and inflammation is a key contributor due to the immune system reacting to excess cholesterol and lipids in the walls of blood vessels. Different subsets of immune cells have opposing roles in atherosclerosis, some contribute to the build-up of plaques, and others protect against it but with a western diet, protective cells change to damaging cells, causing more inflammation and HDL -- the good cholesterol -- actually helps shield the protective cells against the damaging changes that occur during atherosclerosis plaque development.

Bananas

Green bananas are a good source of potassium and resistant fiber.

Postmenopausal women who eat foods higher in potassium are less likely to have strokes and die than women who eat less potassium-rich foods. See Potassium.

Barley

Eating barley or foods containing barley significantly reduced levels of two types of 'bad cholesterol' associated with cardiovascular risk, a research paper has found. Barley is higher in fiber, has twice the protein and almost half the calories of oats. Barley reduced both low-density lipoprotein, or LDL, and non-high-

---

[221] Nutr Rev. 2017 Sep 1;75(9):718-730. doi: 10.1093/nutrit/nux035. Revisiting the safety of aspartame.

[222] "Sucralose promotes metabolic dysregulation and intracellular ROS accumulation" ENDO 2018; Abstract SUN-071.

density lipoprotein, or non-HDL, by 7%. incorporate barley into existing recipes, using it as a substitute for rice or even on its own -- just like oatmeal.[223]

BBQ

Marinate: Marinating food for a while before grilling limits the formation of potential carcinogens. Beer, wine or vinegar work fine.

Char is potentially carcinogenic. Clean plate. Don't char meat, poultry or fish.

Clean plate: Scrape, brush then wipe with a paper towel to get rid of debris.

Smoke and fire: Open flames produce heterocyclic amines from meat proteins. Smoke, especially from burning fat, contains polycyclic aromatic hydrocarbons. These two groups of chemicals have been linked to various cancers. Use a solid clean grill plate and cook longer at lower temperature.

Grilling intensifies the flavor of fruits and vegetables

Keep meat plate, especially pooled blood, separate from other food and don't use again.

High Temperature and BBQ Cooking

One suspect that has been extensively studied as potentially increasing the risk for cancer is the high-temperature cooking of meat, such as barbequing, grilling, frying, and roasting, during which the meat is charred and can form carcinogens. But after more than 30 years of study, this link has not been refuted or confirmed in any clear way. It cannot be said with absolute certainty that the risk is increased due to carcinogens formed in burned meat. If there was a strong association it would have been seen by now, but a mild or moderate effect cannot be excluded. To fry or barbeque meat, the heat should be turned down and any burned portions should be cut off when it's finished. Cooking meat sufficiently to kill bacteria without charring and microwaving meat for a few minutes and pouring off the juices before cooking it on the grill to reduce the precursors of cancer-causing compounds is also recommended.[224]

---

[223] A systematic review and meta-analysis of randomized controlled trials of the effect of barley β-glucan on LDL-C, non-HDL-C and apoB for cardiovascular disease risk reductioni-iv. European Journal of Clinical Nutrition, 2016; DOI: 10.1038/ejcn.2016.89

[224] American Association for Cancer Research (AACR) 100th Annual Meeting: Presented April 21, 2009

A prospective analysis of 62,581 participants of the Prostate, Lung, Colorectal, and Ovarian multicenter screening trial, looked at 208 cases of pancreatic cancer and found that individuals who preferred very well done steak were almost 60% more likely to develop pancreatic cancer than those who ate their steak less well done or who did not eat steak at all. When the researchers considered overall consumption and doneness preferences, this rose to a 70% higher risk for pancreatic cancer.[225]

Adding spices to burgers and steaks dramatically reduces carcinogenic compounds known as heterocyclic amines. Cooking meats with natural antioxidants decreases or eliminates HCAs on meat. Consuming dietary carcinogens has been associated with different cancers in humans, and last year one of the HCAs was shown to cause prostate cancer in rats. There is even evidence that other chemicals formed during cooking or grilling can enhance the onset of type 2 diabetes. Previous research has shown that grilled beef is a major source of dietary HCAs when cooked at 375 degrees F (190.5 degrees C) and above.[226]

Cooking[227]

Study results of open-flame and/or high-temperature cooking (grilling/barbequing, broiling, or roasting) and doneness preferences (rare, medium, or well-done) of red meats, chicken, and fish suggest that, independent of the amount of meat consumption, open-flame and/or high-temperature cooking and high doneness level for both red meats and white meats are associated with an increased risk of hypertension.

Beetroot

Beetroot is rich in nitrates. When ingested, scientists believe our body converts nitrates into nitric oxide, a chemical thought to lower blood pressure. A well-conducted review of the current evidence from 2013 concluded that beetroot juice was associated with a modest reduction in blood pressure. Another well-conducted review from 2013 found that inactive and recreationally active individuals saw "moderate improvements" in exercise performance from drinking beetroot juice. However, there was very little effect on elite athletes. A 2014 study looked at the effects of beetroot juice on cyclists and found the juice had a modest

---

[225] ACCR press release: University of Minnesota School of Public Health, in Minneapolis.

[226] Adapted from the spring 2007 Food Safety Consortium News- letter, Editor: David Edmark. For the complete article, go to http:// www.uark.edu/depts/fsc/news-pdf/news.spring07.pdf

[227] AHA EPI 2018 Home, March 21, 2018

but significant increase in terms of their time trial scores; on average there was a 16 second improvement.

Beetroot juice

- Beetroot juice rich in nitrates did not enhance muscle blood flow or vascular dilation during exercise, researchers found that it did "de-stiffen" blood vessels under resting conditions, potentially easing the workload of the heart[228]
- Dietary nitrate in the form of daily beetroot juice significantly reduced elevated blood pressure compared with placebo in hypertensive patients over 4 weeks who drank 250 mL of the juice daily and suggests a role for dietary nitrate as an affordable, readily available adjunctive treatment in the management of patients with hypertension. Reductions of 7.7 to 8.1 mm systolic and 2,4 to 3.8 mm diastolic were recorded and there was no evidence for a declining nitrate effect over time[229]
- Beet juice is a dietary source of the molecule nitrate. When converted in the body, nitrate can dilate the blood vessels and increase blood flow, both important factors for exercise performance. Healthy male subjects who drank beet juice for 15 days had lower blood pressure and more dilated blood vessels at rest and during exercise. Blood vessels also dilated more easily, and the heart consumed less oxygen during exercise with beet juice consumption[230]
- Dietary nitrate may improve muscle performance in elite athletes and drinking concentrated beet juice-high in nitrates increases muscle power in patients with heart failure[231]

Berries

Berries are high in flavonoids, especially anthocyanins, and improve cognition in experimental studies. Greater long-term intakes of berries and flavonoids are associated with slower rates of cognitive decline in older women. Higher intake

---

228 *Applied Physiology, Nutrition, and Metabolism*, 2014; 1 DOI: 10.1139/apnm-2014-0228
229 Dietary nitrate provides sustained blood pressure lowering in hypertensive patients: A randomized, phase 2, double-blind, placebo-controlled study. *Hypertension* 2014; DOI: 10.1161/HYPERTENSIONAHA.114.04675.
230 Effects of Chronic Dietary Nitrate Supplementation on the Hemodynamic Response to Dynamic Exercise. *American Journal of Physiology - Regulatory, Integrative and Comparative Physiology*, 2015; ajpregu.00099.2015 DOI: 10.1152/ajpregu.00099.2015
231 Acute Dietary Nitrate Intake Improves Muscle Contractile Function in Patients With Heart FailureCLINICAL PERSPECTIVE. *Circulation: Heart Failure*, 2015; 8 (5): 914 DOI: 10.1161/CIRCHEARTFAILURE.115.002141

of flavonoids, particularly from berries, appears to reduce rates of cognitive decline in older adults.[232]

Blueberries

A study in 2012 of 93,000 women found those who ate three or more portions of blueberries and strawberries a week had a 32% lower risk of a heart attack compared with those who ate berries once a month or less. However, the study could not prove that these fruits definitely caused the lower risk. Eating blueberries may improve thinking and memory skills in older adults with mild cognitive impairment (MCI) as were found in two human blueberry studies of 47 adults aged 68 years and older in one study and 94 adults aged 62 to 80 years in the other. The beneficial effects of blueberries could be due to the presence of anthocyanins, flavonoids shown to improve cognition in animals.[233] In the Nurses' Health Study a half a cup of blueberries two to three times a week was shown to delay the onset of cognitive decline.

Healthy people aged 65-77 who drank concentrated blueberry juice every day showed improvements in cognitive function, blood flow to the brain and activation of the brain. There was also evidence suggesting improvement in working memory. Just 12 weeks of consuming 30ml of concentrated blueberry juice every day, brain blood flow, brain activation and some aspects of working memory were improved.[234]

Breakfast

- A 2016 study of New York City's serving free breakfast inside classrooms found no evidence it boosted student achievement.
- Breakfast promoted as the most important meal was a 1920s advertising scam to sell more bacon and then carried on by the cereal manufacturers.235

---

[232] Ann Neurol. 2012 Jul;72(1):135-43. doi: 10.1002/ana.23594. Epub 2012 Apr 26. Dietary intakes of berries and flavonoids in relation to cognitive decline.

[233] Presented March 13 at the 251st National Meeting and Exposition of the American Chemical Society (ACS), in San Diego, California.

[234] Enhanced task related brain activation and resting perfusion in healthy older adults after chronic blueberry supplementation. Applied Physiology, Nutrition, and Metabolism, 2017; DOI: 10.1139/apnm-2016-0550

[235] American Psychological Association, Psychoanalysis shapes consumer culture Or how Sigmund Freud, his nephew and a box of cigars forever changed American marketing. By Lisa Held December 2009, Vol 40, No. 11

- In Japanese breakfast intake was inversely associated with risk for stroke, especially for cerebral hemorrhage, suggesting that breakfast may reduce of morning blood pressure236

Broccoli

Eating more non-starchy vegetables, such as broccoli, is associated with a reduced risk of some cancers (including mouth, throat and stomach cancers), according to a good quality 2007 review (PDF, 1.8Mb) of the evidence on cancer prevention by the World Cancer Research Fund. It is possible that some of the compounds in broccoli may have health benefits, but clinical trials are needed to investigate this further. Eating leafy green vegetables supplies significant amounts of sulfoquinovose (SQ) sugars, which good bacteria, fungi and other organisms feed on limiting the ability of bad bacteria to colonize the gut by shutting them out and may protect our gut and promote health.[237]

An anti-cancer compound found in broccoli and cabbage, indole-3-carbinol (I3C), stops cell growth lowering the activity of an enzyme associated with rapidly advancing cancer.[238] When a diluted solution of various brassicas, including broccoli was dropped on cancer cells growing on a petri dish, Bok Choi proved to be the most potent killer of these cancer cells. A new broccoli variety "Benefort", has been bred to contain three times more naturally occurring compound glucoraphanin, and reduces blood LDL-cholesterol levels by around 6%[239]

Eating broccoli three to five times per week can lower the risk of many types of cancers. Consuming a high-fat, high-sugar diet and having excess body fat is linked with the development of nonalcoholic fatty liver disease (NAFLD), which can lead to diseases such as cirrhosis and liver cancer. A new study shows that including broccoli in the diet may protect against liver cancer, as well as aid in countering the development of NAFLD. Previous research shows that eating broccoli freshly chopped or lightly steamed is the best way to get to the vegetables'

---

[236] Stroke January 5th 2016 Yasuhiko Kubota, MD, Osaka University Graduate School of Medicine, Osaka, Japan.
[237] YihQ is a sulfoquinovosidase that cleaves sulfoquinovosyl diacylglyceride sulfolipids. Nature Chemical Biology, 2016; DOI: 10.1038/nchembio.2023
[238] ScienceDaily (Dec. 14, 2008)
[239] Diet rich in high glucoraphanin broccoli reduces plasma LDL cholesterol: Evidence from randomised controlled trials. Molecular Nutrition & Food Research, 2015; DOI: 10.1002/mnfr.201400863

cancer-fighting compound, sulforaphane. Other brassica vegetables, such as cauliflower or Brussel sprouts, may have the same effect.[240]

Consumption of phenolic compounds in broccoli is associated with a lower risk of coronary heart disease, type 2 diabetes, asthma, and several types of cancer. Phenolic compounds are flavorless and stable, so the vegetables can be cooked without losing health-promoting qualities.

Flavonoids spread through the bloodstream, reducing inflammation through their antioxidant activity. We have to get them from our diets so we need to eat Brassicas every three or four days to lower the risk of cancers and other degenerative diseases.[241]

Butter

Patients who consumed the most butter after a heart attack had x 3 times the risk of dying within 42 months compared to those eating the Mediterranean Diet.[242] Butter is still not recommended. When cheese was added to a low fat diet the cholesterol and lipid levels didn't alter but added butter did elevate them.[243]

Calcium

The 2016 joint clinical guideline from the National Osteoporosis Foundation (NOF) and the American Society for Preventive Cardiology (ASPC) states that dietary and supplemental calcium are safe for cardiovascular health when consumed in recommended amounts. The recommendation applies to calcium consumed either alone or with vitamin D that does not exceed the National Academy of Medicine's tolerable upper intake limit of 2000 to 2500 mg/day.

However, a ten-year follow-up from the Multi-Ethnic Study of Atherosclerosis (MESA) shows no excess cardiovascular risk with dietary calcium intake but suggests calcium supplements may be associated with a higher risk of coronary

---

[240] Dietary Broccoli Lessens Development of Fatty Liver and Liver Cancer in Mice Given Diethylnitrosamine and Fed a Western or Control Diet. Journal of Nutrition, 2016; 146 (3): 542 DOI: 10.3945/jn.115.228148

[241] QTL analysis for the identification of candidate genes controlling phenolic compound accumulation in broccoli (Brassica oleracea L. var. italica). Molecular Breeding, 2016; 36 (6) DOI: 10.1007/s11032-016-0497-4

[242] JAMA 2000;284 Dec 13

[243] Cheese intake in large amounts lowers LDL-cholesterol concentrations compared with butter intake of equal fat content. Am J Clin Nut;94:1479-84, 2011.

artery calcification (CAC).[244] It would seem safest to get your calcium from natural foods rather than supplements.

Calories

Not all calories are equal, and the health benefits of low-carbohydrate or low-fat diets depend more on the specific (high quality-nutrient) foods consumed than the carbohydrates–fats distribution.[245]

CBD

Many people attest that this non-psychoactive component of the cannabis plant—which is readily available in gummies, tinctures, and capsules—relieves anxiety, insomnia, and a host of other ills and chronic pain.

CBD cannot be marketed as a supplement, and its overall legality is complicated. (In the USA it depends on the plant source and the state.) CBD has been frustratingly difficult to study, says Jahan Marcu, PhD, the former chief scientific officer for Americans for Safe Access. Most of the research has been done on animals or has involved doses that aren't available on the market. The FDA has cautioned that not enough is known about CBD's safety and has pointed to potential risks, such as liver injury.

It's also a challenge to find trustworthy products, says Marcu. He was one of the researchers on a study published in *JAMA* in 2017 that discovered that only a third of the 84 CBD extracts they tested contained what the labels claimed.

Because there are no established dosages, it makes sense to start at a very low dose and monitor your reaction.

Chamomile tea

Drinking chamomile tea was associated with a decreased risk of death from all causes in Mexican-American American women.[246]

---

[244]Calcium intake from diet and supplements and the risk of coronary artery calcification and its progression among older adults: 10-year follow-up of the Multi-Ethnic Study of Atherosclerosis (MESA). *J Am Heart Assoc* 20161; DOI:10.1161/jaha.116.003815.

[245] *Shan Z et al. JAMA Intern Med 2020 Jan 21*

[246] University of Texas Medical Branch at Galveston. "Drinking chamomile decreases risk of death in older Mexican American women." ScienceDaily. ScienceDaily, 20 May 2015. <www.sciencedaily.com/releases/2015/05/150520160312.htm>.

Cheese

The "French paradox" is why the French have low CVD rates despite a diet high in saturated fats. perhaps its the wine and lifestyle but high cheese consumption may explain it. Cheese eaters had higher fecal levels of butyrate linked to a reduction in cholesterol.[247] The French eat 24 kg a year and have a third the heart attack rate of the British and Americans who eat 13 kg annually. Most cheese contains 30 to 40% fat of which most is saturated. Only 1% is cholesterol. Cheese has a protective effect on heart disease and mortality.[248]

Processed Cheese: Not recommended. It is made by treating cheese with chemicals or boiling and spinning so the fat and the milk blend. It is sterile, and often comes in thin slices separated by plastic strips, or in plastic tube sticks or a squeeze bottle sometimes colored a violent orange. Often used in kids' lunches (mother thinks she is providing healthy food) and pizzas.

Chili

People who ate chili peppers regularly had less mortality over a median 8.2 years compared to peers who didn't eat them or only rarely did so. This was observed after adjustment for age, sex, and caloric intake.[249]

- PEITC phenylethyl isothiocyanate, found in these, has anti-cancer properties[250]
- Dietary capsaicin -- the active ingredient in chili peppers -- produces chronic activation of a receptor on cells lining the intestines of mice, triggering a reaction that ultimately reduces the risk of colorectal tumors[251]
- In a large prospective study, an inverse association between consumption of spicy foods and total mortality, after adjusting for potential confounders. Compared with those who ate spicy foods less than once a week, those who consumed spicy foods almost every day had a 14% lower risk of death. Inverse associations were also observed for deaths due to cancer, ischemic heart diseases, and respiratory diseases. The associations were consistent in

---

[247] Metabolomics Investigation To Shed Light on Cheese as a Possible Piece in the French Paradox Puzzle. *Journal of Agricultural and Food Chemistry*, 2015; 63 (10): 2830 DOI: 10.1021/jf505878a
[248] Recent Observational Research. Curr Nutr Reo;3:130-38 (15 Mar 2014).
[249] *Journal of the American College of Cardiology*. Dec. 24, 2020
[250] A. Assoc Ca Research 19/04/05
[251] Ion channel TRPV1-dependent activation of PTP1B suppresses EGFR-associated intestinal tumorigenesis. *Journal of Clinical Investigation*, 2014; DOI: 10.1172/JCI72340

men and women while in women it was also significantly associated with a reduced risk of death due to infections[252]

Update 2020:

Contrary to some previous findings that it may enhance cognitive function, a high intake of hot chili peppers is associated with an increased risk of cognitive decline, new research shows. A large longitudinal study found a high chili intake was positively associated with lower cognitive scores and doubling of the risk of self-reported memory loss.

Authors note: In this latter study the participants ingested an incredible amount of chilis (50g) daily by Western standards.

- According to an extensive population-based study published in BMJ in 2015, "Compared with those who ate spicy foods less than once a week, those who consumed spicy foods 6 or 7 days a week showed a 14 percent relative risk reduction in total mortality."
- In a large adult Mediterranean population, regular consumption of chili pepper is associated with a lower risk of total and CVD death independent of CVD risk factors or adherence to a Mediterranean diet. People who ate chili peppers regularly had less mortality over a median 8.2 years compared to peers who didn't eat them or only rarely did so. This was observed after adjustment for age, sex, and caloric intake:
    - All-cause mortality
    - Cardiovascular disease (CVD) mortality
    - Ischemic heart disease mortality
    - Cerebrovascular death

Notably, cancer deaths weren't lower with more consumption of chili peppers[253]

---

252 Consumption of spicy foods and total and cause specific mortality: population based cohort study *BMJ* 2015; 351 doi: http://dx.doi.org/10.1136/bmj.h3942 (Published 04 August 2015) Cite this as: *BMJ* 2015;351:h3942

253 J Am Coll Cardiol 2019; DOI: 10.1016/j.jacc.2019.09.068.
Secondary Source Journal of the American College of Cardiology

Chili Antidote - Milk[254]

Capsaicin is the chemical compound found in chili peppers that makes them taste hot. Milk and other dairy products like sour cream or even ice cream have a protein in it that replaces the capsaicin on the receptors on your tongue. It's really the quickest way to alleviate the burning feeling. Carbohydrates also replace the capsaicin on the receptors, just not as effectively as milk; things like bread or sugar with sugar the better of the two. That's why we see the traditional Mexican desserts like flan and sopapillas with honey. These are made from breads, sugars and milk. Alcohol and water won't work. They both just wash the capsaicin around your mouth. Neither will block it.

Chinese Herbs

uzen-taiho-to (shi quan da bu tang) is a most popular herbal formula in China and Japan. Its 10 component herbs include cinnamon, ginseng, licorice and an assortment of other roots and fungi that are ground into a fine powder and consumed as a tea-like broth. Now research suggests the remedy's immune-boosting effects are due, at least in part, to of Rahnella aquatilis bacteria growing on the Angelica roots but the amount of bacteria on a plant's roots may vary.[255]

Chocolate

Eating up to 100g of (dark) chocolate a day may reduce the risk of coronary heart disease, stroke and cardiovascular death.

Higher chocolate intake was associated with an 11% lower risk of cardiovascular disease and a 25% lower risk of cardiovascular death compared to no chocolate intake. People who ate the most chocolate (up to 100g per day) had a 22% lower risk of stroke compared to chocolate abstainers. People who ate more chocolate had a 29% decreased risk of coronary heart disease, 21% reduced risk of stroke (across five studies) and 45% reduced risk of cardiovascular death (across three studies) compared to people who ate smaller amounts of chocolate.

Chocolate contains flavonoid antioxidants, which may have a beneficial effect on endothelial function.

---

[254] New Mexico State University (NMSU). "Milk works best to extinguish the heat from chile peppers." ScienceDaily. ScienceDaily, 19 July 2016. <www.sciencedaily.com/releases/2016/07/160719094751.htm>.

[255] Federation of American Societies for Experimental Biology (FASEB) 2016

Interestingly, non-chocolate eaters had the highest BMI, highest CRP and highest levels of inactivity among the participants.[256]

Cholesterol

Foods that fight high cholesterol

Changing what you eat can lower your cholesterol and improve the armada of fats floating through your bloodstream. Fresh fruits and vegetables, whole grains, and "good fats" are all part of a heart-healthy diet. But some foods are particularly good at helping bring down cholesterol.

How? Some cholesterol-lowering foods deliver a good dose of soluble fiber, which binds cholesterol and its precursors in the digestive system and drags them out of the body before they get into circulation. Others provide polyunsaturated fats, which directly lower LDL. And those with plant sterols and stanols keep the body from absorbing cholesterol. Here are 5 of those foods:

Oats. An easy way to start lowering cholesterol is to choose oatmeal or a cold oat-based cereal like Cheerios for breakfast. It gives you 1 to 2 grams of soluble fiber. Add a banana or some strawberries for another half-gram. *Barley* is even better.

Beans. Beans are especially rich in soluble fiber. They also take a while for the body to digest, meaning you feel full for longer after a meal. That's one reason beans are a useful food for folks trying to lose weight. With so many choices — from navy and kidney beans to lentils, garbanzos, black-eyed peas, and beyond — and so many ways to prepare them, beans are a very versatile food.

Nuts. A bushel of studies shows that eating almonds, walnuts, peanuts, and other nuts is good for the heart. Eating 2 ounces of nuts a day can slightly lower LDL, on the order of 5%. Nuts have additional nutrients that protect the heart in other ways.

Foods fortified with sterols and stanols extracted from plants gum up the body's ability to absorb cholesterol from food. Companies are adding them to foods ranging from margarine and granola bars to orange juice and chocolate. They're also available as supplements. Getting 2g of plant sterols or stanols a day can lower LDL cholesterol by about 10%.

---

[256] Heart 2015; online 15 June.

Fatty fish. Eating fish two or three times a week can lower LDL in two ways: by replacing meat, which has LDL-boosting saturated fats, and by delivering LDL-lowering omega-3 fats. Omega-3s reduce triglycerides in the bloodstream and also protect the heart by helping prevent the onset of abnormal heart rhythms.

Fish oil. While oil from actual fatty fish such as salmon and sardines contain omega-3 fatty acids which are heart healthy, fish oil does not seem to have the same impact.

Hawthorne. The leaves, berries, and flowers of this plant are used to make medicines. It may lower cholesterol.

Red yeast rice. This Chinese medicine has been marketed in the United States as a supplement that's said to lower cholesterol levels. Some red yeast rice products contain a chemical that's identical to the active ingredient in lovastatin. But an independent analysis of 12 red yeast rice products found that although all claimed to have 600 milligrams (mg) of the active ingredient in each capsule, the actual content varied between 0.1 mg and 10.9 mg. In addition, one-third of the products were contaminated with a potentially toxic compound called citrinin, which can cause kidney failure.

Four ways to eat your way to lower cholesterol

Many people can reduce cholesterol levels simply by changing what they eat. For example, if you are a fan of cheeseburgers, eating less meat (and leaner cuts) and more vegetables, fruits, and whole grains can lower your total cholesterol by 25% or more. Cutting back on saturated fat (found in meat and dairy products) and trans-fat (partially hydrogenated oils) can reduce cholesterol by 5% to 10%.

Here are four steps for using your diet to lower your cholesterol.

1. Stick with unsaturated fats and avoid saturated and trans fats. Most vegetable fats (oils) are made up of unsaturated fats that are healthy for your heart. Foods that contain healthy fats include oily fish, nuts, seeds, and some vegetables. At the same time, limit your intake of foods high in saturated fat, which is found many meat and dairy products, and stay away from trans fats. These include any foods made with "partially hydrogenated vegetable oils."

2. Get more soluble fiber. Eat more soluble fiber, such as that found in oatmeal and fruits. This type of fiber can significantly lower blood cholesterol levels when eaten as part of a healthy-fat diet.

3. Include plant sterols and stanols in your diet. These naturally occurring plant compounds are similar in structure to cholesterol. When you eat them, they help limit the amount of cholesterol your body can absorb. Plant sterols and stanols are found in an increasing number of food products such as spreads, juices, and yogurts.

4. Adopt the Newtrition Diet

Choline[257]

Choline is an essential dietary nutrient, critical to brain health, particularly during fetal development. The primary sources of dietary choline are found in beef, eggs, dairy products, fish, and chicken, with much lower levels found in nuts, beans, and cruciferous vegetables, such as broccoli but the amount produced by the liver on a vegetarian diet is not enough to meet the requirements of the human body.

Cinnamon

Cinnamon may cool your body by up to two degrees, according to animal studies and may also contribute to a general improvement in overall health.[258] But get the Ceylon and not the Cassia species.

Citrus : oranges

- Citrus fruits can reduce the risk of Ca of mouth, larynx and stomach by up to 50% and stroke by 20%

- Eat one more / day on top of recommended

- A compound found in oranges, grapefruit, and other citrus fruit may modestly reduce stroke risk among women. Women with the highest levels of flavanone in their diet were 19% less likely to have an ischemic stroke during 14 years of follow-up than those with the least flavanone intake. The main source of these antioxidants is citrus fruit and juice. Vitamin C has gotten most of the praise for the protective effect of citrus found in prior stroke studies, but in this Study, the vitamin didn't correlate with total or ischemic stroke or attenuate the link to flavanones.

---

[257] BMJ Nutrition, Prevention & Health, 2019; bmjnph-2019-000037 DOI: 10.1136/bmjnph-2019-000037

[258] Potential of in vivo real-time gastric gas profiling: a pilot evaluation of heat-stress and modulating dietary cinnamon effect in an animal model. *Scientific Reports*, 2016; 6: 33387 DOI: 10.1038/srep33387

Eating the whole fruit would likely be a better way to boost intake, the researchers suggested[259]

- Oranges: Have the highest level of antioxidants in Citrus with anti-inflammatory, anti-tumor and anti-coagulation properties

- Oranges and other citrus fruits contain plenty of vitamins and substances, such as antioxidants (flavanones found in oranges, limes and lemons were hesperidin, eriocitrin and eriodictyol). These fruits also help prevent harmful effects of obesity in mice fed a Western-style, high-fat diet. The high-fat diet without the flavanones increased the levels of cell-damage markers while the flavones reduced this damage by around 50%[260]

Update: See oranges

Cocoa / chocolate

Cocoa is not a chocolate bar. Chocolate has added ingredients and processing, which reduce the number and type of flavonols (natural substances that can reduce the risk of disease) but which increase calories (cocoa itself has very few) and possibly change the response of gut bacteria to the cocoa. A few tablespoons of unsweetened cocoa powder sprinkled onto oatmeal would be better. Large-scale epidemiological studies have found that people whose diets include dark chocolate have a lower risk of heart disease than those whose diets do not. But it hasn't been clear how these flavonols could be affecting the human body, especially the heart.

- 10 yr. study found 45 to 50% lower risk of CVS & all-cause mortality
- Daily cocoa lowered both systolic and diastolic BPs
- Arm arteries dilated & aortic stiffness decreased by 7% within 3 hrs. after 100g[261]
- Improves endothelial function and improve insulin sensitivity
- Subtype flavonoids: flavonols or catechins (flavan-3-ols) are procyanidins and can inhibit platelets, LDL oxidation and raise HDL

---

[259] "Dietary flavonoids and risk of stroke in women" *Stroke* 2012; DOI: 10.1161/STROKEAHA.111.637835.

[260] American Chemical Society. "Citrus fruits could help prevent obesity-related heart disease, liver disease, diabetes." ScienceDaily. ScienceDaily, 21 August 2016. <www.sciencedaily.com/releases/2016/08/160821093054.htm>.

[261] Am J HT June 2005

- Does not explain the reduction in all-cause mortality
- Must be at least 60% cocoa
- Milk chocolate has only 20% cocoa. White chocolate has nil.
- Dark unsweetened = >75% [262]
- People of the San Blas Islands who consumed 900mg of flavonoids a day (cocoa) when compared with mainland Panama had 9.2 deaths from CVS disease compared with 83.4 and 4.4 deaths from cancer compared with 68.4 deaths per 100,000[263]
- Cocoa Flavanols May Reverse Age-Related Memory Decline: Age-related memory decline may be reversed with high doses of naturally occurring cocoa flavanols. This was not about Alzheimer's disease, which is a fatal brain disease but specifically about cognitive decline in normal aging[264]
- An EEG study shows chocolate can increase brain characteristics of attention and significantly affect blood pressure levels. Historically, chocolate has been recognized as a vasodilator, meaning that it widens blood vessels and lowers blood pressure in the long run, but chocolate also contains some powerful stimulants. The results for the participants who consumed 60% cacao chocolate showed that the brain was more alert and attentive after consumption. Their blood pressure also increased for a short time. Regular chocolate with high sugar and milk content won't be as good; it's the high-cacao content chocolate that has these effects[265]
- Vasodilation was significantly improved in both age groups (<35 years and 50-80 years of age) that consumed flavanols over the course of the study (by 33% in the younger age group and 32% in the older age group over the control intervention). In the older age group, a statistically and clinically significant decrease in systolic blood pressure of 4 mmHg over control was also seen.
- Flavanols significantly improves several of the hallmarks of cardiovascular health significantly increasing flow-mediated vasodilation by 21%. Increased flow-mediated vasodilation is a sign of improved endothelial function and has been shown by some studies to be associated with decreased risk of developing CVD. In addition, taking flavanols decreased blood pressure (systolic by 4.4 mmHg, diastolic by 3.9 mmHg), and improved the blood cholesterol profile by decreasing total cholesterol (by 0.2 mmol/L), decreasing LDL cholesterol (by 0.17 mmol/L), and increasing HDL cholesterol (by 0.1 mmol/L). The Framingham Risk Score found that flavanol

---

[262] Arch Int Med 2006;166:411-417

[263] Int J med Sc 2007;4:53-8

[264] *Nat Neurosci.* Published online October 26, 2014

[265] The Acute Electrocortical and Blood Pressure Effects of Chocolate. Neuro Regulation, 2015 Northern Arizona University. "Eat dark chocolate to beat the midday slump?." ScienceDaily. ScienceDaily, 8 May 2015. <www.sciencedaily.com/releases/2015/05/150508140302.htm

intake reduced the 10-year risk of being diagnosed with CVD by 22% and the 10-year risk of suffering a heart attack by 31%[266]

- A study has found 40 g / day of dark chocolate could help give sports enthusiasts an extra edge in their fitness training. The study found that after eating dark chocolate, bike riders used less oxygen when cycling at a moderate pace and also covered more distance in a two-minute flat-out time trial[267]
- In a small study of peripheral artery disease (PAD) patients over age 60, those who drank a beverage containing flavanol-rich cocoa three times a day for six months were able to walk up to 42.6 meters further in a 6-minute walking test.[268]

Coca Cola

Two major campaigns from Coca-Cola were targeted at teenagers and mothers and used social media influencers and celebrities—including Olympic athletes—to make products seem healthier.[269]

This is just the latest in the incredible saga of Coke and Pepsi sponsorship.

Cancer Council NSW has revealed eight out of nine food and beverage sponsors of children's sports development programs in Australia are classified as unhealthy. Brands including McDonald's, Schweppes, Gatorade and Nutrigrain are all competing for brand exposure in kids' sport.

Coconut Oil - see oils

Coffee – Caffeine

Reading all these studies **Newtrition's advice** is to limit coffee to three or four normal cups a day and less if you have blood pressure.

---

[266] Cocoa flavanol intake improves endothelial function and Framingham Risk Score in healthy men and women: a randomised, controlled, double-masked trial: the Flaviola Health Study. British Journal of Nutrition, 2015; 1 DOI: 10.1017/S0007114515002822

[267] Dark chocolate supplementation reduces the oxygen cost of moderate intensity cycling. Journal of the International Society of Sports Nutrition, 2015; 12 (1) DOI: 10.1186/s12970-015-0106-7

[268] American Heart Association.

[269] BMJ 2019; 367 doi: https://doi.org/10.1136/bmj.l7022

Filtered Best

Strong and convincing evidence of a link between coffee brewing methods, heart attacks, and longevity. Unfiltered coffee contains substances which increase blood cholesterol. Using a filter removes these and makes heart attacks and premature death less likely.[270]

The case for:

Earlier this year, the Dietary Guidelines Advisory Committee (DGAC) released a report as follows:[271]

It stated that up to five cups of coffee per day, or up to 400 mg of caffeine, is not associated with long-term health risks. Not only that, they highlighted observational evidence that coffee consumption is associated with reduced risk for several diseases, including type 2 diabetes, cardiovascular disease (CVD), and neurodegenerative disorders. The body of data suggesting that moderate coffee—and, in all likelihood, tea—consumption is not only safe but beneficial in a variety of mental and medical conditions is growing fast.

A 2012 study of over 400,000 people, published in the *New England Journal of Medicine*, reported that coffee consumption is associated with a 10% reduction in all-cause mortality at 13-year follow-up. A large meta-analysis published in the *American Journal of Epidemiology* in 2014 also reported significant reductions in all-cause as well as CVD-related mortality associated with consuming three to four cups of coffee per day. It's important to note that much of the evidence on the potential health effects of coffee, caffeine, and other foods and nutrients is associational and doesn't prove causality—observational investigations come with limitations and often rely on error-prone methods such as patient questionnaires. However, the sheer volume of existing observational data linking coffee and/or caffeine with various health benefits—as well as, in many cases, evidence of a dose response—suggests that the most widely consumed stimulant in the world has positive influences on our health.

When caffeine is ingested via coffee, enduring blood pressure elevations are small and cardiovascular risks may be balanced by protective properties. Coffee beans contain antioxidant compounds that reduce oxidation of low-density lipoprotein (LDL) cholesterol, and coffee consumption has been associated with reduced concentrations of inflammatory markers. Moderate coffee intake is associated with a lower risk for coronary heart disease as far out as 10 years, and data suggest

---

[270] European Journal of Preventive Cardiology, April 22nd, 2020
[271] Scientific Report of the 2015 Dietary Guidelines Advisory Committee

that an average of two cups per day protects against heart failure. Finally, a study presented during a poster session at the Heart Rhythm Society 2015 Scientific Sessions counters the long-held dogma that patients with arrhythmias should avoid caffeine, finding no association between the compound and premature atrial or ventricular contractions.

According to a 2011 meta-analysis, consuming between one and six cups per day reportedly cut stroke risk by 17%. A 22%-25% risk reduction was seen in a large sample of Swedish women followed for an average of 10 years. And while coffee's impact on stroke risk in those with CVD is still in question, a meta-analysis presented at the 2012 European Meeting on Hypertension and Cardiovascular Protection found that one to three cups per day may protect against ischemic stroke in the general population. A 2013 study of over 80,000 Japanese adults without CVD reported that those who drank coffee or green tea for a mean duration of 13 years had a 20% lower risk for stroke than those who seldom drank the beverages.

It appears to confer benefit to other aspects of so-called "metabolic syndrome," the dangerous cluster of hypertension, hyperglycemia, abnormal lipid levels, and increased body fat. Numerous studies have linked regular coffee drinking with improved glucose metabolism, insulin secretion, and a significantly reduced risk for diabetes. Most recently, findings from a long-term study published this year suggest that coffee drinkers are roughly half as likely to develop type 2 diabetes as are nonconsumers, even after accounting for smoking, high blood pressure, and family history of diabetes. High levels of serum amyloid and C-reactive protein, both inflammatory markers, preceded the onset of diabetes in non–coffee drinkers, suggesting that coffee's anti-inflammatory properties might confer its protective effects. Experts have suggested that coffee's inverse correlation with diabetes might also be in part due to its containing chlorogenic acid, a plant compound with antioxidant properties thought to reduce glucose absorption.

Evidence suggests that moderate to heavy coffee consumption can reduce the risk for numerous cancers, including endometrial (> 4 cups/day),prostate (6 cups/day), head and neck (4 cups/day), basal cell carcinoma (> 3 cups/day), melanoma, and breast cancer (> 5 cups/day). The benefits are thought to be at least partially due to coffee's antioxidant and antimutagenic properties.

Beyond the short-term mental boost it provides, coffee also appears to benefit longer-term cognitive well-being. A 2012 study reported that patients with mild cognitive impairment and plasma caffeine levels of > 1200 ng/mL—courtesy of approximately three to five cups of coffee per day—avoided progression to dementia over the following 2-4 years. On a related note, a study from last year reported that caffeine consumption appears to enhance memory consolidation. Corresponding studies in mice suggest that caffeine suppresses enzymes involved in amyloid-beta production, while coffee consumption boosts granulocyte colony-stimulation factor, interleukin-10, and interleukin-6 levels, cytokines thought to contribute to the reported benefits. Caffeinated coffee has long been thought to be neuroprotective in Parkinson disease (PD)—recent work found that variants in the glutamate-receptor gene *GRIN2A* affect PD risk in coffee drinkers—as well as in multiple sclerosis. Furthermore, drinking coffee may prevent the formation of Lewy bodies, a signature pathologic finding in PD.

Depression

A 2011 study suggests that a boost in coffee consumption might also benefit our mental health: Women who drank two to three cups of coffee per day had a 15% decreased risk for depression compared with those who drank less than one cup per week. A 20% decreased risk was seen in those who drank four cups or more per day. Newer work also suggests that regular coffee drinking may be protective against depression. The short-term effect of coffee on mood may be due to altered serotonin and dopamine activity, whereas the mechanisms behind its potential long-term effects on mood may be related to its antioxidant and anti-inflammatory properties, factors that are thought to play a role in depressive illnesses.

Liver Disease

The liver might help break down coffee, but coffee might protect the liver (in some cases). Evidence suggests that coffee consumption slows disease progression in patients with alcoholic cirrhosis and hepatitis C and reduces the risk of developing hepatocellular carcinoma. A 2012 study reported that coffee intake is associated with a lower risk for nonalcoholic fatty liver disease (NAFLD), while work published in 2014 found that coffee protects against liver fibrosis in those with already established NAFLD

Coffee intake might also relieve dry-eye syndrome by increasing tear production, reduce the risk for gout, and potentially fight infection. Coffee and hot tea consumption were found to be protective against one of the medical community's most concerning bugs, methicillin-resistant *Staphylococcus aureus* (MRSA). While it remains unclear whether the beverages have systemic antimicrobial activity, study participants who reported any consumption of either were approximately half as likely to have MRSA in their nasal passages.

Greek Coffee, endothelial function and Longevity

The elderly inhabitants of Ikaria, the Greek island, boast the highest rates of longevity in the world. Researchers investigated links between coffee-drinking habits and the subjects' endothelial function. The endothelium is a layer of cells that lines blood vessels, which is affected both by aging and by lifestyle habits (such as smoking).

Subjects consuming mainly boiled Greek coffee had better endothelial function than those who consumed other types of coffee. Even in those with high blood pressure, boiled Greek coffee consumption was associated with improved endothelial function, without worrying impacts on blood pressure.

"Boiled Greek type of coffee, which is rich in polyphenols and antioxidants and contains only a moderate amount of caffeine, seems to gather benefits compared to other coffee beverages,[272]

- Caffeine is the world's most used stimulant
- People are more likely to agree with persuasive arguments after consuming caffeine[273]
- A study found that coffee consumption lowered all-cause mortality by over 10% at 13-year follow-up[274]
- Coffee prolongs life by a new dose-response meta-analysis of prospective studies. The largest risk reductions were seen for four cups per day for All-Cause Mortality and three cups per day for death from cardiovascular disease. Coffee consumption was not associated with death from cancer[275]
- The first study to examine links between coffee brewing methods and risks of heart attacks and death has concluded that filtered brew is safest. For death from cardiovascular disease, filtered brew was associated with a 12% decreased risk of death in men and a 20% lowered risk of death in women compared to no coffee. The lowest mortality was among consumers of 1 to 4 cups of filtered coffee per day.[276]
- Coffee Linked to 26% Drop in Colorectal Cancer Risk[277]
- Regular coffee consumption (caffeinated or decaffeinated, boiled black coffee, black espresso, instant coffee, and filtered coffee) is inversely

---

[272] Consumption of a boiled Greek type of coffee is associated with improved endothelial function: The Ikaria Study. Vasc Med, March 18, 2013 DOI: 10.1177/1358863X13480258

[273] Europe J Soc Psych 5 June 2006

[274] Association of coffee drinking with total and cause-specific mortality. N Engl J Med. 2012;366:1891-1904

[275] American Journal of Epidemiology 2014, doi:10.1093/aje/kwu194

[276] European Journal of Preventive Cardiology

[277] Cancer Epidemiol Biomarkers Prev. 2016;25:634-639.

correlated to colorectal cancer risk. Overall coffee consumption was associated with 26% lower odds of developing colorectal cancer, drinkers vs nondrinkers

- Higher coffee consumption was associated with lower odds of developing colorectal cancer
- Coffee has been proposed as a protective agent against colorectal cancer because several of its components affect the physiology of the colon. These compounds include caffeine, melanoidins, diterpenes, and polyphenols. Protection may arise from changes to the microbiome, antioxidant effects, antimutagenic effects, reduction of bile acid secretion, and improved bowel functions such as motility and capacity
- A study looked into a number of genes that affect our desire for coffee. If you have the special coffee genes, you may be drinking more coffee than those not having the genes. It was found that the coffee genes are surprisingly not associated with a risk of developing type 2 diabetes or obesity. This suggests that drinking coffee neither causes nor protects against these lifestyle diseases[278]
- There is growing evidence suggesting that coffee consumption may be inversely associated with CVD risk. There is some dose-effect of coffee -- a moderate amount (<5 cups a day) looks slightly more beneficial than a small amount. There was also an observed "lag time" in between when coffee consumption was measured and Coronary Artery Calcium (CAC) measurements (on average, 7-8 years between the two measurements)
- Coffee drinking seems to have a protective effect in Japanese women. Over 10 years of follow-up, inverse associations between coffee consumption and death from all causes and from heart disease were seen in women, but not in men[279]
- People older than 65 who had more than four servings a day of caffeine in coffee, tea, cola or chocolate had less than half the risk of dying of heart disease than people who had less[280]
- Moderate coffee intake was associated with a lower risk for coronary heart disease[281]
- Coffee beans contain antioxidant compounds that reduce oxidation of low-density lipoprotein (LDL) cholesterol and coffee consumption has been

---

[278] University of Copenhagen The Faculty of Health and Medical Sciences. "Coffee not associated with lifestyle diseases." ScienceDaily. ScienceDaily, 9 July 2015. <www.sciencedaily.com/releases/2015/07/150709132454.htm>.

[279] Journal of Nutrition 2010;140:1007-13, doi:10.3945/jn.109.109314

[280] Am J Clin Nutr 2007;85(2):392-8

[281] Coffee consumption and risk of coronary heart diseases: a meta-analysis of 21 prospective cohort studies. Int J Cardiol. 2009;137:216-225

associated with reduced concentrations of inflammatory markers[282, 283,284,285,286,287]

- Coffee drinkers were less likely to have calcium in their coronary arteries than nondrinkers. The relationship was U-shaped, with the lowest levels occurring in people who drank 3 or 4 cups daily. In a sample of more than 25,000 people in South Korea.[288]
- An average of 2 cups a day may protect against heart failure.[289]
- Heavy long-term coffee drinking did not raise the risk of heart disease[290]
- Between 1 and 6 cups a day reportedly cut stroke risk by 17%.[291]
- A 22% to 25% risk reduction in strokes was seen in Swedish women followed for an average of 10 years.[292]
- A meta-analysis found that 1 to 3 cups a day may protect against ischemic stroke in the general population.[293]
- No association was found it causing Blood Pressure (whereas sugary soft drinks did)[294]
- Coffee may interfere with anti-hypertensive drug treatment and raise BP slightly.[295]
- 7 cups or more a day more than halves the risk of Type 2 Diabetes.[296] But 4 cups optimum.

---

[282] Coffee consumption and risk of stroke: a dose-response meta-analysis of prospective studies. Am J Epidemiol. 2011;174:993-1001.

[283] Coffee consumption and risk of coronary heart diseases: a meta-analysis of 21 prospective cohort studies. Int J Cardiol. 2009;137:216-225.

[284] Coffee drinking induces incorporation of phenolic acids into LDL and increases the resistance of LDL to ex vivo oxidation in humans. Am J Clin Nutr. 2007;86:604-609.

[285]. In vitro antioxidant activity of coffee compounds and their metabolites. J Agric Food Chem. 2007;55:6962-6969.

[286] Inhibition of human low-density lipoprotein oxidation by caffeic acid and other hydroxycinnamic acid derivatives. Free Radic Biol Med. 1995;19:541-552.

[287]Coffee intake and cardiovascular disease: virtue does not take center stage. Semin Thromb Hemost. 2012;38:164-177.

[288]Association of coffee drinking with total and cause-specific mortality. N Engl J Med 2012 May 17; 366:1891. (http://dx.doi.org/10.1056/NEJMoa1112010) -

[289]Habitual coffee consumption and risk of heart failure: a dose–response meta-analysis. Circ Heart Fail.
2012;DOI:10.1161/CIRCHEARTFAILURE.112.967299. http://circheartfailure.ahajournals.org

[290] JAMA 250406

[291]Coffee consumption and risk of stroke: a dose-response meta-analyosis of prspective studies. Am J Epidemiol. 2011;174:993-1001.

[292]Coffee consumption and risk of stroke in women. Stroke. 2011;42:908-912

[293] Moderate coffee consumption is associated with lower risk of stroke: meta-analysis of prospective studies. J Hypertension. 2012;30 (e-Supplement A):e107.

[294] JAMA 2005;294:2330-35

[295] A J Clin Nutr 20007;86:457-64

[296] Int J of Obesity 2006 Apr 25

- A large 2014 meta-analysis, an inverse dose-response relationship was demonstrated between diabetes risk and consumption of coffee, decaffeinated coffee, and tea
- Another meta-analysis confirmed these findings and showed that the effect was stronger in women, nonsmokers, and people with a body mass index of <25 kg/m. Evidence suggests that moderate to heavy coffee consumption can reduce the risk for numerous cancers: endometrial (> 4 cups/day),[297] Coffee helps to protect against breast cancer, a number of research studies have shown. A new study is added to that research, confirming that coffee inhibits the growth of tumors and reduces the risk of recurrence in women who have been diagnosed with breast cancer and treated with the drug tamoxifen.[298] A dose-response meta-analysis of prospective studies found the largest risk reductions were seen for four cups per day for All-Cause Mortality (16%) and three cups per day for death from cardiovascular disease (16% to 26%). Coffee consumption was not associated with death from cancer. [299] There would seem to be both fast & slow metabolizers which alters persons reaction(s)
- Prostate (6 cups/day),[300] head and neck (4 cups),[301,302] basal cell carcinoma (> 3 cups),[303] and estrogen receptor-negative breast cancer (> 5 cups).[304] Ca liver > 2 cups.[305]
- Coffee consumption, including decaf, instant and espresso, was found to decrease the risk of colorectal cancer in a study that showed that even moderate coffee consumption, between one to two servings a day, was associated with a 26% reduction in the odds of developing colorectal cancer after adjusting for known risk factors. Moreover, the risk of developing colorectal cancer continued to decrease to up to 50% when participants drank more than 2.5 servings of coffee each day. The indication of decreased risk

---

[297] A prospective cohort study of coffee consumption and risk of endometrial cancer over a 26-year follow-up. Cancer Epidemiol Biomarkers Prev. 2011;20:1-9. Wilson KM, Kasperzyk JL, Rider JR, et al

[298] Caffeine and caffeic acid inhibit growth and modify estrogen receptor (ER) and insulin-like growth factor I receptor (IGF-IR) levels in human breast cancer. *Clinical Cancer Research*, 2015; DOI: 10.1158/1078-0432.CCR-14-1748

[299]American Journal of Epidemiology 2014, doi:10.1093/aje/ kwu194).

[300] Coffee consumption and prostate cancer risk and progression in the Health Professionals Follow-up Study. J Natl Cancer Inst. 2011;8;103:876-884.

[301] Coffee and cancers of the upper digestive and respiratory tracts: meta-analyses of observational studies. Ann Oncol. 2011;22:536-544.

[302] Coffee and tea intake and risk of head and neck cancer: pooled analysis in the international head and neck cancer epidemiology consortium. Cancer Epidemiol Biomarkers Prev. 2010;19:1723-1736.

[303] SIncreased caffeine intake is associated with reduced risk of Basal cell carcinoma of the skin. Cancer Res. 2012;72:3282-3289.

[304] Coffee consumption modifies risk of estrogen-receptor negative breast cancer. Breast Cancer Res. 2011;13:R49.

[305] Association of coffee and caffeine consumption with fatty liver disease, nonalcoholic steatohepatitis, and degree of hepatic fibrosis. Hepatology. 2012;55:429-436

was seen across all types of coffee, both caffeinated and decaffeinated. Coffee contains many elements that contribute to overall colorectal health and may explain the preventive properties. Caffeine and polyphenol can act as antioxidants, limiting the growth of potential colon cancer cells. Melanoidins generated during the roasting process have been hypothesized to encourage colon mobility. Diterpenes may prevent cancer by enhancing the body's defense against oxidative damage. Nevertheless, while the evidence certainly suggests this to be the case, we need additional research before advocating for coffee consumption as a preventive measure.[306]

- There is evidence that drinking > 4 cups of caffeinated coffee a day reduces the recurrence rate of Cancer of the Colon (CaC) post-operatively.
- 2 cups of coffee or tea seem to slow alcoholic liver disease[307]
- There is an ingredient that seems to protect against cirrhosis especially alcoholic cirrhosis[308]
- Coffee may help prevent gallstone disease[309]
- Higher coffee & caffeine intake is associated with a reduced incidence of Parkinson's[310]
- Women who drank 2 to 3 cups of coffee / day had a 15% decreased risk for depression compared with those who drank less than 1 cup per week. A 20% decreased risk was seen in those who drank 4 cups or more a day.[311,312,313,314]
- Women (but not men) who drank more than 3 cups of coffee/tea a day had less cognitive decline than those who drank less. (Less decline in verbal retrieval and visulospatial memory).[315]
- Powdered caffeine, easily bought online, contains roughly the same amount of caffeine as 25 cups of coffee in one teaspoon of it which is more than four times the amount that appears safe to consume in a day and has been blamed

---

[306] Coffee Consumption and the Risk of Colorectal Cancer. Cancer Epidemiology Biomarkers & Prevention, 2016; 25 (4): 634 DOI: 10.1158/1055-9965.EPI-15-0924
[307] Gastroenerology Dec 2005
[308] Arch Int Med 2006;166:1190-95
[309] JAMA 1999;281:2106-12
[310] JAMA 2000;283:2674-79
[311] Coffee, caffeine, and risk of depression among women. Arch Intern Med. 2011;171:1571-1578.
[312] Association of high-sensitivity C-reactive protein with de novo major depression. Br J Psychiatry. 2010;197:372-377.
[313] Oxidative stress in psychiatric disorders: evidence base and therapeutic implications. Int J Neuropsychopharmacol. 2008;11:851-876.
[314] Coffee drinking linked to less depression in women. New York Times. February 13, 2012. http://well.blogs.nytimes.com/2011/09/26/coffee-drinking-linked-to-less-depression-in-women/ Accessed January 11, 2012.
[315] Neurology Aug 2007

for at least two deaths and numerous hospitalizations for overdose nationwide USA in 2014.[316]

- Drinking coffee and taking naps objectively improved night -ime driving[317]
- Long-term consumption of coffee is associated with reduced risk for gout in men older than 40 years[318]
- Coffee intake may relieve dry-eye syndrome by increasing tear production.[319]
- Coffee can cause withdrawal effects-fatigue, grumpiness, headaches, incite or worsen anxiety, insomnia, and tremor and potentially elevate glaucoma risk.
- There is no association between coffee consumption and an increased risk of atrial fibrillation, according to research which included a meta-analysis of four other studies, making it the largest study its kind, involving nearly 250,000 individuals over the course of 12 years. Moderate coffee consumption has been associated with a reduced risk of coronary heart disease and stroke.[320]
- In a 2015 analysis which included nearly 210,000 U.S. health professional participants who drank one to five cups of coffee (decaf or regular) daily had slightly lower risk for all-cause mortality than nondrinkers. Results from this and previous studies indicate that coffee consumption can be incorporated into a healthy lifestyle.[321]
- High consumption of coffee may decrease the risk of developing MS. Caffeine, one component of coffee, has neuroprotective properties, and has been shown to suppress the production of proinflammatory cytokines, which may be mechanisms underlying the observed association. However, further investigations are needed to determine whether exposure to caffeine underlies the observed association and, if so, to evaluate its mechanisms of action.[322]
- A study evaluated coffee consumption in 5,000 patients with Colorectal Cancer (CRC) vs. 4,000 controls. Findings suggested the existence of an inverse correlation which was also observed with decaffeinated coffee. The

---

[316]The perils of powdered caffeine and alcohol."ScienceDaily, 18 Feb <www.sciencedaily.com/releases/2015/02/150218122106.htm>.

[317] Ann Int Med 2006;144:792-8

[318] Prospective study Arthritis Rheum. 2007;56:2048-54

[319]Caffeine increases tear volume depending on polymorphisms within the adenosine A2a receptor gene and cytochrome P450 1A2. Ophthalmology. 2012;119:972-978

[320] Coffee consumption is not associated with increased risk of atrial fibrillation: results from two prospective cohorts and a meta-analysis. *BMC Medicine*, 2015; 13 (1) DOI: 10.1186/s12916-015-0447-8

[321] Association of Coffee Consumption with Total and Cause-Specific Mortality in Three Large Prospective Cohorts. DOI: 10.1161/CIRCULATIONAHA.115.017341

[322] J Neurol Neurosurg Psychiatry. 2016;87(5):454-460.

study even found a dose-response trend between the number of daily cups of coffee and the protective effect on both colon and rectum.[323]

2020 Update

Caffeine boosts problem-solving ability but not creativity.

While the cognitive benefits of caffeine -- increased alertness, improved vigilance, enhanced focus and improved motor performance -- are well established it did not help creativity. In addition to the results on creativity, caffeine did not significantly affect working memory, but test subjects who took it did report feeling less sad.[324]

The case against

In a study of 18-to-45-year-olds with untreated stage 1 hypertension, "moderate coffee drinkers" who drank one to three espressos a day were three times as likely to have a CV event (mostly a heart attack) within a decade as those who did not drink coffee. Moreover, "heavy coffee drinkers" who drank four or more espressos a day were four times as likely to have a CV event as abstainers. These findings from the Hypertension and Ambulatory Recording Venetia Study (HARVEST) were presented as a poster at the European Society of Cardiology (ESC) 2015 Congress.[325]

Drinking more than four cups of coffee per day does more than increase the risk of the jitters, a new study suggests. Researchers report that heavy coffee consumption, defined as more than 28 cups of coffee per week, is associated with an increased risk of all-cause mortality among men. For men and women 55 years of age and younger, the association between heavy coffee consumption and all-cause mortality is more pronounced. In a multivariate analysis, men who drank more than 28 cups of coffee had a statistically significant 21% increased risk of all-cause mortality. In women, the risk was not statistically significant. In men younger than 55 years of age, drinking more than 28 cups per week was associated with a 56% increased risk of death compared with nondrinkers. In younger women, such heavy consumption increased the risk of death 113% compared with those who did not drink coffee. Overall, there was no association

323 Source: http://cebp.aacrjournals.org/content/25/4/634.abstract
324 University of Arkansas
325 Coffee Tied to MI Risk in Younger Adults With Mild Hypertension. Medscape. Sep 08, 2015.

Type 2 Diabetes

Filtered coffee has a positive effect in terms of reducing the risk of developing type 2 diabetes. But boiled coffee does not have this effect,[326]

And Finally, the Risks

As is often the case, with benefits come risks, and coffee consumption certainly has negative medical and psychiatric effects to consider. Besides the aforementioned potential increase in blood pressure, coffee can incite or worsen anxiety, insomnia, and tremor and potentially elevate glaucoma risk. Also, given the potential severity of symptoms, caffeine withdrawal syndrome is included as a diagnosis in the DSM-5 (the Psychiatric Manual of Diagnosis).

Cranberries

Do not prevent or treat urinary tract infections (UTI) in women.[327]

Curcumin

Curcumin is a naturally occurring compound found in the spice turmeric that has been used for centuries as an Ayurvedic medicine treatment for such ailments as allergies, diabetes and ulcers. Anecdotal and scientific evidence suggests curcumin promotes health because it lowers inflammation, but it is not absorbed well by the body. Most curcumin in food or supplements stays in the gastrointestinal tract, and any portion that's absorbed is metabolized quickly. Curcumin powder was mixed with castor oil and polyethylene glycol in a process called nano-emulsion (think vinaigrette salad dressing), creating fluid teeming with microvesicles that contain curcumin. This process allows the compound to dissolve and be more easily absorbed by the gut to enter the bloodstream and tissues.[328]

Author's NOTE: This study was done on mice. Castor oil tastes vile. Perhaps, if people want to try curcumin, which does seem to have benefits, then another oil

---

[326] Chalmers University of Technology. "Filtered coffee helps prevent type 2 diabetes, show biomarkers in blood samples." ScienceDaily. ScienceDaily, 19 December 2019. <www.sciencedaily.com/releases/201

[327] JAMA 27 Oct 2016

[328] Oral Administration of Nano-Emulsion Curcumin in Mice Suppresses Inflammatory-Induced NFκB Signaling and Macrophage Migration. PLoS ONE, 2014; 9 (11): e111559 DOI: 10.1371/journal.pone.0111559

could be used, perhaps EVOO. Activated curcumin is now available which claims to be x30 times stronger with enhanced absorption.

Curcurmin (tumeric) may protect against dementia.

Combining curcumin, the active ingredient in curry dishes and silymarin, a component of milk thistle, inhibited the spread of colon cancer cells and increased cancer cell death but concentrations of curcumin and silymarin that are too high could be harmful. It's safer to get your curcumin from foods that contain turmeric, such as curry, rather than taking high doses of the compound.[329]

Curcumin-Tumeric

While studies in humans are still in very early stages, lab and animal studies have shown promising effects of curcumin in the fight against cancer. Curcumin "interferes with several important molecular pathways involved in cancer development, growth and spread," according to the American Cancer Society, even killing cancer cells in the lab setting and shrinking tumors and boosting the effects of chemotherapy in animals. It exerts potent anti-inflammatory effects, and these anti-inflammatory effects seem to be quite protective against some form of cancer progression. However, curcumin has additional anti-cancer effects that are independent of its anti-inflammatory effects and thus is a heavily researched molecule for both cancer prevention and treatment.

Update

Curcumin is a compound that suppresses oxidative stress and inflammation, both key pathological factors for Alzheimer's, and it also helps remove amyloid plaques, small fragments of protein that clump together in the brains of Alzheimer disease patients.

The failure of the body to easily absorb curcumin has been a thorn in the side of medical researchers seeking scientific proof that curcumin can successfully treat cancer, heart disease, Alzheimer's and many other chronic health conditions.

Now, researchers have shown that curcumin can be delivered effectively into human cells via tiny nanoparticles.

---

[329] Curcumin Sensitizes Silymarin to Exert Synergistic Anticancer Activity in Colon Cancer Cells. Journal of Cancer, 2016; 7 (10): 1250 DOI: 10.7150/jca.15690

The researchers have shown in animal experiments that nanoparticles containing curcumin not only prevents cognitive deterioration but also reverses the damage. This finding paves the way for clinical development trials for Alzheimer's.[330]

Dairy

Higher consumption of low-fat milk and yogurt was associated with lower risk of frailty (slow walking speed and weight loss). Increasing low-fat yogurt and milk might prevent frailty in older adults[331]

Milk consumption has fallen about 40% since 1975 in the USA but consuming more dairy overall. According to the U.S. Department of Agriculture, the average American ate and drank about 9% more dairy in 2018 than consumed per person in 1975, eating more cheese and yogurt but drinking a lot less milk. But because it takes more milk to make products like cheese and yogurt, dairy consumption is up overall. With Global warming dairy farming has been identified as hard on the environment. The current dietary guidelines for dairy are based on the idea that we need milk to help meet daily calcium requirements, but calcium can be found from other foods and it is felt milk is not necessary for good health.[332]

Dates

The combination of pomegranate juice and dates along with their pits provided maximum protection against atherosclerosis (plaque buildup or hardening of the arteries), which can cause a heart attack or stroke, in a trial performed on arterial cells in culture, as well as in atherosclerotic mice. The combination reduced oxidative stress in the arterial wall by 33% and decreased arterial cholesterol content by 28%. People at high risk for cardiovascular diseases, as well as healthy individuals, could benefit from consuming the combination of half a glass of pomegranate juice (4 ounces), together with 3 dates. Ideally, the pits should be ground up into a paste and eaten as well, but even without the pits, the combination is better than either fruit alone.[333]

Dates, however, are incredibly high in sugar.

---

[330] University of South Australia. "Curcumin is the spice of life when delivered via tiny nanoparticles: Treatment for Alzheimer's and genital herpes." ScienceDaily. ScienceDaily, 5 March 2020. <www.sciencedaily.com/releases/2020/03/200305132144.htm>.

[331] Alberto Lana, PhD; Fernando Rodriguez-Artalejo, MD, PhD; Esther Lopez-Garcia, PhD J Am Geriatr Soc. 2015;63(9):1852-1860.

[332] February 13, 2020 N Engl J Med 2020; 382:644-654 DOI: 10.1056/NEJMra1903547

[333] Atherogenic properties of date vs. pomegranate polyphenols: the benefits of the combination. Food Funct., 2015; DOI: 10.1039/C4FO00998C

Diabetes: It's the weight loss that cures[334]

2300 people with proven prediabetes were recruited to see if one of two different diets prevented developing TD2 but participants had to lose 8% of their body weight in order to qualify for the next phase.

The alternatives were high protein with a low glycemic index, or moderate protein with a moderate glycemic index. The expectation was that participants on the moderate-protein diet with activity would drop the rate of type 2 diabetes to approximately 15%, and those on the high-protein diet would drop it even further, to about 10%. It was very exciting, then, that only 4% developed type 2 diabetes, but it was disappointing that there was no difference between the diets.

It was thought the initial weight loss was a real determinant of success.

Diet Drinks

PLOS Medicine warns that there is scant evidence that so called diet (artificially sweetened) drinks help people lose weight and that they should not be recommended as part of a healthy diet.[335] However, it would seem they are better than high-sugar drinks such as colas, sodas and fruit juices. To lose weight people have to gradually cut down on liking sweet foods and drinks and move on to healthy substitutes.

Eggs

1 egg / day is unlikely to have substantial overall impact on CHD or stroke risk in healthy people[336]

Eating a salad with a variety of colorful vegetables provides several unique types of carotenoids, including beta-carotene, lutein, zeaxanthin and lycopene. Adding eggs to a salad with a variety of raw vegetables is an effective method to improve the absorption of carotenoids, which are fat-soluble nutrients that help reduce inflammation and oxidative stress.

Eggs, a nutrient-rich food containing essential amino acids, unsaturated fatty acids and B vitamins, may be used to increase the nutritive value of vegetables. The lipid contained in whole eggs enhances the absorption of all these carotenoids.

---

[334] PREVIEW Nutrients 2017 Jun. 9(6):632

[335] Artificially sweetened beverages and the response to the global obesity crisis. PLoS Med2017;356:e1002195. doi:10.1371/journal.pmed.1002195. pmid:28045913.

[336] JAMA 1999;2811387-94

People obtain more of the health-promoting carotenoids from raw vegetables when cooked whole eggs were also consumed. Eggs, a nutrient-rich food containing essential amino acids, unsaturated fatty acids and B vitamins, may be used to increase the nutritive value of vegetables.

All salads were served with three grams of canola oil. The second salad had 75 grams of scrambled whole eggs and the third 150 grams of scrambled whole eggs. The absorption of carotenoids was 3.8-fold higher when the salad included three eggs compared to no eggs.

Many salad dressings contain about 140-160 calories per serving, about two tablespoons. One large whole egg is about 70 calories and provides 6 grams of protein. People are at a greater risk of putting too many calories on a salad because they don't always know proper portion sizes for salad dressings, but you do know the portion size of an egg[337]

A meta-analysis suggested reducing intake to prevent diabetes 2[338]

An Oxford university study of 418,000 people over 12 years found eggs increased hemorrhagic strokes. Every extra 0.7oz of eggs (about half a small egg) consumed a day was linked to a 25 per cent higher risk of hemorrhagic stroke.[339]

Update

CONFLICTING ADVICE[340]

A large study in the BMJ found no association between egg intake and risk of incident cardiovascular disease except for those with diabetes 2 (who did have a positive association between higher intake of eggs and cardiovascular risk).

However, a meta-analysis of randomized clinical studies involving dietary interventions showed that higher egg consumption led to higher serum concentrations of low-density lipoprotein (LDL) cholesterol, extending earlier findings. Since high LDL cholesterol is a causal factor in cardiovascular disease risk.

337Effects of egg consumption on carotenoid absorption from co-consumed, raw vegetables. *American Journal of Clinical Nutrition*, 2015; DOI: 10.3945/ajcn.115.111062

338Egg consumption and risk of type 2 diabetes: a meta-analysis of prospective studies First published January 6, 2016, doi: 10.3945/ ajcn.115.119933

339 European Heart Journal, ehaa007, https://doi.org/10.1093/eurheartj/ehaa007 Published: 24 February 2020

340 Research, doi: 10.1136/bmj.m513

The conclusion is that daily eggs, in the Western diet of refined, ultra-processed added sugar, red meat, are not recommended but OK with the Mediterranean Diet (but not for those with diabetes 2).

These authors examined habitual egg intake (assessed by food frequency questionnaires) and risk of cardiovascular disease over decades of follow-up in an updated individual level analysis of three prospective US cohorts: The Nurses' Health Study (I and II), and the Health Professionals' Follow-Up Study). Data were then pooled for a summary estimate.

In over 215 000 women and men who were free of major chronic disease at baseline, the researchers found no association between egg intake and risk of incident cardiovascular disease (defined as fatal or non-fatal myocardial infarction, coronary heart disease, and stroke).[341]

If frequent egg consumption is occurring in the context of a typical Western dietary pattern (high levels of refined grains, added sugars, red and processed meats, and ultra-processed foods), the best evidence for cardio- protection supports shifting one's overall dietary pattern to a Dietary Approaches to Stop Hypertension (DASH) or Mediterranean diet.

A recent meta-analysis of randomized clinical studies involving dietary interventions showed that higher egg consumption led to higher serum concentrations of low-density lipoprotein (LDL) cholesterol, extending earlier findings. Since high LDL cholesterol is a causal factor in cardiovascular disease risk.

Emulsifiers

Emulsifiers, used in margarine, mayonnaise, creamy sauces, candy, ice cream, packaged processed foods, packaged bread and baked goods are ubiquitous but mice experiments reveal they may promote the inflammatory bowel diseases ulcerative colitis and Crohn's disease as well as the metabolic syndrome. The study involved two widely used emulsifiers, polysorbate 80 and carboxymethylcellulose.[342]

---

[341] The BMJ (doi:10.1136/bmj.m513).

[342] Nature 2015. Study Links Common Food Additives to Crohn's Disease, Colitis. *Medscape*. Feb 25, 2015.

EPA Icosapent ethyl (*Vascepa,* Amarin): Unique benefits[343]

There would appear to be unique benefits specific to icosapent ethyl (*Vascepa,* Amarin), a high-strength formulation of purified eicosapentaenoic acid (EPA) as found in the REDUCE-IT Trial.

A high dose of icosapent ethyl (4 g daily) reduced the rate of cardiovascular events by 25% over a median of 4.9 years of follow-up.

These benefits appear to be mediated only through EPA levels and are specific for EPA and can't be generalized to other EPA formulations beyond icosapent ethyl or to the other omega-3 fatty acid, docosahexaenoic acid (DHA). Nor can these benefits be got from eating fish,

Fat

Grass fed fat on meat is yellow (as is the fat in our own bodies). This is arguably healthier than the 'pure' white fat found on grain and lot fed cattle.

Fiber - Resistant Starch

Eating more dietary fibre improves life expectancy, although food processing may remove these benefits. Not all foods that contain fibre are created equal -- while whole grains are an important source of fibre, their benefits may be diluted when heavily processed. Wholegrain foods are now widely perceived to be beneficial, but increasingly products available on the supermarket shelves are ultra-processed.

Adequate fiber intake - 30 g per day - is important for a healthy, balanced diet, reducing the risk of a range of chronic diseases. Resistant starch is a type of dietary fiber that increases the production of short chain fatty acids in the gut, and there have been numerous studies reporting its impact on different health outcomes. There is consistent evidence that it can aid blood sugar control. It has also been suggested that it can support gut health and enhance satiety via increased production of short chain fatty acids. Some resistant starch occurs in bananas, potatoes, grains, and legumes, and some are produced or modified commercially and incorporated into food products[344]

---

[343] *REDUCE-IT: CV Benefit of Icosapent Ethyl Directly Related to EPA Levels - Medscape - Apr 02, 2020.*

[344] Health effects of resistant starch. *Nutrition Bulletin*, 2017; DOI: 10.1111/nbu.12244

An Oxford University study of 418,000 people over 12 years found higher consumption of both dietary fiber and fruit and vegetables was strongly associated with lower risks of ischemic stroke making it 23 per cent less likely.

Every third of an ounce more intake of fiber a day – the equivalent of two cups of chopped carrots. Fruit and vegetables were associated with a 13 per cent lower risk for every 7oz (200g) eaten a day.[345]

A *Lancet* study commissioned by the World Health Organization found that for every 8 g increase in dietary fiber eaten per day, total deaths and incidences of coronary heart disease, type 2 diabetes, and colorectal cancer decreased by 2-19%. Risks of stroke and breast cancer were also reduced.2 Choosing foods with fiber also makes us feel fuller, helps digestion, and prevent constipation.

"The evidence from prospective studies is remarkably consistent that a higher intake of fiber is related to lower risk of type 2 diabetes, cardiovascular disease and weight gain," Dr. Walter Willett, professor of nutrition and epidemiology at Harvard School of Public Health 2019.

Don't take Fiber Supplements

The dietary guidelines recommend a daily fiber intake for adult men is 33.6 grams per day and 38 grams for women. Sadly, the average fiber intake is 17 grams, and only 5 percent of people meet the adequate daily intake

Fiber supplements are lacking in essentials One of the main drawbacks of any supplement is that it lacks vitamins, minerals, and protective antioxidants that you get when you eat high-fiber foods such as vegetables, fruits, whole grains, beans, and lentils.

Fish

- Overwhelming advice is to eat more oily fish
- But a most recent review found evidence was "weak with moderate inconsistency' 'confounders may not have been adequate'[346]
- Farmed salmon fed vegetable oils decrease beneficial effects
- High intake = >80g/d
- Low = <10g/d

---

[345] *European Heart Journal*, ehaa007, https://doi.org/10.1093/eurheartj/ehaa007
Published: 24 February 2020

[346] BMJ 2006

- Higher consumption in women associated with a lower risk of CHD [347]
- Non-fried fish x 3 /wk. led to a 50% reduction in fatal IHD & 58% arrhythmias but not if fried[348]
- Consumption associated with a reduction in the risk of hepatocellular carcinoma. Mollusks and crustaceans come top, with a 14% reduction[349]
- People who ate baked or broiled fish (not fried) at least once a week, regardless of how much omega-3 fatty acid it contains, had greater grey matter brain volumes in areas of the brain responsible for memory (4.3%) and cognition (14%). The high heat in frying fish destroyed the beneficial omega-3 fatty acids[350],[351]
- Daily fish *oil* offers no benefit for primary or secondary prevention of coronary heart disease. However, *dietary* intake of fish was found to be of benefit for protection against heart disease and stroke and was associated with lower incident rates of heart failure in addition to lower sudden cardiac death, stroke and myocardial infarction.
- Recommendations are to eat two to three servings of fish, including oily fish such as salmon, blue-eye trevally, blue mackerel, herring, canned salmon, sardines and some varieties of canned tuna each week to reduce their risk of heart disease. It also recommends people consume some plant-based omega-3s each day, such as a handful of walnuts or by using soya bean, canola or flaxseed oil[352]
- Eating seafood is linked to a reduced risk of dementia-associated brain changes in people who carry the ApoE4 (but not all E4s) gene variation, which increases the risk for Alzheimer's disease[353]
- Mercury from fish appears to pose little risk for aging people but in pregnancy can cause cognitive problems in babies[354]

Fish Oil (also see vitamins & supplements)

- A meta-analysis of 20 randomized trials (69,000 patients) found ω-3 fatty acid supplementation did not lower risk for death, myocardial

---

347 (Nurse's H Study ~85,000 1980-94) JAMA 2002;287:1815-21
348 Circulation 2003;107:1372-77
349 Annals of Oncology (2013, doi:10.1093/ annonc/mdt168).
350 *Am J Prev Med.* Published online July 29, 2014.
351 Regular Fish Consumption and Age-Related Brain Gray Matter Loss. *American Journal of Preventive Medicine*, 2014; DOI: 10.1016/j.amepre.2014.05.037
352 Heart, Lung and Circ 2015; online 13 Apr
353 JAMA. 2016;315(5):489-497. doi:10.1001/jama.2015.19451
354 JAMA. 2016;315(5):489-497. doi:10.1001/jama.2015.19451

infarction or stroke with follow-ups ranging from 1 to 6 years.355

- Italian researchers then conducted an industry-supported trial (The 12,500 participants) that is a hybrid of primary and secondary prevention. ω-3 fatty acid supplementation did not lower the incidence of any secondary endpoints356.
- Daily fish oil offers no benefit for primary or secondary prevention of coronary heart disease. However, intake of fish was consistently found to be of benefit for protection against heart disease and stroke and was associated with lower incident rates of heart failure in addition to lower sudden cardiac death, stroke and myocardial infarction.
- Recommendations are to eat two to three servings of fish, including oily fish such as salmon, blue-eye trevally, blue mackerel, herring, canned salmon, sardines and some varieties of canned tuna each week to reduce their risk of heart disease. It also recommends people consume some plant-based omega-3s each day, such as a handful of walnuts or by using soya bean, canola or flaxseed oil357
- Examination of the contents of 32 fish oil supplements on the market in New Zealand, half of which were made in Australia, found only three products contained quantities of omega-3 fatty acids (EPA and DHA) that were equal to or higher than that stated on the label. In addition, new research suggests, the oil in fish oil supplements is in many cases was nearly rancid due to oxidation, potentially causing harm. On average, capsules contained 68% of the claimed content and two brands had only one-third of the claimed content358
- However, it would seem the profile is similar to that in fish.
- Taking a high dose of omega-3 fatty acids from fish oil daily for six months after a heart attack improved the function of the heart and reduced scarring in the undamaged muscle359.
- The n−3 LCPUFAs (Long Chain Polyunsaturated fatty Acids)— mainly eicosapentaenoic acid (EPA) and docosahexaenoic acid (DHA) — are the active components of fish oils. The n−3 LCPUFAs are essential, and since humans do not produce them to any great extent, they must be added to our diet.

---

[355] JAMA 2012; 308:1024.

[356] The Risk and Prevention Study Collaborative Group. n-3 fatty acids in patients with multiple cardiovascular risk factors. N Engl J Med 2013 May 9; 368:1800. (http://dx.doi.org/10.1056/NEJMoa1205409)

[357] Heart, Lung and Circ 2015; online 13 Apr

[358] *Scientific Reports 2015; online 21 Jan*

[359] Effect of Omega-3 Acid Ethyl Esters on Left Ventricular Remodeling After Acute Myocardial InfarctionClinical Perspective. *Circulation*, 2016; 134 (5): 378 DOI: 10.1161/CIRCULATIONAHA.115.019949

- These n−3 LCPUFAs are substrates for biosynthesis of potent mediators that resolve inflammation and infection.
- These specialized pro-resolving mediators are present in placenta and human milk and, in preclinical experimental models, two types of these pro-resolving mediators, resolvins and protectins, decrease airway inflammation, mucus metaplasia, and hyperreactivity and promote host defense against respiratory infection.
- Epidemiologic studies have linked maternal fish intake during pregnancy to reductions in allergic disorders in their offspring
- Airway mucosal levels of n−3 LCPUFAs are lower in patients with asthma than in those without asthma and pro-resolving mediators within the lung are under-produced in patients with severe and uncontrolled asthma.
- Several studies have shown a lower incidence of allergic sensitization among infants born to mothers who supplemented with fish oil than among infants born to mothers who did not, as well as a lower prevalence of allergic disorders, including food allergies, atopic dermatitis, and wheezing illnesses in the first year of life,8 with possible persistence until later in life.

2020 Update

Contradicting some of the above studies[360]

Britons who took fish oil supplements -- and not the prescription pharmaceutical-grade kind -- lived longer on average and were less likely to develop cardiovascular disease (CVD) years down the line, according to a large prospective cohort study.

U.K. Biobank participants who reported habitual supplementation with store-bought omega-3 fatty acid-rich fish oil pills had better outcomes over 8 to 9 years of follow-up:

- All-cause mortality: adjusted HR 0.87 (95% CI 0.83-0.90)
- CVD mortality: adjusted HR 0.84 (95% CI 0.78-0.91)
- Overall CVD events: adjusted HR 0.93 (95% CI 0.90-0.96)

The inverse relationship between fish oil supplements and CVD risk persisted after adjustment for sex, age, income, diet, and alcohol consumption, and other variables.

---

[360] Associations of habitual fish oil supplementation with cardiovascular outcomes and all causmortality: evidence from a large population based cohort study
BMJ 2020; 368 doi: https://doi.org/10.1136/bmj.m456 (Published04March2020)Cite this as: BMJ 2020;368:m45

Two systematic reviews found that omega 3 supplements may slightly reduce coronary heart disease mortality and events, but slightly increase risk of prostate cancer. Both beneficial and harmful effects are small.

If 1,000 people took omega 3 supplements for around four years, three people would avoid dying from heart disease, six people would avoid a coronary event (such as a heart attack) and three extra people would develop prostate cancer.[361]

Fish Oil Supplements Are Associated with Better Testicular Function

Healthy young men who took fish oil supplements had higher semen volume and total sperm count than those who did not.[362]

Folate

No evidence it prevents CAC but some evidence it may make high-grade adenomas worse[363]

Fructose

The liver converts fructose very efficiently into fat. People who consume too much high-fructose food can in time become overweight and develop high blood pressure, dyslipidaemia with fatty liver and insulin resistance -- symptoms named the metabolic syndrome. In addition, a previously unknown molecular mechanism has been discovered that points to fructose as a key driver of uncontrolled growth of the heart muscle, a condition that can lead to fatal heart failure.

Fruits (& Seeds)

Fruits and vegetables were classified in four-color groups:

Green, including dark leafy vegetables, cabbages and lettuces
Orange/Yellow, which were mostly citrus fruits
Red/Purple, which were mostly red vegetables
White, of which 55% were apples and pears

---

[361] British Journal of Cancer and the Cochrane Database of Systematic Reviews. February 29, 2020
[362] Jensen TK et al. JAMA Netw Open 2020 Jan 17
[363] JAMA 2007 Jun 6; 297:2351-9.

Fresh fruit associated with lower risk of heart attack and stroke

Study of 500,000 Chinese adults confirms benefits of eating fruit

People who eat fresh fruit on most days are at lower risk of heart attack and stroke than people who rarely eat fresh fruit, according to new research. The findings come from a seven-year study of half a million adults in China, Fruit is a rich source of potassium, dietary fiber, antioxidants, and various other potentially active compounds, and contains little sodium or fat and relatively few calories. The study found that fruit consumption (which was mainly apples or oranges) was strongly associated with many other factors, such as education, lower blood pressure, lower blood glucose, and not smoking. But, after allowing for what was known of these and other factors, a 100g portion of fruit per day was associated with about one-third less cardiovascular mortality and the association was similar across different study areas and in both men and women.[364]

Fruit & veg diets

- No proven benefit in reducing risk of any Ca
- Reduced risk of gall stone formation [365]
- Reinforcing the mantra about five servings of fruits and vegetables a day, a meta-analysis in *The BMJ* showed that each additional serving cut all-cause mortality by 5% and cardiovascular death by 4%. But after five a day, no further survival benefit accrued.
- Daily fruit consumption cuts the risk of cardiovascular disease (CVD) by up to 40% were the findings from the seven-year follow-up study of nearly 0.5 million people in the China Kadoorie Biobank[366]
- Copenhagen General Population Study (CGPS) and City Heart Study showed that those who ate the most fruit and vegetables had a 13% lower risk of CVD and a 20% lower risk of all-cause mortality compared with those that ate these foods only rarely[367]
- Two servings of fruit and three of vegetables are associated with a lower risk of death from any cause, particularly from cardiovascular disease, but beyond five portions appears to have no further effect. Each fruit or vegetable serving was associated with a 4% reduction in cardiovascular mortality. (A serving

---

364 Fresh Fruit Consumption and Major Cardiovascular Disease in China. *New England Journal of Medicine*, 2016; 374 (14): 1332 DOI: 10.1056/NEJMoa1501451

365 A J Epidem 15 Jul 2004

366 European Society of Cardiology. "Fruit consumption cuts cardiovascular disease risk by up to 40 percent." Science Daily, 1 September 2014 <www.sciencedaily.com/releases/2014/09/140901123545.htm>.

367 Kobylecki CJ, Afzal S, Smith GD, Nordestgaard BG. Genetically high plasma vitamin C, intake of fruit and vegetables, and risk of ischemic heart disease and all-cause mortality: a Mendelian randomization study. *Am J Clin Nutr* 2015; 101:1135-1143

was defined as roughly 80 g, or 2.8 oz., of fruit or vegetable.) Sixteen studies involving a total of 833,234 participants and 56,423 deaths were analyzed[368]

- Infants do significantly better on developmental tests when their mothers consume more fruit during pregnancy[369]

Fruit Juice - avoid

When carbohydrates are consumed the digestive system breaks the carbs down into glucose, which enters the bloodstream and raises the blood sugar stimulating the pancreas to produce the hormone insulin, a signal to the body cells to absorb the glucose so it can be used immediately as energy or stored in the liver and muscles for later use. Repeatedly eating foods that cause surges in blood sugar makes the pancreas work harder. Over time, that can lead to insulin resistance and an increased risk of Type 2 diabetes.

Refined grain products like white bread, crackers, and cookies, which tend to be low in fiber, deliver large amounts of carbohydrates per serving and are digested very quickly, raising blood sugar and insulin levels. Sugars enter into the bloodstream especially rapidly when you consume carbohydrates in liquid form, such as in sugary sodas / soft drinks.

The quality and physical form of carbohydrates are critical, which means favoring whole foods over processed foods and added sugars. That includes favoring whole fruit over fruit juice: Fruit juices can contain fiber, but some of that fiber is broken down in the juicing process, reducing the metabolic benefit compared with intact fruit.

To minimize spikes in insulin, it's best to eat fruit whole. That's because with whole fruit the cell walls remain intact. This is how fiber can offer the greatest benefit, because the sugars are effectively sequestered within the fiber scaffolding of the cells, and it takes time for the digestive tract to break down those cells. Four apples may contain the same amount of sugar as 24 ounces of soda, but the slow rate of absorption minimizes the blood sugar surge.

But see "Orange Juice".

---

368 Fruit and vegetable consumption and mortality from all causes, cardiovascular disease, and cancer: systematic review and dose-response meta-analysis of prospective cohort studies. *BMJ*, 2014; 349 (jul29 3): g4490 DOI: 10.1136/bmj.g4490

369 Cognitive Enhancement in Infants Associated with Increased Maternal Fruit Intake During Pregnancy: Results from a Birth Cohort Study with Validation in an Animal Model. *EBioMedicine*, 2016; DOI: 10.1016/j.ebiom.2016.04.025

Garlic

- No form of garlic given over 6 months 6 days a week had any effect on cholesterol or other plasma lipids in adults with moderate hyper-cholesterolaemia[370]
- Raw garlic reduced cholesterol, triglyceride, glucose in lab rats. Boiled garlic didn't[371]
- Several trials of varying quality show that garlic protects against colorectal cancer[372]
- Numerous studies have suggested garlic reduces the incidence of gastric and colon cancer but there are study limitations, including the accuracy of reporting the amounts and frequency of garlic consumed, and the inability to compare data from studies that used different garlic products and amounts make an overall conclusion about garlic and cancer prevention extremely difficult. Since many of the studies looking at garlic use and cancer prevention have used multi-ingredient products, it is unclear whether garlic alone or in combination with other nutritional components may have the greatest effect.
- The USA National Cancer Institute does not recommend any dietary supplement for the prevention of cancer, but recognizes garlic as one of several vegetables with potential anticancer properties. Because all garlic preparations are not the same, it is difficult to determine the exact amount of garlic that may be needed to reduce cancer risk. Furthermore, the active compounds present in garlic may lose their effectiveness with time, handling, and processing. The World Health Organization's (WHO) guidelines for general health promotion for adults is a daily dose of 2 to 5 g of fresh garlic (approximately one clove), 0.4 to 1.2 g of dried garlic powder, 2 to 5 mg of garlic oil, 300 to 1,000 mg of garlic extract, or other formulations that are equal to 2 to 5 mg of allicin.
- Studies using high concentrations of garlic extracts have been associated with improved blood circulation, healthier cholesterol levels and lower blood pressure, all of which reduce the risk of cardiovascular disease. However, current evidence does not support the use of garlic supplements to improve health

---

[370] Arch Int Med 2007;167:346-53
[371] J Nutr 2006;136:800-2S
[372] J Nutrit 2007;137:2264

Garlic Breath

Try yoghurt mixed with parsley
Raw apple or lettuce may help reduce garlic breath[373]

Ginger

May help prevent or treat nausea and vomiting from motion sickness, pregnancy, and cancer chemotherapy. It is also used to treat mild stomach upset, to reduce pain of osteoarthritis. Preliminary studies suggest that ginger may lower cholesterol and help prevent blood from clotting. That can help treat heart disease where blood vessels can become blocked and lead to heart attack or stroke. Other studies suggest that ginger may help improve blood sugar control among people with type 2 diabetes. More research is needed to determine whether ginger is safe or effective for heart disease and diabetes.

Grains

Whole grains are defined as the 'intact, ground, cracked or flaked kernel after the removal of the inedible parts such as the hull and husk'.

Whole grains. In their natural state growing in the fields, whole grains are the entire seed of a plant. This seed (which industry calls a "kernel") is made up of three key edible parts – the bran, the germ, and the endosperm – protected by an inedible husk that protects the kernel from assaults by sunlight, pests, water, and disease. Whole grains may be eaten whole, cracked, split or ground (Kibbled just means to crush or grind coarsely). They can be milled into flour or used to make breads, cereals and other processed foods. If a food label states that the package contains whole grain, the "whole grain" part of the food inside the package is required to have the same proportions of bran, germ, and endosperm as the harvested kernel does before it is processed.

Whole Grains - 3 basic components:

1. Outer layer	=	Bran
2.Inner layer	=	Germ
3. Starch layer	=	Endosperm

---

[373] Deodorization of Garlic Breath by Foods, and the Role of Polyphenol Oxidase and Phenolic Compounds. *Journal of Food Science*, 2016; DOI: 10.1111/1750-3841.13439

Bran

The bran is the multi-layered outer skin of the edible kernel. It contains important antioxidants, B vitamins and fiber.

The Germ

The germ is the embryo, with the potential to sprout into a new plant. It contains many B vitamins, some protein, minerals, and healthy fats.

The Endosperm

The endosperm is the germ's food supply, which provides essential energy to the young plant so it can send roots down for water and nutrients and send sprouts up for sunlight's photosynthesizing power. The endosperm is by far the largest portion of the kernel. It contains starchy carbohydrates, proteins and small amounts of vitamins and minerals.

Whole grains are healthier

Whole grains contain all three parts of the kernel.

Refining normally removes the bran and the germ, leaving only the endosperm. Without the bran and germ, about 25% of a grain's protein is lost, along with at least seventeen key nutrients.

Processors add back some vitamins and minerals to enrich refined grains, so refined products still contribute valuable nutrients.

But whole grains are healthier, providing more protein, more fiber and many important vitamins and minerals.

Processing, as in white bread, removes bran & germ which takes away the vitamins, nutrients & fiber

Diets rich in whole grains such as whole grain breads, popcorn, barley, bulgur confer 18% to 30% lowered risk of heart disease

So, add bran or eat whole grain breads[374]

16 g / serving	= excellent
8 - 15 g / serving	= good

[374] A J Nutrition Dec 2004

Dehusking / Refining of Grains

Refining consists of when the bran and germ are stripped off and all that is left is nutrient poor starch in the form of white flour. Grains were originally refined to extend their shelf life. However, Grains consist of fiber-rich bran and nutrient-rich germ, which is lost in the refining.

Wheat is the most eaten grain in Western diets and 98% of this wheat is eaten in the form of white flour.

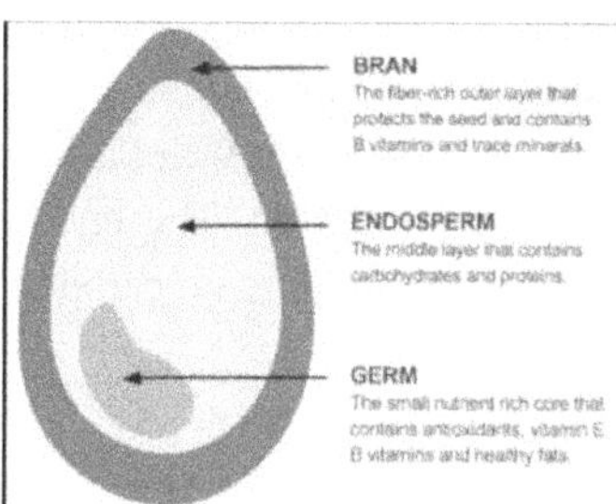

% of Nutrients Lost by Refining

Nutrient	loss
Protein	25%
Fiber	95%
Calcium	56%
Copper	62%
Iron	84%
Manganese	82%
Phosphorous	69%
Potassium	74%
Selenium	52%
Zinc	76%
Vitamin B1	73%
Vitamin B2	81%
Vitamin B3	80%
Vitamin B5	56%
Vitamin B6	87%
Folate	59%
Vitamin E	95%

'Enriching' only chemically adds 5 of the lost 25 nutrients back

Higher Whole-Grain Intake Is Associated with Lower Mortality

During 25 years of follow-up, cardiovascular-related mortality was 15% lower among those who ate the most whole grains (including popcorn!).

Each 28-gram serving of whole grains per day was associated with a 5% reduction in overall death risk and a 9% reduction in death from cardiovascular causes[375]

It was estimated that every serving (28 g/d) of whole grain consumption was associated with a 5% lower total morality or a 9% lower CVD mortality, whereas the same intake level was nonsignificantly associated with lower cancer mortality. Similar inverse associations were observed between bran intake and CVD mortality whereas germ intake was not associated with CVD mortality.

Analysis also found that replacing one serving of refined grains with a serving of whole grains each day was associated with an 8% lower mortality from cardiovascular causes.

Replacing one serving of red meat with whole grains daily, reduced CVD mortality risk by 20%.

High whole grain intake has been associated with a lower risk for colorectal cancer in numerous studies.

Whole grain consumption was associated with lower mortality due to colorectal cancer in men, but no significant associations with mortality due to lung cancer, prostate cancer, or breast cancer found.

The observation that bran, but not germ, was consistently associated with reduced CVD mortality was a new and significant finding.

Adding bran to the diet, in addition to eating whole grain foods with bran, was associated with lower mortality.

Whole grain breakfast is associated with a longer healthier life[376]

Whole grains protect against Diabetes 2 by 21%[377]

---

[375] JAMA Intern Med 2015 Jan 5;
[376] Am J Clin Nutrit 2003;77:594-9
[377] PloS Med 2007;4:1385-95 Am J Clin Nutrit 2003;77:622-9

Over 80% of the UK are not eating enough whole grains[378]

How much whole grain do we need to eat?

In the US, the recommended daily intake is defined as 'at least 3-5 servings a day' where a serving is 16g, and in Denmark they go further to suggest a 'minimum intake of 75g a day'.

Three servings (around 48g) is equivalent to:

- 3 slices of whole meal bread
- A bowl of porridge or wholegrain breakfast cereal and a slice of whole meal toast
- A portion of whole grain rice/pasta/quinoa or other whole grains

Suggest

Replacing white rice and pasta for brown or eating porridge or a wholegrain cereal for breakfast or three slices of whole meal bread a day (Not just brown colored bread)

- Rye bread and other wholegrain foods contain a particular group of bioactive health-promoting substances benzoxazinoids, or BX for short, which pass through the gut wall and circulate in the body in different chemical forms such that eating a diet rich in BX compounds made certain immune system cells react more strongly to some types of bacteria.[379]
- Data from more than 74,000 women from the Nurses' Health Study and more than 43,000 men from the Health Professionals Follow-Up Study found that eating more whole grains is associated with up to 9% lower overall mortality and up to 15% lower CVD-related mortality. For each serving of whole grains (28g/day), overall mortality dropped by 5%, and by 9% for CVD-related mortality. The study also found that bran, a component of whole grain foods, was associated with similar beneficial effects. Bran intake was linked with up to 6% lower overall mortality and up to 20% lower CVD-related

---

[378] Low whole grain intake in the UK: results from the National Diet and Nutrition Survey rolling programme 2008-2011. British Journal of Nutrition, April 2015 DOI: 10.1017/S0007114515000422 Whole grain intake and its association with intakes of other foods, nutrients and markers of health in the National Diet and Nutrition Survey rolling programme 2008–11. British Journal of Nutrition, 2015; 1 DOI: 10.1017/S0007114515000525

[379] Cereal phytochemicals with putative therapeutic and health-protecting properties. Molecular Nutrition & Food Research, 2015; 59 (7): 1324 DOI: 10.1002/mnfr.201400717

mortality. Eating more whole grains is associated with a lower risk of major chronic diseases, such as type 2 diabetes and CVD.

- Swapping just one serving of refined grains or red meat per day with one serving of whole grains was linked with lower CVD-related mortality: 8% lower mortality for swapping out refined grains and 20% lower mortality for swapping out red meat.
- In contrast, the researchers found no association between eating whole grains and lowered cancer-related mortality.[380]
- Increased intake reduces chronic disease and premature mortality.[381]

Benefits: Whole grains reduce the incidence of All-Cause Mortality, cardiovascular disease and total cancer.

Types: Whole grain bread, breakfast cereals added bran. Little effect with refined grains white rice

A slice of 100 percent whole grain bread contains about 16 grams of whole grains, and current dietary guidelines recommend 48 grams or more of whole grains daily. Reductions in risks were observed up to 210 - 225 g/day (7 servings)

CHD, stroke, CVD = 0.81
total cancer = 0.85
all causes = 0.83
respiratory diseases = 0.78
diabetes = 0.49
infectious diseases = 0.74
CNS diseases = 1.15
all non-cardiovascular, non-cancer causes = 0.78

A risk ratio < 1 suggests a reduced risk in the exposed group.

Green Leafy Vegetables

There is evidence that eating green leafy vegetables and other foods rich in vitamin K, lutein, folate and beta-carotene (including brightly colored fruits and vegetables) can help to keep the brain healthy to preserve functioning.[382]

---

[380] The study appears online January 5, 2015 in JAMA Internal Medicine.
[381] BMJ 2016;353:i2716
[382] Federation of American Societies for Experimental Biology (FASEB). "Eating green leafy vegetables keeps mental abilities sharp." ScienceDaily. ScienceDaily, 30 March 2015. <www.sciencedaily.com/releases/2015/03/150330112227.htm>.

Hamburgers

Home-made hamburgers are healthy good food if made with the right ingredients (lean meat, wholemeal/multigrain bun, plenty of salad) with 18g fat vs. 30g for commercial hamburgers.

Adding spices reduces cancer risk from meat.

Home Cooking Best

At fast-food restaurants, 70 percent of the meals Americans consumed were of poor dietary quality in 2015-16. At full-service restaurants, about 50 percent were of poor nutritional quality, an amount that remained stable over the study period. The remainder were of intermediate nutritional quality.

Less than 0.1 percent of all the restaurant meals consumed over the study period were of ideal quality.

- Restaurant meals accounted for 21 percent of Americans' total calorie intake.
- Full-service restaurant meals represented 9 percent of total calories consumed.
- Fast-food meals represented 12 percent of total calories consumed.
- Fast-food breakfasts increased from just over 4 percent to nearly 8 percent of all breakfasts eaten in America.[383]

Homocysteine

Nonfasting total homocysteine levels are an independent risk factor for incident stroke in elderly persons.[384]

Honey

Postoperative administration of honey after tonsillectomy significantly reduces pain and promotes wound healing[385]

---

383 Journal of Nutrition 2 Feb 2020

384 Nonfasting Plasma Total Homocysteine Levels and Stroke Incidence in Elderly Persons: The Framingham Study

385 The efficacy of honey for ameliorating pain after tonsillectomy: a meta-analysis European Archives of Oto-Rhino-Laryngology (Dec 2014)

Inulin

Available by eating chicory root, Jerusalem artichokes, other foods or it can be bought as a faintly sweet fine powder. Inulin is not absorbed from the gastrointestinal tract, It is considered to be a soluble fiber. It has been implicated in reducing visceral fat.

Isoflavones

Consuming tofu, which is high in isoflavones, more than once a week was associated with a 18% lower risk of heart disease, compared to a 12% lower risk for those who ate tofu less than once a month.[386]

Kombucha

Despite all the health claims nutrition experts say there's not enough scientific evidence yet to support most of them.

Labels[387]

A study that examined millions of grocery store purchases in the United States found that dubious claims about sugar, salt and fat were common. Many fruit juices that claimed to be low in sugar, for example, tended to have added sugars and more sugar than comparable juices with no claims on them. Some breakfast cereals labeled low in calories had more calories than the cereals that did not make calorie claims. And sports, energy, tea and coffee drinks with low-sodium claims had almost 17 percent more sodium than similar products with no sodium claims on them.

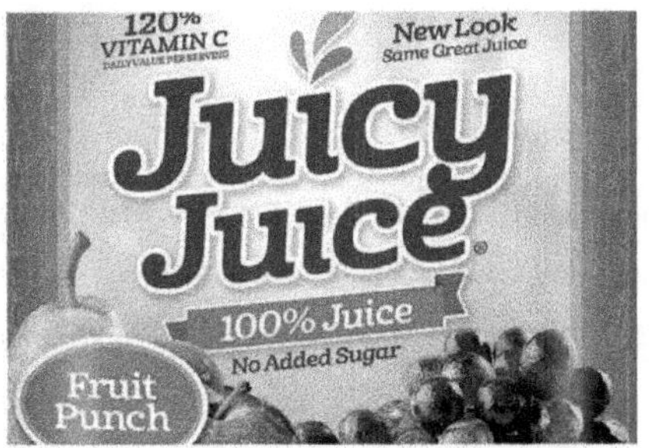

Many contain less than 2% of the fruit pictured on their labels.

---

[386] American Heart Association

[387] J Acad Nutr Diet. 2018 Jun;118(6):1130. doi: 10.1016/j.jand.2018.04.018

Legumes and Pulses

The Food and Agricultural Organization of the United Nations uses the term 'pulse' to describe crops harvested for their dry grains, such as lentils or chickpeas. They suggest the term 'legume' includes these dry grains, as well as fresh peas, beans and crops mainly grown for oil extraction, such as soya beans and peanuts. Distinctions are small so it's easy to see why they are used interchangeably.

Lentils & peanuts

- Can reduce CVD by 20%[388]

Linoleic acid (Omega 6) linked to lower mortality in older men

A higher proportion of linoleic acid in adipose tissue was associated with a 10% lower risk of death. The proportion of polyunsaturated fatty acids in adipose tissue reflects the individual's intake of these fatty acids over the long term, and this appears to be particularly true of linoleic acid, which is the most common polyunsaturated fatty acid occurring in sunflower, rapeseed (canola) and other vegetable oils, in soft table and cooking fats (margarine), nuts and seeds. Linoleic acid is known to reduce the content of bad cholesterol in the blood.

The consumption of linoleic acid in the US diet began to increase around 1969 and paralleled the introduction of soybean oil as the major commercial additive to many processed foods

With regard to Omega 3 fats, however, this study showed no clear association with a risk of cardiovascular disease or mortality.[389]

Low fat diets

Total fat, specific fats or cholesterol did not seem associated with an increased risk of stroke in men[390]

No benefit in reducing risk for Colorectal nor Breast Ca[391]

---

[388] Arch Int Med 2001;161:2573-78

[389] Association of Adipose Tissue Fatty Acids With Cardiovascular and All-Cause Mortality in Elderly Men. JAMA Cardiology, 2016 DOI: 10.1001/jamacardio.2016.2259

[390] BMJ 2003;327:777-82

[391] JAMA 2006;295:643-54

~50,000 post-menopausal women showed no CVS benefit from a low fat, high vegetable, fruit & grain diet over 8yrs[392]

Magnesium – 'The Calming Mineral'

Magnesium has been blamed for almost everything from heart arrhythmias and attacks, anxiety, leg cramps, fatigue and on and on. The problem is that only 1% is not bound in body tissues and so blood levels are not an accurate measure. AWHO report of 2009 stated that 75% of Americans consumed less than needed.[393] Foods high in magnesium include dark leafy greens such as kale, spinach, nuts, oily fish, beans, lentils, legumes, avocado, yoghurt, bananas, dried fruit, dark chocolate (i.e. the diet recommended in this book). Alcohol can quadruple its excretion[394] and protein pump inhibitors and over-the-counter medications lower body levels. A 400mg daily supplement may be worth a trial. If you feel better, take it. Magnesium is involved in some 300 regulatory enzyme systems controlling bone, muscle, protein, nerve, DNA, glucose and energy metabolism.

Magnesium is a necessary co-factor in over 300 enzyme reactions and has an important role in glucose metabolism and insulin sensitivity.[395] Magnesium and insulin have a reciprocal relationship. Insulin helps regulate the transport of magnesium cation from the extracellular to intracellular space for use in glucose metabolism. As part of glucose metabolism, magnesium promotes many of the enzymatic reactions in glycolysis. Magnesium deficiency causes insulin resistance—that is, more insulin than normal is required to metabolize glucose. As a result, the presence of hypomagnesemia and glucose intolerance can feed a comorbid cycle of insulin resistance caused by hypomagnesemia and reduced serum magnesium caused by insulin resistance.[396] Hypomagnesemia is a common laboratory abnormality in patients with type 2 diabetes, suggesting that increasing magnesium intake could be beneficial for glucose control. Thus, it may be reasonable to advise patients who are at risk for diabetes to increase magnesium intake.

---

[392] JAMA 2006;295:655-66

[393] World Health Organization. Calcium and Magnesium in Drinking Water: Public Health Significance. Geneva: World Health Organization Press; 2009.

[394] JahMagnesium basics. Clin Kidney J. 2012;5 Suppl 1:i3-i14.

[395] Magnesium metabolism in type 2 diabetes mellitus, metabolic syndrome and insulin resistance. Arch Biochem Biophys. 2007;458:40-47.

[396] Hypomagnesemia in Type 2 Diabetes: A Vicious Circle? Diabetes. 2016;65:3-13.

Meat:

Also see Protein - Centerfold

On October 26th 2015 the International Agency for Research on Cancer (IARC) announced that the consumption of both red meat and processed meat was associated with an increased risk of cancer. The specialist institution of the World Health Organization (WHO) reviewed more than 800 studies and classified red meat as 'probably carcinogenic to humans' (Group 2A) and processed meat as 'carcinogenic to humans' (Group 1), with sufficient evidence that its consumption can cause colorectal cancer.

Then a study published late 2015 in The Lancet Oncology stated that the substances responsible for this potential carcinogenicity would be generated by the meat processing itself, such as salting, fermentation, curing and smoking, or when the meat is heated to high temperatures releasing substances suspected of being carcinogenic such as nitrous compounds, polycyclic aromatic hydrocarbons (PAHs) and heterocyclic aromatic amines, among others.

However, a study published in Environmental Research indicates that the IARC made no reference to environmental pollutants that were already known to be present in raw or unprocessed meat. Therefore, scientists at the Rovira i Virgili University (URV) have analyzed the role of these compounds, which include polychlorinated naphthalenes, toxic trace elements, and perfluoroalkylated substances (PFAs), among others.

The risks to consumer health are related to micropollutants -generated by human activity through breeding or veterinary treatments- or toxins induced by the processing itself. The potential environmental toxins include inorganic elements such as arsenic, cadmium, mercury, lead, PAHs, PFAs, dioxins, pesticides and other persistent organic pollutants (POPs), such as polychlorinated biphenyls (PCBs), industrial chemicals which are viewed as one of the twelve most harmful pollutants produced by humans, according to the United Nations Environment Program. Most of these substances are fat-soluble, so any food with high fat contents accumulates higher levels of micropollutants than plant matter. PCBs and other POPs accumulate in the fatty parts of meat because they are fat soluble. Reduced consumption of meat fats will reduce the intake of PCBs. On the other hand, eating meat with a high fat content can result in a significant exposure to PCBs.

To check how cooking processes affect the presence of pollutants in meat, researchers analyzed in the laboratory the effects of frying, grilling, roasting or boiling on the concentration of various environmental, organic and inorganic pollutants present in beef steaks, pork loin, chicken breast and drumstick - which contains fewer organic pollutants than red meat - and lamb steak and chops. The results showed that different types of cooking influence the concentration of toxins differently depending on the meat product. For example, POPs hardly undergo any changes between cooked and raw meat. Being organic substances, the study argues that only cooking processes that release or eliminate fat from meat would tend to reduce the total concentration of these pollutants in the cooked meat.

Probably not the meat but the processing which produces carcinogens such as heterocyclic amines and polycyclic aromatic hydrocarbons[397]

It is recommended to reduce the daily intake of fat from meat, which would prevent not only cardiovascular risks, but also carcinogens, especially those associated with exposure to some environmental pollutants in the meat. But the concentrations of hazardous substances depend not only on the way food is prepared, but even more so on the original content of toxins in the food itself before cooking. In fact, not all meat is equally contaminated from the source but depends on precisely where and how the animals have been reared. Clean air and pastures can give meat with very low levels of environmental pollutants. Overall, the level of contamination in raw and unprocessed meat is below that of fish and seafood, although it is much higher than that of fruits, vegetables and legumes. The contamination depends heavily on the content of fat, a key tissue in the accumulation of carcinogenic POPs.[398]

All-cause mortality is higher for those who eat meat, particularly red or processed meat, on a daily basis, a review of large-scale studies involving more than 1.5 million people has found. This study found a 3.6-year increase in life expectancy for those on a vegetarian diet for more than 17 years, and that all-cause mortality is higher for those who eat meat.[399]

However, Regents Professor of meat sciences in the Department of Animal Science at Texas A & M university, Dr Stephen Smith, after studying marbling in cattle in the US, Australia, Japan, Korea and China over 30 years, has found that as cattle fatten to lay down marbling, the fat in the meat muscle itself, the fat

---

397 Ca Research Centre Hawaii 19/04/0

398 Carcinogenicity of consumption of red and processed meat: What about environmental contaminants? *Environmental Research*, 2016; 145: 109 DOI: 10.1016/j.envres.2015.11.031

399 *Journal of the American Osteopathic Association*, 2016; 116 (5): 296 DOI: 10.7556/jaoa.2016.059

replaces the saturated fat with oleic acid raising good HDL and lowering bad LDL.[400]

Processed meats: Include:

- *Bacon*
- *Sausage*
- *Hot dogs*
- *Ham*
- *Bologna*
- *Salami*
- *Luncheon meat*

Heavy consumption of processed meats like sausages and hot dogs increases the risk of pancreatic Ca by 67%

British love for sausages and bacon outweighs health concerns

The WHO said 50g of processed meat a day increased the chance of certain cancers by 18%, putting it in the highest risk ranking with alcohol, asbestos, arsenic and cigarettes. Despite this bacon for breakfast in 2015 increased by 14.3% on the year before, according to Kantar World panel data but total sales of processed meats fell by 2.1% over the year. Almost 6% more sausages were being eaten at breakfast compared with the previous year despite overall sales falling by 2.9%. Egg consumption at breakfast was up by 18% over the past two years while supermarket sales of ready-to-eat cereals – still the nation's most popular breakfast – fell by £52.6 million in a year.

---

400 Australian Wagyu Association conference May 2016

Meat – Red

Includes:

- *Bacon*
- *Sausage*
- *Hamburgers*
- *Cheeseburgers*
- *Meatloaf*
- *Casserole, stew, pot pie*
- *Minced beef*
- *Beef (steaks, roasts, sandwiches, stew)*
- *Liver, pork, luncheon meat*

Red meat & cancer:

- Long term high intake of red meat is associated with an increase in colorectal cancer
- Processed meat is even more risky
- Two very large studies (38,000 male health workers, 84,000 nurses) showed that just eating one extra serving a day increased the risk of death by 13% for red meat and 20% for processed meats[401]
- Another (450,000) found a 10% increased mortality risk with red meat and 40% for processed[402]
- Long-term intake of fish & poultry is inversely associated with risk of both proximal & distal colon Ca[403]
- Grass fed beef is up to 65% lower in saturated fat
- Ensure your meat is grass fed, has not been 'finished off' in a feed lot
- Reduce consumption to x 2 weekly
- Vegetable protein 30% better for protecting against CHD[404] But the animal protein in these studies is lot fed 'red meat' i.e. with > saturated fat
- Eat only grass-fed lean meat with normal yellow fat and not white fat, which means it, is grain lot fed.
- This minimises mad-cow disease, heart problems, cancer and even anti-biotic resistance.
- High intake *Men* = *3 oz / 160 g / day*

---

[401] Red meat consumption and mortality: results from two prospective cohort studies (9 Apr 2012)
[402] BMC Med(7 Mar 2013);11;63.doi:10.1186/1741-7015-11-6. Meat consumption and mortality-results from the European Prosective Investigation into Cancer and Nutrition.
[403] JAMA 2005;293:172-82. JNCI 2005 97;12:906-16
[404] Mayo Clinic A J Epidem Feb 2005

- Women = 2 oz (2oz = large hamburger)
- *Low intake* = *< 20 g/day*
- Consumption of resistant starch may help reduce colorectal cancer risk associated with a high red meat diet. Resistant starch includes bananas that are still slightly green, cooked and cooled potatoes [such as potato salad], whole grains, beans, chickpeas, and lentils[405]

Red meat and Kidney Failure

Red meat may increase the risk for kidney disease and eventually kidney failure and replacing some red meat in the diet with other types of protein - whether chicken, fish, eggs or vegetable sources - might dramatically reduce that risk. Participants who ate the largest amount of red meat had about a 40% greater risk of developing kidney failure compared with people consuming the lowest amounts of meat.[406]

The EPIC study

This is the European Prospective Investigation into Cancer and Nutrition, another prospective cohort study, so it isn't randomized. It was big, 448,568 people from ten different European countries. These people were followed for a median time of 12.7 years, and during follow-up 26,344 of them died. Red meat was found to pose no detectable risk, as judged by all-cause mortality. But this wasn't even mentioned in the headline conclusions.

Conclusions: Analysis supports a moderate positive association between *processed* meat consumption and mortality, in particular due to cardiovascular diseases, but also to cancer.

Red Meat and Heart Disease

- Red meat can harm the heart because of the way one of its nutrients is broken down by gut bacteria, by digesting the meat compound, L-carnitine, the bugs generate metabolites that promote hardening and narrowing of the arteries. Previously identified one of the danger metabolites was trimethylamine-N-oxide (TMAO). Now the latest research has uncovered a second, gamma-butyrobetaine, produced by the microbes at a rate 1000 times higher than TMAO formation. Both contribute to atherosclerosis, the build-up of hard fat

---

[405] Dietary Manipulation of Oncogenic MicroRNA Expression in Human Rectal Mucosa: A Randomized Trial. Cancer Prevention Research, 2014; 7 (8): 786 DOI: 10.1158/1940-6207.CAPR-14-0053

[406] J Am Soc Nephrol 2016.

and mineral deposits on the walls of arteries that can lead to heart attacks and strokes.

- People should be wary of taking supplements that contain gamma-butyrobetaine. The compound is used in fat-burning and body-building products.[407]
- Researchers assessed intake of red meat and other protein sources among nearly 90,000 premenopausal women. During 20 years of follow-up women in the top quintile of red meat consumption (1.6 servings/day) had a 22% increased breast cancer risk, compared with women in the bottom quintile (0.2 servings/day). Swapping out red meat for poultry or legumes one meal a day was associated with significant risk reductions.[408]

Research found a modest increased risk of total, cancer, and cardiovascular mortality among both men and women who were in the highest quintile of red meat intake (66-68 g/1000 kcal), compared with those in the lowest quintile (about 9 g/1000 kcal. Similar results were found when comparing the highest and lowest quintiles of processed meat intake. Conversely, white meat consumption had an inverse association with total and cancer mortality in both sexes (*P*0.001). However, there was a small increase in risk of cardiovascular mortality in men who ate more white meat.[409]

Reducing red meat consumption while eating more plant and dairy protein could lower the risk of developing and dying from coronary heart disease, according to two Harvard studies.

Middle-aged Americans who ate the most plant protein were 27% less likely to die of any cause and 29% less likely to die of coronary heart disease compared to those who ate the least amount of plant protein.

People who replaced one serving per day of red or processed meat with foods such as nuts, whole grains, or dairy were up to 47% less likely to have coronary heart disease than those who didn't replace a serving of meat.[410]

TMAO is produced in the gut when certain bacteria digest animal products, primarily red meat. A small Australian study found individuals consuming the

---

[407] Cell Metabolism 2014; 20(5):799–812

[408] BMJ

[409] Sinha R, et al "Meat intake and mortality" Arch Intern Med 2009; 169(6): 562-71.

[410] Presented at the American Heart Association's Epidemiology and Prevention and Lifestyle and Cardiometabolic Health Scientific Sessions 2020, March 3-6, 2020

popular Paleo diet had significantly higher levels of TMAO in their bloodstream compared to a cohort eating more traditional diets.

New research examined data from a large longitudinal study known as the Nurses' Health Study, which followed over 100,000 nurses for a decade. This data offers some of the first insights into the long-term relationship between TMAO blood levels and cardiovascular health.

Over 10 years a distinct link between increased TMAO levels and coronary heart disease (CHD) was detected. Women with the largest TMAO blood level increase across the 10-year period displayed a 63-percent higher risk of CHD.

Long-term increases in TMAO were associated with higher CHD risk, and repeated assessment of TMAO over 10 years improved the identification of people with a higher risk of CHD. Diet may modify the associations of ΔTMAO with CHD risk.[411]

Red Meat, Poultry Linked to Slightly Higher Risk for CVD Events, CV Death analysis supports that greater consumption of processed meat, unprocessed red meat, and, unexpectedly, poultry — but not fish — is significantly associated with a small increased risk of incident cardiovascular disease (CVD), which included cardiovascular deaths.

Moreover, the large six-cohort study finds that a higher intake of processed meat and unprocessed red meat, but not poultry or fish, significantly correlates with a small increase in the risk of all-cause mortality.

The analysis reports increased relative risks for these associations ranging from approximately 3% to 7% and increased absolute risks of less than 2% during a follow-up period that lasted up to 30 years.[412]

Microwaving

Microwave cooking is probably the best method for vegetables to preserve their vitamins, minerals and micronutrients some of which are broken down by heat or are leached out with boiling, but because microwave cooking is shorter it preserves more. Microwaving essentially heats up the water content in the food. Microwave vegetables using a small amount of water.

---

[411] Is Our Diet Turning Our Gut Microbiome Against Us?*
Journal of the American College of Cardiology, Volume 75, Issue 7, 25 Feb 2020, Pages 773-5
[412] JAMA Intern Med. Published online February 3, 2020. doi:10.1001/jamainternmed.2019.6969

Do not microwave take away or margarine containers or such, nor film-wrap, which then may liberate and leech Endocrine Disrupting Chemicals especially BPA.

Milk

Milk consumption is an interesting adaptation in the human race since the advent of agriculture and lactase persistence in adults—meaning you can digest lactose into adulthood—has evolved six separate times over the past 6000 years. Clearly there's an evolutionary population advantage to it. Milk consumption may help explain why modern humans are so much taller than other hominids.

People started avoiding dairy in part as reaction to the "China study," a large epidemiologic study that reported a correlation between dairy and cancer. But this is one of those cases where we take a correlational study and go crazy with it and its data have also been called into question.

Milk is reasonably nutrient dense and that is not pro- or anti-dairy.

(Other) "Milks"[413]

After cow's milk, which is still the most nutritious, soy milk comes out a clear winner.

Soy milk

The most balanced nutritional profile. Has been a substitute for cow's milk for 4 decades. Widely consumed for its health benefits linked to the anti-carcinogenic properties of phytonutrients present in the milk known as isoflavones.
Concerns, however, are the 'beany flavor' and the presence of anti-nutrients (substances that reduce nutrient intake and digestion).

Rice milk

Sweet taste and relatively little nutrition. Lactose free and can act as an alternative for patients with allergy issues caused by soybeans and almonds.

---

413 McGill University. "Nutritionally-speaking, soy milk is best plant-based milk: Closest to cow's milk in range of nutrients it offers." ScienceDaily. ScienceDaily, 29 January 2018. <www.sciencedaily.com/releases/2018/01/180129131311.htm>.

Concerns, apart from the high carbohydrate count, is that consumption of rice milk without proper care can result in malnutrition, especially in infants.

Coconut milk

No protein and few calories, but most of them from fat. Widely consumed in Asia and South America. Nutritional values are reduced if stored for over 2 months.

Almond milk

Complementary sources of food needed to provide essential nutrients. Almonds have a high content of monounsaturated fatty acids (MUFA) that are considered helpful in weight loss and weight management. MUFA also helps in reduction of low-density lipoprotein (bad cholesterol).

Cow's milk benefits & drawbacks

A wholesome, complete food, providing all major nutrients like fat, carbohydrates and proteins. Can help humans by providing a wide range of host-defence proteins because various beneficial anti-microbial effects are found in both human and bovine milks. (E.g., a study shows that in the case of infants, consumption of cow's milk has considerably reduced risk of fever and respiratory infections.)

Cow's milk allergy & lactose intolerance

One of the most common allergies among infants and children affecting 2.2-3.5% of children (a greater percentage than those who are affected by peanuts and tree nut allergies). As many as 35 % of these infants outgrow being allergic to milk by the age of 5-6, and this may increase to 80% by age 16.

Lactose intolerance, due to the absence or deficiency of the enzyme lactase in the digestive tract, affects somewhere between 15-75 % of all adults depending on race, food habits and gut health. Some studies have suggested that 80 % of people of African origin and 100 % of those of Asian and Indigenous American origin are lactose intolerant.

It is thought Lactase Persistence occurred in those races that migrated to the colder climates, evolved white skin and needed more calcium because of a lack of vitamin D (less sun). As such lactase persistence is 100% in the Irish and Finns.

Mushrooms

A University of Florida study shows increased immunity in people who ate a cooked shiitake mushroom every day for four weeks.[414]

Nitrites and nitrates in foods can be converted in the body to N-nitroso compounds, shown to cause stomach cancer in lab animals.

Nitrates

Nitrates, found in highest concentrations in leafy green vegetables such as spinach and beetroot, are converted in the body to nitric oxide which relaxes and widens blood vessels and affects how efficiently cells use oxygen. Manufacturers have liquified beetroots and concentrate the nitrate into beetroot juice "shots."

Nitrites

The less nitrite added to processed meat, the lower the levels of potentially carcinogenic nitrosamines formed in the products. Nitrite is used for preservation of processed meats (bacon, sausage, ham and deli meats). Cooking processed meat increases certain nitrosamines.[415]

Today better processing practices allow not using nitrites. Nitrates and Nitrites are naturally occurring in all fruits and vegetables. The Nitrites used in commercial meats is chemically processed. It isn't the NO2 and NO3 you have to worry about, but rather the high temperature of frying (as in stir fried vegetables) that create nitrosamines that are carcinogenic. One view is that you might as well give up green vegetables if you are worried about using celery as a curing agent for which it is often used).

Nooch

Nutritional Yeast has no health benefits. Any vitamin B12 is added.

Nutmeg

Nutmeg contains at least two psycho-active chemicals, myristicin and elemicin, which have serious side effects. Use sparingly as it is meant to be used.

---

414 Consuming Lentinula edodes (Shiitake) Mushrooms Daily Improves Human Immunity: A Randomized Dietary Intervention in Healthy Young Adults. Journal of the American College of Nutrition, 2015; 1 DOI: 10.1080/07315724.2014.950391

415Technical University of Denmark (DTU). "Less nitrite in meat products reduces levels of nitrosamines." ScienceDaily. ScienceDaily, 6 November 2014.

Nutrient Loss

Nutrients last longer than appearance in cut fruit. Loss after 6 days:

* Mango, strawberry, watermelon <5%
* Pineapple 10%
* Kiwi 12%
* Cantaloupe 25%

Nuts (also see Peanuts – below)

Nuts have become an essential ingredient of **Newtrition Micronutrient Foods:** A number of studies have linked nut consumption to reduced risk of cardiovascular disease (CVD), total cancer, All-Cause Mortality and mortality from respiratory disease, diabetes and infections.

Analysis of 29 published world studies of 819,000 participants, including more than 12,000 cases of coronary heart disease, 9,000 cases of stroke, 18,000 cases of cardiovascular disease and cancer, and more than 85,000 deaths.

Quantity	**Entity**	**% Reduction**
20g	CAD	29
	CVD	21
	Cancer	15
	Respiratory Disease	52
	Diabetes	39
	Infectious Disease	75
	Premature death 22[416]	

20g = Best amount = or 15 walnut or pecan halves or 2 doz almonds a day. Eating more did not donate any further benefit.

Nuts lower triglycerides and cholesterol in the blood.

Anti-Cancer Effects[417]

Nine types of tree nuts and peanuts commonly available in the United States were evaluated for total phenolic and flavonoid contents, antioxidant, and anti-proliferative activities. Walnuts had the highest total phenolic and flavonoid contents and also possessed the highest total antioxidant activity of vitamin C.

---

416 Nut consumption and risk of cardiovascular disease, total cancer, all-cause and cause-specific mortality: a systematic review and dose-response meta-analysis of prospective studies. BMC Medicine, 2016; 14 (1) DOI: 10.1186/s12916-016-0730-3

417 LWT - Food Science and Technology Volume 42, Issue 1, 2009, Pages 1–8

They were also tested for their anti-proliferative effect on human cancer cell proliferation, growing in petri dishes. If water was dripped on these cancer cells as a control, nothing happened, whereas:

- Walnuts, pecans, and peanuts caused a dramatic drop in cancer proliferation at just tiny doses.
- Almonds were twice as protective, halving cancer cell growth at only half the dose as pine nuts, cashews, and macadamias.
- Hazelnuts, pistachios and Brazil nuts had little anti-cancer effect

A 30-year-long large Harvard study found that:

People who ate a small handful (approximately 1 ounce or 28 grams) of nuts seven times per week or more were 20% less likely to die for any reason, compared to those who avoided nuts.

Eating nuts at least five times per week was associated with a 29% drop in mortality risk from heart disease, and an 11% drop in mortality risk from cancer. Even those who ate nuts only occasionally — less than once a week — had a 7% reduction in mortality.

Dutch researchers found that people who ate just 10 grams of nuts each day had a 23 percent lower risk of death from any cause. This study went on for 10 years and included more than 120,000 men and women between the ages of 55 and 69.

Five servings a week of any type of nuts, including peanuts, cuts the chances of death from prostate cancer by 34%[418]

Peanuts and tree nuts contain a number of healthful components including magnesium, fiber, L-arginine, antioxidants and unsaturated fatty acids such as α-linolenic acid.

Epidemiological studies have associated nut consumption with a protective effect against Pancreatic Cancer[419]

A study confirms a link between peanut and nut intake and lower mortality rates, but finds no protective effect for peanut butter. Men and women who eat at least 15 grams of nuts or peanuts per day have a lower risk of dying from several major causes of death than people who don't consume nuts or peanuts. A higher intake

---

[418] Harvard Medical School Study British Journal of Cancer June 2016.
[419] Diet and Pancreatic Cancer Prevention: Cancers (Basel). 2015 Dec; 7(4): 2309–2317. Published online 2015 Nov 23. doi: 10.3390/cancers7040892

was not associated with further reduction in mortality risk. The reduction in mortality was strongest for respiratory disease, neurodegenerative disease, and diabetes, followed by cancer and cardiovascular diseases. The effects are equal in men and women. This study was carried out within the Netherlands Cohort Study, which has been running since 1986 among over 120,000 Dutch 55-69 year old men and women[420]

Eating tree nuts appears to help reduce triglycerides and blood sugars.[421]In large cohort studies, nut consumption was associated inversely with 30-year mortality. These findings are consistent with a randomized trial in which a Mediterranean diet with substantial nut intake was associated with lower risk for adverse cardiovascular events[422]

Almonds:

May lower LDL [423] but results idiosyncratic and individual

Can reduce the risk of heart disease by keeping blood vessels healthy. Almonds contain a range of beneficial substances such as vitamin E, healthy fats, fiber which increases the sense of fullness, and flavonoids the combination of all these nutrients working together to create the overall health benefits rather than just one particular nutrient in isolation may explain the effect[424]

Almonds reduced LDL and central adiposity, important risk factors for cardiometabolic dysfunction, while maintaining HDL concentrations. Daily consumption of almonds (1.5oz.), substituted for a high-carb snack, may be a simple dietary strategy to prevent the onset of cardiometabolic diseases in healthy individuals[425] Greater intake was associated with lower biomarkers of inflammation that may help explain benefits[426]

---

[420] Relationship of tree nut, peanut, and peanut butter intake with total and cause-specific mortality: a cohort study and meta-analysis. International Journal of Epidemiology, June 2015

[421] Effect of Tree Nuts on Glycemic Control in Diabetes: A Systematic Review and Meta-Analysis of Randomized Controlled Dietary Trials. PLoS ONE, 2014; 9 (7): e103376 DOI: 10.1371/journal.pone.0103376

[422] NEJM JW Gen Med Mar 12 2013 Allan S. Brett, MD Reviewing Bao Y et al., N Engl J Med 2013 Nov 21; 369:2001

[423] JAMA 2003;290:502-10

[424] KAn almond-enriched diet increases plasma α-tocopherol and improves

[425] "Effects of Daily Almond Consumption on Cardiometabolic Risk and Abdominal Adiposity in Healthy Adults With Elevated LDL-Cholesterol: A Randomized Control Trial" JAMA 2015; DOI: 10.1161/JAHA.114.000993.

[426] Associations between nut consumption and inflammatory biomarkers. American Journal of Clinical Nutrition, 2016; DOI: 10.3945/ajcn.116.134205

Peanuts / Groundnuts

Previous studies have shown that individuals who consume peanuts more than two times a week have a lower risk of coronary heart disease. Another study showed that including them as a part of a high fat meal improved the post-meal triglyceride response and preserved endothelial function and maintained normal vascular function whereas the high fat-matched control meal impaired vascular function acutely. Peanut consumption was shown to be atheroprotective as a part of high fat meal.[427]

Walnuts;

Substituting walnuts for part of monosaturates in Mediterranean diet further lowered Total & LDL in hypercholesterolaemics[428]

- Eating walnuts may change gut bacteria in a way that suppresses colon cancer, in mice studies. Other studies have shown walnuts have promise warding off diseases connected to diet and lifestyle, including heart disease, diabetes and neurological disorders. But because the studies were done only in mice, more testing needs to be done in humans before walnuts can be unequivocally recommended as a cancer-prevention agent. However, the chief researcher isn't waiting, he says, "I try to eat walnuts every day."[429]
- Walnuts significantly improved diet quality, endothelial function, and cholesterol without negatively affecting blood pressure or glucose levels with about 56 g of walnuts per day - a handful. Walnuts are uniquely nutritious, so they may confer benefits that other nuts do not. Compared with most other nuts, walnuts have a higher content of polyunsaturated fatty acids. But walnuts also have a high-energy density, so there's the possibility that it contributes to a positive energy balance and to weight gain. The walnut diets neither significantly improved nor worsened body mass index, percent body fat, percent body water, or visceral fat.[430]
- Women who ate a dozen walnut halves twice a week reduced their risk of becoming frail or needing care when elderly.[431]
- Previous research has linked walnuts to a lower risk of heart attacks and diabetes and boosting sex drive and cutting levels of IGF-1 implicated in

---

427 Federation of American Societies for Experimental Biology (FASEB). "Adding peanuts to a meal benefits vascular health." ScienceDaily. ScienceDaily, 30 March 2015. <www.sciencedaily.com/releases/2015/03/150330112230.htm>.

428 Ann Int Med 2000;132:538-46

429 Effects of walnut consumption on colon carcinogenesis and microbial community structure. Cancer Prevention Research, 2016; DOI: 10.1158/1940-6207.CAPR-16-0026

430 BMJ Open Diab Res Care 2015;3:e000115 doi:10.1136/bmjdrc-2015-000115

431 Nurses' Health Study. Journal of Nutrition 2016

breast and prostate cancer and may reduce the risk of Alzheimer's Disease, delay its onset and slow its progression.

- Walnuts contain twice the anti-oxidants than any other commonly eaten nut.

Oats

Oats contain large amounts of the soluble fiber beta-glucan. Considerable evidence suggests that beta-glucan can lower high levels of cholesterol in the blood and has anticoagulant properties, making it heart-friendly. A 2007 US study found eating 6g of oat beta-glucan per day for six weeks was enough to cause a significant reduction in total and LDL (bad) cholesterol, as well as improving bowel health.

Replacing one weekly serving of eggs or white bread with oatmeal was specifically associated with a 5% lower risk of ischemic stroke from blockages in small arteries, the researchers note.[432]

Oils

Olive Oil

- Olive Oil is made up of several fatty acids. The main one (80%) is Oleic acid which is a monosaturate, then palmitic (saturated) then linoleic acid (polyuunsaturated along with some 30 phenol compounds and hundreds of other compounds.
- There are different grades from extra-virgin, virgin, light to just olive oil. Only use Extra-virgin which has more beneficial ingredients and completely unprocessed. Thereafter heat and chemicals are used which progressively denude the pristine olive oil of its beneficial compounds.
- **Caution:** In 1997 and 1998 Olive oil was the most adulterated agricultural product in the European Union and this practice is especially common in Italy where it is often incorrectly branded. *'Profits are comparable to cocaine trafficking with none of the risks'* with even big firms involved. There is little reassurance that this has changed with 87,000 adulterated litres labelled EVOO but mostly soybean oil seized in New Jersey in 2006[433]
- 2015: In November seven of Italy's best-known olive oil companies were investigated for allegedly passing off inferior oil as extra virgin to sell at a third more

432 Stroke, online December 12, 2019.
433 New Yorker Aug 13, 2007

- 2016: It would seem the Italians are incorrigible: An undercover operation code named Mamma Mia seized $20 million of olive oil in a scam in which Spanish and Greek oil was passed off as Extra-Virgin Italian Olive Oil[434]
- Olive oil is good for your heart, but it was unclear which components were the helpful ones – the monosaturated fat Oleic Acid or the antioxidant polyphenol content, or both. A trial has confirmed that using Extra Virgin Olive Oil, which is unprocessed, is better due to its higher concentration of polyphenols which boost HDL compared with refined (processed) Olive Oil. Olive oil contains 30 to 40 anti-oxidants which protect it against frying so it can be used 10 times (whereas PUFAs – vegetable oils - should only be used only once)[435] In the most recent and definitive test I can find (Dr McCubbin Glasgow) only Olive oil (any type not just Extra Virgin) at 20 ml a day (on salads etc or raw) reduced heart disease whereas Safflower or Canola/Rape seed did not.
- Extra virgin - cold pressed pulp only
- Does not apparently lower total cholesterol as much as PUFA, which reduce good HDL.
- EVOO lowers LDL & raises HDL
- Contains 30 to 40 anti-oxidants which protect it against frying so it can be used x 10 times (whereas PUFAs should only be used x 1)
- In vitro tests demonstrated some cancer inhibiting effects[436]
- OO is more than a monosaturated fat. Its phenolic content can also provide benefits for plasma lipid levels and oxidative damage[437]
- Benefits of unsaturates
- Less gallstone disease (men)[438]
- Oil on salads dissolve the fat-soluble vitamins and micronutrients to allow absorption into the body e.g. lycopene, alpha and beta carotene

Update 2020[439]

Greater olive oil consumption was tied to lower cardiovascular disease (CVD) risk but substituting plant-based oils for animal fats in general could also be helpful for most people.

---

434 Nick Squires, London Daily Telegraph,4th February 2016
435 Ann Int Med 2006;145:333-41
436 Int J Ca 20 Oct 2005
437 Ann Int Med 2006;145:333-341
438 Ann Int Med 2004;141:514-22
439 Journal of the AmericanCollege of Cardiology March 31, 2020 | Vol. 75 No. 12
439 J Am Coll Cardiol. Published online March 5, 2020.

Comparing those who ate the most vs the least olive oil (people who ate at least 1/2 tablespoon of olive oil per day vs those who consumed olive oil less than once per month), it was found that the former group had the following improvements in outcomes over 24 years of follow-up:

- Lower risk of CVD (fatal and non-fatal strokes and myocardial infarctions): HR 0.86 (95% CI 0.79-0.94)
- Lower risk of coronary heart disease (CHD): HR 0.82 (95% CI 0.73-0.91)
- No significant reduction in total or ischemic stroke risk

Previous research studied EVOO in unnatural settings, like in a laboratory or in a microwave but it can also be used to cook at high temperatures. for deep-frying, pan-frying / sautéing, roasting, or stir-frying.

High heat can break down the polyphenols, thereby diminishing the beneficial health effects of EVOO. After sautéing at 120°C, the number of polyphenols decreased by 40%. At 170°C, the number of polyphenols decreased by 75%. Time did not seem to play a significant factor in overall polyphenol degradation.

But even though EVOO broke down at high heat, it still maintained enough polyphenols and antioxidants to be considered healthy by the European Union (EU). The EU considers an oil to be healthy if it can prevent the formation of bad cholesterol.[440]

Olive oil in the Mediterranean diet may be the key to improving lifespan and mitigating aging-related diseases. Consuming olive oil is not enough to elicit all of the health benefits. Studies suggest that when coupled with fasting, limiting caloric intake and exercising, the effects of consuming olive oil will be most pronounced. The way it works is it first has to get stored in microscopic lipid droplets, which is how our cells store fat. And then, when the fat is broken down during exercising or fasting the benefits are released.[441]

---

[440] Lozano-Castellón J, Vallverdú-Queralt A, Rinaldi de Alvarenga J, Illán M, Torrado-Prat X, Lamuela-Raventós R. Domestic Sautéing with EVOO: Change in the Phenolic Profile. Antioxidants. 2020;9(1):77. doi:10.3390/antiox9010077
Extra olive virgin oil keeps healthy properties when used for cooking. EurekAlert!. https://www.eurekalert.org/pub_releases/2020-02/uob-eov022720.php. Published 2020. Accessed March 7, 2020.

[441] Molecular Cell, Minnesota Medical School,2020

Soya Bean Oil

Soyabean Oil is ubiquitous in the American Diet as a common ingredient in vegetable oil blends and processed foods. It has been said that if you eat in an American restaurant you will be eating soya bean oil, and which is most likely genetically modified. It contains high amounts of linoleic acid, which seems to provoke fat deposition. It is also used in cattle feed.

Soybean oil caused more obesity and diabetes than fructose in mice. In the U.S. the consumption of soybean oil has increased greatly in the last four decades. As a result of these studies, nutritional guidelines were created that encouraged people to reduce their intake of saturated fats, commonly found in meat and dairy products, and increase their intake of polyunsaturated fatty acids found in plant oils, such as soybean oil. Implementation of those guidelines, as well as an increase in the cultivation of soybeans in the United States, has led to a remarkable increase in the consumption of soybean oil, which is found in processed foods, margarines, salad dressings and snack foods. Soybean oil now accounts for 60% of edible oil consumed in the United States. That increase in soybean oil consumption mirrors the rise in obesity rates in the United States in recent decades. But mice on a soybean oil-enriched diet gained almost 25% more weight than the mice on the coconut oil diet and 9% more weight than those on the fructose-enriched diet. And the mice on the fructose-enriched diet gained 12 percent more weight than those on a coconut oil rich diet

Coconut Oil

Is high in saturated fats but low in linoleic acid. There is a current vogue to sing its 'health benefits' but it is 86.5 g/100g of saturated fat and clinical cardiologists do not recommend it.

Coconut Oil is the latest fad. The enthusiasm for the claims makes it difficult to discern the facts. A few years ago, the Samoans were the fattest people on earth, and this was attributed to their high ingestion of coconut oil.

The claims do not match the facts: The claim that it helps weight loss is not supported by any trials. One small trial of 40 women found it was no better than soybean oil.

Eight clinical trials and 13 observational studies of coconut oil found coconut oil raises LDL levels more than other vegetable oils, but not as much as butter does. There is also no evidence that it helps prevent Alzheimer's Disease.

There is interest in the mid-chain acids but there are no definitive results to date. Time will tell.

Update 2020

Coconut Oil Bad

Coconut oil should not be used as a regular cooking oil. Coconut oil may be viewed as one of the most deleterious cooking oils that increases risk for cardiovascular disease. Even in comparison with palm oil, another tropical oil with high saturated fat content, coconut oil increased LDL cholesterol. Replacing coconut oil with nontropical unsaturated vegetable oils, especially those rich in polyunsaturated fat, will have a health benefit.

Advertisements give the impression that purportedly beneficial constituents other than saturated fat compensate for its adverse effects on LDL cholesterol. 72% of Americans viewed coconut oil as a healthy food.

Yet, controlled trials in humans are not available that support beneficial actions of the components of coconut oil on cardiovascular disease risk factors or mechanisms.

Coconut oil contributes to cardiovascular disease because its saturated fat content increases plasma low-density lipoprotein

A systematic review, published in 2016, identified 7 trials that tested the effect of coconut oil on LDL cholesterol. In these trials, coconut oil was compared with oils that had a high content of unsaturated fats.[3] Significant detrimental effects were found in 6 of them. The latest meta-analysis found that coconut oil significantly increased plasma LDL cholesterol and high-density lipoprotein (HDL) cholesterol, and had no effect on triglycerides, body weight, body fat, and markers of glycemia and inflammation in comparison with nontropical vegetable oils.

The Truth About Coconut Oil and Cardiovascular Risk[442]

Coconut oil is associated with higher cholesterol levels compared with other vegetable oils in a meta-analysis.

---

[442] Neelakantan N et al. Circulation 2020 Jan 13

Evidence is cracking open some of the health claims made about coconut oil. Combining the findings from 16 published studies, it was found that use of coconut oil was associated with increases in low-density lipoprotein (LDL) and total cholesterol levels, potentially placing people at higher risk for cardiovascular disease.

Compared to nontropical olive, soybean, or canola oil, high consumption of coconut oil substantially increased LDL cholesterol. Consuming 3 to 4 tablespoons of coconut oil daily was associated with an estimated 10-mg/dL increase — about a 9% jump — in LDL levels.

Cooking Oil Choices

Whatever you do make sure they are cold-pressed. Many are "refined" which makes them more heat stable but potentially damaging for health.

Heating oils produces Aldehyde implicated in causing Cancer.

Corn and Sunflower produce high levels while Olive Oil has low and Butter / Lard produce the least aldehyde. Overall mono - saturates best - Olive Oil.

Olive oil withstands the heat of the fryer or pan better than several seed oils to yield more healthful food. The researchers deep- and pan-fried raw potato pieces in four different refined oils -- olive, corn, soybean and sunflower -- and reused the oil 10 times. They found that olive oil was the most stable oil for deep-frying at 320 and 374 degrees Fahrenheit, while sunflower oil degraded the fastest when pan-fried at 356 degrees. They conclude that for frying foods, olive oil maintains quality and nutrition better than seed oils[443]

Researchers have studied the changes that take place in fish lipids and in the oil during frying processes, and have concluded that using extra virgin olive oil is the best choice[444]

---

[443] Journal of Agricultural and Food Chemistry, 2014; 62 (42): 10357 DOI: 10.1021/jf503146f
[444] The influence of frying technique, cooking oil and fish species on the changes occurring in fish lipids and oil during shallow-frying, studied by 1H NMR. Food Research International, 2016; 84: 150 DOI: 10.1016/j.foodres.2016.03.033

Extra virgin olive oil – most recommended

Ideal for salad dressings, eating with bread and drizzling over dishes. high quality EVOO can reach smoke points at temperatures of between 200-215 degrees, making it a healthy option for most types of cooking, including oven baking.

Olive Oil lowered the risk of cardiovascular disease whereas in another Canola / Rape Oil, considered a viable alternative, did not.[445]

Also see the PREDIMED Study

A large 2020 study found that higher olive oil intake was associated with a lower risk of CHD and total CVD in two large prospective cohorts of US men and women. The substitution of margarine, butter, mayonnaise, and dairy fat with olive oil could lead to lower risk of CHD and CVD.[446]

Analysis of data from the long running Nurses' Health and Health Professionals Follow Up studies in the US finds that, after making adjustments for other dietary and lifestyle factors, risk of coronary heart disease in people with higher intakes of olive oil was 20% lower than in people who didn't consume it (JACC doi:10.1016/j.jacc.2020.02.036).

Avocado oil

Unrefined extra virgin avocado oil due to its unusually high smoke point (up to 250 degrees), makes it ideal for high-temperature grilling, pan-roasting, frying vegetables such as brussels sprouts and drizzling over home-made pizzas. But it costs about four times the price of EVOO.

Macadamia oil

Known for its mildly nutty to gloriously buttery flavor, High in monounsaturates (about 80 per cent), it's more stable than many other polyunsaturated fats and has a high smoke point of between 210C and 234 degrees. Best for Pan-frying fish, veal and salad dressings.

Sunflower oil

Best use deep-frying dishes such as tempura and chips.

---

[445] Impact of a 6-wk olive oil supplementation in healthy adults on urinary proteomic biomarkers of coronary artery disease, chronic kidney disease, and diabetes (types 1 and 2): a randomized, parallel, controlled, double-blind study. First published November 19, 2014, doi: 10.3945/ ajcn.114.094219 Am J Clin Nutr ajcn.094219

[446] J Am Coll Cardiol 2020 Apr 21

Sesame oil

Typically, it's equally high in monounsaturated and polyunsaturated fats

Given its strong flavor, it's best used as an additive, particularly to Asian dishes such as stir-fries. It's also an excellent addition to marinades and sauces.

Peanut oil

Similar to macadamia oil with predominantly monounsaturated fats, this fragrant oil has a relatively high smoke point at about 230 degrees and is neutral in flavor. Best for Asian cooking, especially stir-fries.

Canola oil

High in monounsaturates, low in saturated fat and has plenty of omega-3s.

Best use? a good all-purpose cooking oil. It does become unstable after heating, so never reuse.

Flaxseed oil

This is not a cooking oil. Also known as linseed oil, with a fatty acid profile higher in polyunsaturated fats it's packed with the highest amount of plant-based omega-3s of all these oils but can develop "off" flavors, so buy in small quantities and store in a cool, dark place, such as the fridge. Tends to be a dietary supplement oil.

Soya Bean Oil

See above

Rice bran oil

Extracted from the bran and the germ, this neutral-tasting oil has a low viscosity and a relatively high smoke point (around 260 degrees) making it ideal for roasting and cooking subtle ingredients, such as seafood. It has an unusual mix of fatty acids - roughly half-and-half monounsaturated and polyunsaturated - and some good plant sterols but it's industrially processed, not mechanically extracted (or "cold-pressed") Don't be confused by packaging con that talks about being "extra cold-filtered" - it's got nothing to do with being cold pressed.

Best use? High-heat stir-frying or wok-frying.

Coconut oil

Very high in saturated fats at more than 90 per cent but one thing is clear - stay away from hydrogenated coconut oil, which undergoes a process of extreme heat and pressure and the introduction of hydrogen in the presence of a catalyst (usually a metal) to make the oil more stable and last longer. The process makes the oil more viscous, as it will your blood, making your heart work harder. Virgin or extra virgin coconut oil, on the other hand, is a popular vegan replacement for butter in cooking. Best use? Its natural sweetness makes it ideal for baking and certain sauteed dishes. A low smoke point (about 175 degrees) makes it not great for high-temperature cooking, such as deep-frying.

Cottonseed oil

This highly stable but refined oil was often used in chip shops for deep frying (you can use it multiple times before the smoke point is compromised) and said to produce a crisp, attractive chip. A mix of predominantly saturated and polyunsaturated fats cottonseed will never get the Heart Foundation tick (20 per cent is the cut-off).

"Vegetable" oil

This is a stable, refined, plant-based oil but the difficulty is you never really know what it's made of. It could well be 99 per cent canola - it could also be blended with soybean or sunflower. Usually the cheapest option at the supermarket; check the nutrition label on the back to determine specific levels of saturated, monounsaturated and polyunsaturated fats. Best use? Deep-frying and high-temperature cooking. If the saturated fat content is above 20 grams per 100 grams, consider something else. In fact, do yourself a favour and get EVOO.

Palm Oil

Not only is it bad for you but it has led to deforestation in Indonesia, Borneo and Papua-New Guinea with the decimation of Orangutans, 100,000 in Borneo alone in the last 18 years. It started in the 1960s as forests were logged for timber, but now it's palm oil.

Global demand for palm oil has increased more than six-fold since 1990. It's in half of all packaged products on supermarket shelves and impossible to avoid completely (unless you east fresh foods). In Europe palm oil in food can no longer be described simply as vegetable oil and must be clearly labelled, but there is no such law for products such as soap, shampoo and other cosmetics.

The Roundtable on Sustainable Palm Oil (RSPO) – the industry body charged with ensuring registered companies trade only in oil that has not come from deforestation – is failing spectacularly with Greenpeace exposing massive rainforest destruction in Papua allegedly caused by palm oil companies that are subsidiaries of a current RSPO member. Buying from them were big multinationals including Unilever, Nestlé, Pepsico and Mars. It would seem no company can claim the palm oil it uses is 100% "sustainable".

Oranges

Just one serve or 50g a day increased plasma ascorbic acid and reduced mortality risk by 20%[447]

Men who drank orange juice every day were 47 percent less likely to develop poor thinking skills than the men who drank less than one serving per month. This association was mainly observed for regular consumption of orange juice among the oldest men.[448]

Researchers studying a molecule found in sweet oranges and tangerines called nobiletin, have shown it to drastically reduce obesity and reverse its negative side-effects. But why it works remains a mystery.

Note: Pure fruit juice e.g. orange, have a high natural sugar content and, remarkably and disappointingly, have been found to be associated with a higher rate of cancers. Eat the whole fruit as the fiber drags this sugar through.

Oysters

Oysters and other mollusks are very high in nutrients, including B12, which is commonly deficient in people consuming vegan or vegetarian diets and is necessary for myelin and neurotransmitter function.

Pasta

When cooked pasta is chilled its composition changes to form resistant fiber which is far better for us. When it is reheated, it is better still.

---

[447] Lancet 2001; 357; 657

[448] American Academy of Neurology. Changzheng Yuan, ScD, of Harvard T.H. Chan School of Public Health in Boston

Peppermint Tea

Improved long-term memory, working memory and alertness[449]

Peppers

Peppers, a nicotine-containing vegetable in the same family as tobacco, were associated with lower relative risk of Parkinson's disease. The effect was mainly noticeable among people who had never smoked, and other vegetables had no association with the neurological disease[450]

Phytoestrogens

Do not help prevent hot flushes

Phytoplankton

Marine phytoplankton are marine algae and often touted as the next important superfood. Claims are that they contain every nutrient that humans need but there are no clinical trials supporting alleged benefits.

Pizza

Perhaps the world's most popular meal but which is the main source in the USA of Saturated fats (14%) and one third of their total calories. One third of young Americans eat it daily. The cheese is usually non-beneficial processed.

Polyphenols

Dietary studies have shown that people who eat the largest amounts of fruit and vegetables have a reduced risk of developing chronic conditions, such as heart disease and cancer. The Institute of Food Research has found evidence for a mechanism by which certain food compounds could help protect health. Polyphenols (epigallocatechin gallate (EGCG) from green tea and procyanidin

---

[449] British Psychological Society annual conference Nottingham 2016:Northumbria University
[450] "Nicotine from edible solanaceae and risk of Parkinson disease" Ann Neurol 2013.

from apples) block a signaling molecule called VEGF, which in the body can trigger atherosclerosis and is a target for some anti-cancer drugs.[451]

Polyphenols in red wine and green tea inhibit cancer growth. There is a signalling pathway that plays a role in not only prostate but also colon, breast and gastric cancers, which these polyphenols disrupt and may lead to future drug development.[452]

More varied and higher phenolic content is found in the skin of the pear than in its flesh or pulp. The study showed that Starkrimson peel had the highest total phenolic content, and that peel extracts had significantly higher total phenolic content than pulp. The pulp extracts of the Bartlett cultivar had higher total phenolics when compared with Starkrimson.[453]

Pomegranates

See 'Dates'. The combination of fresh pomegranate juice and dates with pips reduced cholesterol in experiments.

Pomegranates are rich in micronutrients with potential antioxidant and anti-inflammatory effects but there's little good evidence that the level of nutrients found in the fruit translates into true gains for human health. Among the active ingredients in pomegranates are polyphenols such as ellagitannins, which inhibit the activation of inflammatory pathways, and anthocyanins, which give the fruit its deep red color and also have antioxidant activity. Diets high in these compounds have been linked to a reduced risk for chronic diseases, including heart disease and some cancers. One 2008 study found that pomegranate juice had greater antioxidant activity and polyphenol content than red wine, Concord grape juice, blueberry juice, cranberry juice, acai juice, apple juice and orange juice. Another study found that pomegranate juice and seed extracts had two to three times the antioxidant capacity of either red wine or green tea. Small human trials have found that drinking pomegranate juice on a daily basis may aid cardiovascular health, blood pressure and levels of "good" HDL cholesterol.

---

451 inhibition of VEGFR-2 activation by tight binding of green tea epigallocatechin gallate and apple procyanidins to VEGF: Relevance to angiogenesis. *Molecular Nutrition & Food Research*, 2015; 59 (3): 401 DOI: 10.1002/mnfr.201400478

452 Federation of American Societies for Experimental Biology Science Daily (June 11, 2010)

453 Dietary functional benefits of Bartlett and Starkrimson pears for potential management of hyperglycemia, hypertension and ulcer bacteria Helicobacter pylori while supporting beneficial probiotic bacterial response. *Food Research International*, 2015; 69: 80 DOI: 10.1016/j.foodres.2014.12.014

There is research showing pomegranate extract inhibits the growth of prostate, breast, colon and lung cancer cells in lab cultures. Human trials are now looking at whether pomegranate juice can help slow prostate cancer progression.

Pomegranates may combat aging. They contain ellagitannins as do berries, nuts and acorns which prolong worm life by 42% and mice endurance by 42%. Trials on humans are now in progress but only half of humans can metabolize it into the active compound urolithin A.[454]

A completely natural molecule in pomegranates, Urolithin A, is transformed by microbes in the gut and enables muscle cells to protect themselves against one of the major causes of aging. It re-establishes the cell's ability to recycle the components of the defective mitochondria, otherwise known as mitophagy.[455]

Potassium

Eat more (double to 4.7g). Lowers BP.

High Potassium Foods mg per 100g.

Potassium lowers our Blood Pressure, but it is extracted from foods during processing. The current daily value for potassium is 3.5 grams. The following foods are the best source:

Potassium		**mg/100g**
Dried apricots	=	1162
Salmon	=	628
White Beans	=	561
Dk Leafy Veg Spinach	=	558
Sweet potato	=	542
Baked Potato skin on	=	535
Baked squash	=	437
Avocado	=	485
Mushrooms white	=	396
Bananas	=	358
Yoghurt plain skim	=	255

[454] Nature July 2016

[455] induces mitophagy and prolongs lifespan in C. elegans and increases muscle function in rodents. Nature Medicine, July 2016 DOI: 10.1038/nm.4132

Potatoes

Potatoes Tied to Higher Risk of Type 2 Diabetes; French Fries Worst

Potatoes may increase the risk of type 2 diabetes and replacing them with whole grains may lower this risk. Potatoes contain a large amount of starch and a relatively small amount of fiber, vitamins, minerals, and polyphenols and this lower quality and quantity of carbohydrate is associated with a higher risk of type 2 diabetes. Moreover, when potatoes are served hot their starch becomes more easily digestible and raises blood glucose levels more quickly.

The results showed that participants with a higher consumption of potatoes (baked, boiled, mashed, or French fries) had a significantly higher risk of type 2 diabetes with a 7% increased risk of type 2 diabetes, while those who ate seven or more servings per week had 33% increased risk compared with those who ate less than one serving per week.

The study combined data from three US cohort studies on 70,773 women from the Nurses' Health Study (1984–2010), 87,739 women from the Nurses' Health Study II (1991–2011), and 40,669 men from the Health Professionals Follow-Up Study (1986–2010). Participants who ate French fries had a higher risk of type 2 diabetes.

Participants who increased their potato consumption over time — especially French fries — had an increased risk of diabetes. For every three-servings/week increase, they had a 4% increased risk of diabetes compared with those who ate the same amounts of potatoes over time.

Estimates showed that replacing three servings per week of potatoes (regardless of type) with whole grains would decrease the risk of type 2 diabetes by 12%.

The US national food guide consider potatoes to be a "healthful vegetable." In contrast, the UK national food guid*e* lists potatoes as a cereal[456]

Potatoes and Blood Pressure

Four or more servings a week of baked, boiled, or mashed potatoes was associated with an increased risk of hypertension compared with less than one serving a month in women, but not in men. Higher consumption of French fries was also associated with an increased risk of hypertension in both women and men.

---

[456] *Diabetes Care.* Published online December 17, 2015.

However, consumption of potato chips (crisps) was associated with no increased risk.

Replacing one serving a day of boiled, baked, or mashed potatoes with one serving of a non-starchy vegetable is associated with a decreased risk of hypertension[457]

Prebiotics and Probiotics

Prebiotics are defined as: Non-digestible food ingredients that are marketed to beneficially affect the host by selectively stimulating the growth and/or activity of one or a limited number of bacteria in the colon, and thus improve host health.

There is a huge marketing push because these are not controlled. Probiotics, for instance, have been associated with a wide range of health complications, including "gastrointestinal events such as diarrhea, constipation, nausea, or abdominal pain; respiratory infection, inappropriate immune response in susceptible individuals, deleterious metabolic activities and gene transfer.

Not Good enough[458]

The vast majority of research studies on probiotics, prebiotics, and other interventions to modify the human microbiome report virtually no specific data on possible harms, according to a meta-analysis in the *Annals of Internal Medicine*. Even among studies that reported harms, most were incomplete or otherwise inadequate in doing so, "raising doubts about the confidence we can have in conclusions about the safety of these interventions". In fact, just 2% of the trials adequately reported all the parameters recommended in guidelines for reporting harms.

Doctors may suggest patients try probiotics for a wide range of concerns, particularly as they are available over the counter, but we don't actually have data about whether manipulating the microbiome is a reasonable strategy or not. We have this association, but if we fix the microbiome, do we really fix the condition?

Probiotics Help Reduce BMI

Taking probiotics reduced BMI and body weight by a small amount with the greatest reduction in BMI occurring in overweight adults. Interestingly, ingesting

---

[457] Potato intake and incidence of hypertension: results from three prospective US cohort studies. *BMJ*, 2016; i2351 DOI: 10.1136/bmj.i2351

[458] *Ann Intern Med*. Published online July 16, 2018.

more than one type of probiotic and taking probiotics for 8 weeks or more resulted in increased weight loss.[459]

Probiotic Drinks

Most Probiotic drinks are a waste of money if you are healthy. In 2015 the public spent $33 billion buying them.[460] Kefir, a fermented milk, and Kombuchar, a fermented tea, do seem to add benefit to the gut microbiome.

Oats are cheaper and better.

I would wait for better trials and studies.

Processed Meats and Cancer

Processed Meats: are those that have been salted, cured, smoked, fermented or undergone other processes to preserve them or enhance their flavor.

Some examples are ham, bacon, salami, sausages, hot dogs, frankfurters, corned beef, deli meats and beef jerky.

Processed meats have been clearly linked to colorectal cancer and other negative health outcomes and it is felt the causes are

Nitrates – used as a preservative

Salt - also used as a preservative and flavor enhancer

Cooking method – production of char and hetrocyclic amines

In 2015 the WHO officially classified processed meat as a carcinogen.

Eating just 50 grams of processed meat a day—equivalent to just one hot dog—would raise the risk of getting colorectal cancer by 18 percent over a lifetime. Eating larger quantities raises cancer risk even more. A study published in September 2018 in the journal *Breast Cancer Research and Treatment* combined previous research with new data from over 262,000 British women and found that postmenopausal women who ate the most processed meat (an average of more than nine grams a day or the equivalent of about 1 and a quarter hot dogs a week)

---

459. Effect of probiotics on body weight and body-mass index: a systematic review and meta-analysis of randomized, controlled trials. *International Journal of Food Sciences and Nutrition*, 2016; 67 (5): 571 DOI: 10.1080/09637486.2016.1181156

460 Genome Medicine 2016

had a 21 percent higher risk of breast cancer than those who ate no processed meat.

As with all nutrition studies they are observational finding an *association* between consumption of processed meats and diseases but there is now convincing evidence that a diet habitually high in processed meats does increase the risk of developing colorectal cancer.

Whereas it remains unclear whether processed meat actually contributes to the risk of such as hypertension, heart disease, and chronic obstructive lung disease which is nevertheless suspected.

1. Nitrates: Sodium nitrite and sodium nitrate (which naturally converts to sodium nitrite) are used as preservatives in processed meats because they prevent bacterial growth. Nitrates are also found naturally in a number of foods, including celery, beets, rocket/arugula and other vegetables.

Today it is common to find the statement ‘no added nitrates’ on processed meat products.

Celery Juice: No Added Nitrates

In most instances, products so labelled are manufactured using celery juice or other natural sources of nitrates. But there is no evidence that the nitrates in celery juice act any differently in the body than nitrates added as food-grade chemicals. In fact, unlike food-grade sodium nitrate or nitrite, there is no federal regulation that limits how much celery juice can be added to a processed meat, so it is feasible to actually be consuming more nitrates with a processed meat that says, ‘no added nitrates’. When consumed in vegetables, nitrates are safe, and may even have protective health effects such as improving blood flow. But in meats, nitrites can react during processing, cooking, and storage to form compounds called nitrosamines, which are classified as carcinogens.

Sodium: According to the American Cancer Society, there is good evidence that consuming large quantities of foods preserved by salting is associated with increased risk of stomach, nasopharyngeal, and throat cancers. Deli meats (like pre-packaged turkey and ham slices) are one of the main sources of sodium in the American diet. In fact, six thin slices (two ounces) of deli meat can contain as much as half of the daily recommended sodium intake. Even if all of this sodium does not raise cancer risk, it raises the risk of high blood pressure and heart disease in most people and should be limited none-the-less.

Cooking: There is not enough data to prove that the way meat is cooked affects cancer risk, but it is known that cooking meat (processed or unprocessed) at high temperatures or in direct contact with heat (such as grilling or pan-frying) produces more carcinogenic chemicals than lower-heat, indirect methods like roasting or stewing.

I have pointed out how we all have bias and one of mine is prosciutto which is ham salt and air-cured Prosciutto is a raw, cured ham which is over 2000 years old. Records show that this traditional meat's origin lay in the Italian city of Parma before 100 B.C.

Salt has been used as a preservative for millennia and I find it hard to reconcile that prosciutto has been a source of increased rates of cancer. Nevertheless, I maintain a "watching brief".

One ounce of the average store-bought prosciutto has between 570 and 660 milligrams of sodium. That's between 25 and 29 percent of your daily 2,300-milligram sodium limit.

Serrano Ham (Jamón Serrano) made from the "Landrace" breed of white pig and the much more expensive and entirely different Jamón ibérico from acorn fattened black pigs produce the Spanish rival to prosciutto.

There seems an inference that these Spanish hams may or may not use nitrates but I seem to remember nitrates were introduced following a food-poisoning outbreak in the early 1900s.

Traditionally made prosciutto has no added preservatives and the only ingredients are pork and salt. That said, some cheaper prosciutto products do use nitrates as preservatives. If you want to avoid them, just look for prosciutto which has a PDO certification.

Sodium nitrate is a salt that is often added to jerky, bacon and luncheon meats. Sodium nitrite, on the other hand, is a salt and antioxidant that is commonly used to cure ham and bacon. Both chemicals act as food preservatives and add a red or pink color to processed meats, among other uses.

It is in many foods including bacon, beef jerky, ham, hot dogs, lunch meat, salami, and smoked fish. It creates a distinct flavor, controls lipid oxidation, and acts as an antimicrobial. Sodium nitrate can be found in plants and unregulated drinking water.

Serrano shoulder ham is produced using the most traditional process of salting and curing. It's all natural, made with Mediterranean sea-salt, and contains absolutely NO nitrates, nitrites, antibiotics, preservatives, artificial coloring, glucose or lactose.

The manufacturing process remains similar to Iberico Ham, the main difference lies in the type of pork used. 1. Salting. Traditional production method uses only salt without adding nitrates, although often purified sea salt is mixed with common rock salt.

Manufacturing process for Spanish Hams

1. Salting. Traditional production method uses only salt without adding nitrates, although often purified sea salt is mixed with common rock salt. Sea salt contains many minerals and can create different reactions with meat proteins and fats. The salt is added at 4-7% in relation to the weight of a ham. Using less salt may not prevent the growth of spoilage and pathogenic bacteria and will lower the final quality of the ham. Such an amount of salt immediately draws out some moisture from meat cells and this lowers the water activity of the meat. As a result, a safety hurdle is created, and the meat becomes bacteriologically stable in time. In order to prevent conditions for bacteria to grow, the salting process takes place at 40° F (4° C), 85-95% humidity. A rule of thumb calls for 2 days for each 1 kg of meat, for example the 8 kg (17.6 lbs) ham will be salted for 16 days. After the salting stage hams are thoroughly brushed off to remove excess salt.

2. Equalization. Equalization, sometimes called post-salting takes place at 37-42° F (3-6° C), 85-95% humidity and continues for about 40 days. Equalization is the time after the excess cure has been removed from the product, at the end of the cure contact period until the product is placed in the drying room and the drying period begins.

3. Drying/Ripening. This is the longest stage and lasts 10-12 months. During this stage due to complex reactions between enzymes, meat proteins and fats, the ham develops its characteristic flavor and aroma. With time the ham loses moisture, but the salt remains inside increasing its proportional content. As the ham becomes more stable in time the temperatures are increased which increases the speed of internal reactions and decreases maturation time. The ripening continues in a few cycles: the temperature starts at 53-57° F (12-14° C), 60-80% humidity, and increases up to 75-93° (24-34° C), 70-90% humidity. The ripening takes about 5 months for Serrano Ham and 10 months for Iberico Ham. The high humidity creates better conditions for mold to develop which often happens. After ripening is completed, a thin layer of meat or fat is cut off from the surface of the ham with mold on it.

4. Storing. Then the hams are stored at around 53° F (12° C), 75% humidity for up to a year. For the highest quality Iberico hams, the entire process may take up to 2 years.

Protein

Intake of natural protein, especially fish, is associated with a decreased risk for stroke. A dose-response analysis found that the risk for stroke decreased by 26% for every 20-g per day increment in total protein intake.[461]

Protein Supplements: Sports Drinks - Beware!

Protein has become the new health craze with carbs the enemy. The protein supplement market is booming among the young and healthy, with retail sales of sports nutrition protein powders and other products in the United States alone projected to reach $9 billion by 2020, up from about $6.6 billion in 2016.

Powder supplements that come in all flavors are enormously palatable but provide protein in amounts that far exceed dietary recommendations. The revised Dietary Guidelines for Americans cautioned that some, especially teenage boys and adult men, should "reduce overall intake of protein foods" and eat more vegetables. American men already consume much greater amounts, averaging nearly 100 grams of protein a day.

The only groups that fall short on protein intake are teenage girls, who may not eat properly, and elderly people, who are at risk of losing muscle mass and whose appetites often slacken with age.

The average adult can achieve the recommended intake — 46 grams of protein a day for women, and 56 grams for men — by eating moderate amounts of protein-rich foods like meat, fish, dairy products, beans or nuts every day. There are about 44 grams of protein in a cup of chopped chicken, 20 grams in a cup of tofu or serving of Greek yogurt, and 18 grams in a cup of lentils or three eggs.

Eating excess is not utilized: 300 grams of protein a day doesn't mean you'll put on more muscle than someone who takes in 120 grams a day.

---

461 *Neurology*. Published online June 11, 2014.

Prunes

This study concluded that dried plums did, in fact, appear to promote retention of beneficial microbiota and microbial metabolism throughout the colon, which was associated with a reduced incidence of precancerous lesions[462]

Pulses and Legumes:

The Food and Agricultural Organization of the United Nations uses the term 'pulse' to describe crops harvested for their dry grains, such as lentils or chickpeas. They suggest the term 'legume' includes these dry grains, as well as fresh peas, beans and crops mainly grown for oil extraction, such as soya beans and peanuts. Distinctions are small so it's easy to see why they are used interchangeably.

Pumpkin

A good source of magnesium, manganese, copper, phosphorus, protein, zinc and iron. Zeaxanthin: Helpful against age-related macular degeneration and impaired eyesight. Low in cholesterol and high in Vitamin A. Heart-healthy phytosterols are in pumpkin seeds. Fiber may be a bonus for dieters who want a full feeling.

Resveratrol

Resveratrol had apparent benefits in terms of learning, memory and mood function at least in aged rats[463]

Resveratrol targets SIRT1, the longevity gene, directly at moderate doses and hits other targets at higher ones. Importantly, SIRT1 is required for resveratrol's benefits irrespective of dose.[464]

Rice

Infants who eat foods containing rice have higher urinary levels of arsenic than infants who eat no rice. (Prior studies suggest that exposure to arsenic early in life

---

462"Dried plums can reduce risk of colon cancer, research shows." ScienceDaily. ScienceDaily, 25 September 2015.
www.sciencedaily.com/releases/2015/09/150925131420.htm

463Prevents Age-Related Memory and Mood Dysfunction with Increased Hippocampal Neurogenesis and Microvasculature, and Reduced Glial Activation. *Scientific Reports*, 2015; 5: 8075 DOI: 10.1038/srep08075

464 SIRT1 Is Required for AMPK Activation and the Beneficial Effects of Resveratrol on Mitochondrial Function. *Cell Metabolism*, 2012; 15 (5): 675 DOI: 10.1016/j.cmet.2012.04.003

may have adverse developmental effects.) While not proving causation, the results support the FDA recommendations for infants: don't provide rice as the sole grain and use rice products in moderation.[465] Soaking rice overnight reduces arsenic contamination by 80% and use five times the water as usual.

Rosemary

Rosemary (just the smell) boosted memory by 15%.[466] (Peppermint Tea boosted Long-Term memory).

Sage

Boosted longer alertness

Salmon

Omega 3 fish oil content in farmed salmon has halved in the last 5 years. 130 g of salmon used to contain 3.5g of omega 3 oil, the recommended weekly allowance, but now only delivers 1.75g so now need two servings.

Farmed salmon sadly is fed on other fish in Europe they are mostly anchovies, but anchovies are becoming increasingly in short supply.

Somewhere I was told it takes two and a half times the amount of food for fish to produce a farmed salmon- no wonder there's a shortage.

Salt

Current dietary guidelines for Americans recommend levels below 2300 mg a day. In 2016 the US Food and Drug Administration issued draft guidance to ask the food industry to help Americans gradually reduce average intake to 2300mg / day which would seem apt. The problem is while we can measure our teaspoon of added salt, we simply don't know the amount of salt added to processed foods and this is the main source as in breakfast cereals and bread.

---

465 Eating Rice Products Exposes Infants to Arsenic *Cara Adler, MS, F. Bruder Stapleton, MD reviewing Karagas MR et al. JAMA Pediatr 2016 Apr 25.*

466 British Psychological Society annual conference Nottingham 2016:Northumbria Uni.

Two Major Trials

1. Sodium-Intake, Mortality Relationship Is Linear: TOPH Study

People with the lowest intake of sodium have the lowest rates of total mortality, according to a study spanning more than 20 years. These findings run counter to those of some previous studies that have found a J-curve effect, where people consuming the lowest amounts of sodium seemed also to have increased mortality or sometimes no increased risk. By contrast this study found no disadvantage to ingesting the lowest levels of sodium, as reflected by 24-hour urinary sodium excretion, and a direct linear association between average sodium intake and mortality. It was thought the "J curve studies" included smokers and people who lost weight because they were sick but when these were deleted the J shape went away. Using an accurate measure of usual sodium intake to total mortality over a period of more than 20 years, there was a direct linear relationship, with higher risk at high sodium intake and no evidence of a U or J shape.

In this analysis, for every added 1000 mg/day of sodium (the equivalent of about a half-teaspoon per day), the risk of premature death went up by 12%.[467]

2. Lancet Study

In a pooled analysis of four partially manufacturer-supported studies involving 133,118 individuals from 49 countries (roughly half hypertensive and half normotensive), it was found that the effects differ between those with and without hypertension. Higher sodium intake (sodium excretion, ≥7 g/day) was associated with higher risk for all-cause death and major cardiovascular events only in those with hypertension. Lower sodium intake (excretion, <3 g/day) was associated with increased risk for death and major cardiovascular events in both those with hypertension and those without. This was the J-Curve.[468]

- 80% of salt is in processed foods such as bread, packaged foods, sauces or in restaurant meals.
- It is the Sodium (Na), which is the problem. Na is present in Salt (NaCl) but also in MSG, Baking Soda and Sodium Benzoate also used in food prep

---

[467] Sodium intake and all-cause mortality over 20 years in the Trials of Hypertension Prevention (TOPH *J Am Coll Cardiol* 2016; 68:1609-1617.
How robust is the evidence for recommending very low salt intake in entire populations? *J Am Coll Cardiol* 2016; 68:1618-1621. Editorial
[468] Lancet 2016 May 20. Lancet 2016 May 20.

- 60 to 75% of salt come from processed food. Most of this is in bread, breakfast cereals (e.g. All Bran1g/serve) & cooked meats, restaurant meals, spaghetti sauce & frozen dinners[469]

- 95% of the population are at risk of developing cardiovascular disease (some 42% have it)

- Less salt intake would have a large effect on reducing strokes, heart attacks and heart failure[470]

- Salt represents the greatest preventable cause of hypertension.

- Current guidelines recommend a daily maximum of 2.3 grams of sodium a day — the amount found in a heaped teaspoon of salt — for most people, and less for the elderly or people with hypertension

- In people with high blood pressure, consuming more than seven grams a day increased the risk by 23%, but consuming less than three grams increased the risk by 34%, compared with those who ate four to five grams a day[471]

- The concern today is not in the benefits of 1,500 mg/d versus 2,300 mg/d, but rather reducing dietary intake from 8-10 g per day. 60% to 75% of all sodium intake is built into the manufacture of food so even getting to 4 g/d is the challenge.

- FDA recommended = 2.3 g / day
- Hypertensives = 1.5 g / day
- Av Intake => 4 g/d
- Low = 1.5 g/d
- Intermediate = 2.4
- High = 3.3
- 2.3 g = heaped teaspoon

- Food labels take years to change as Na levels insidiously increase e.g. some potato chips labelled at 15% are now 23%.

- Coke & Pepsi have invested in salty snacks for kids to increase their thirst[472]

---

469 Lancet 2001;358 . BMJ 2004;329:644
470 BMJ 2003;326:222 7.
471 Associations of urinary sodium excretion with cardiovascular events in individuals with and without hypertension: a pooled analysis of data from four studies. The Lancet Published Online: 20 May 2016 DOI: http://dx.doi.org/10.1016/S0140-6736(16)30467-6
472 The Grocer 2001

- DASH (Dietary Approaches to Stop Hypertension)[473]
- Reduce Salt (Na) by 3 g / d drops BP by 5mm & reduces heart attacks by 15% and strokes by 22%; reducing it by 6 g/d reduces heart attacks by 30% and strokes by 44%
- Salt should be iodised appropriately (WHO)
- Roughly 9 in 10 Americans consume more than the recommended daily amount of dietary sodium, according to an analysis of 2009–2012 NHANES data in *MMWR*.
- Read labels - minimise processed foods - usually overloaded
- Fresh food
- Minimize pizza, white bread

Salt Varieties

There are now great vogues for choosing and recommending various salts. Beware most of these are gimmicks and many potentially dangerous. A guide is that, the 'more special' it advertises to be, the more contaminated it may be.

Table salt is arguably best. Thereafter any colored salt claiming to be from some exotic region is only colored by contaminants, some of which could be damaging heavy metals.

Iodine is a good additive as it prevents cretinism.

Sea salt[474]

A study reveals varying levels of mold contamination in commercial sea salts. Among those molds were important food spoilage such as *Aspergillus* and *Penicillium*, and even some notorious producers of mycotoxins.

---

[473] NEMJ 201;344:3-10. Ann Int Med 2001;135:1019-28

[474] Sea salts as a potential source of food spoilage fungi. Food Microbiology, 2018; 69: 89 DOI: 10.1016/j.fm.2017.07.020

This finding contradicts the conventional wisdom that salts are sterile ingredients. The research stressed the importance of understanding the risk of using sea salt during food production.

Selenium

High blood selenium levels are associated with a decreased risk of developing liver cancer.

Selenium (Se) is found in foods like fish, shellfish, meat, milk and eggs; certain South American nuts, such as Brazil nuts, are also good sources of selenium. It is a trace element that occurs naturally in soil and plants and enters the bodies of humans and animals via the food they ingest. European soil has a rather low selenium concentration, in comparison with other areas of the world, especially in comparison to North America. Deficiencies of varying degrees of severity are common among the

general population and are the reason why German livestock receive selenium supplements in their feed.[475]

People are advised to get their levels done before embarking on any supplementation.

Sirtuins

Sirtuins are known as housekeeping genes and regulate numerous cellular and organismal functions, including metabolism, cellular death, inflammation, and longevity. The main role of sirtuins is to selectively regulate the activity of many key genes responsible for metabolism, cell defense, reproduction and other functions. Sirtuins (SIRT1) also modulates brain plasticity and memory formation functions. Scientist observed that Sirtuins (SIRT6) regulates the telomere length.

Sirtfoods

Foods that contain high levels of sirtuin activators are known as 'sirtfoods'. Sirtfoods include kale, olives, green tea, fish oil, onions, cocoa, blackcurrants, turmeric, citrus fruits, miso soup, capers, parsley, tofu and other soy products,

475 Prediagnostic selenium status and hepatobiliary cancer risk in the European Prospective Investigation into Cancer and Nutrition cohort. Am J Clin Nutr., 2016 DOI: 10.3945/ajcn.116.131672

extra-virgin olive oil and apples. The top ten sirtuin foods are blackcurrants, green tea, dark chocolate, kale, olives, capers, parsley, onions, turmeric, omega-3 fish oil.

Soft Drinks - Sugar Sweetened beverages (SSB), Sodas

Are a very great contributor to osteoporosis, obesity and dental decay.

Also see Fructose poisoning and sugar

Drinking more than one soft drink a day (even zero calorie, diet sodas) is associated with a higher risk of developing the Metabolic Syndrome.[476]

Recipients of Grants from Coke-Cola d 2013:

- The American College of Cardiology received $3.1 million.
- The American Academy of Family Physicians received $3.5 million
- The American Academy of Pediatrics received nearly $3 million
- The American Cancer Society received $2 million
- The Academy of Nutrition and Dietetics received $1.7 million

Soy

Several types of soy products are widely consumed, such as tofu (soybean curd), natto (soybean fermented with *Bacillus subtilis*), and miso (soybean fermented with *Aspergillus oryzae*). It is, however, still unclear whether different soy products, especially fermented soy products, are associated with specific health effects

Soy protein & isoflavones (phytoestrogens) have been touted to be beneficial to CVS, but 22 randomised trials found:

- No significant effects on LDL, HDL, triglycerides, lipoprotein or BP
- No lessening of menopausal symptoms
- No evidence re Ca breast, prostate[477]
- But may be cardioprotective in postmenopausal women

---

[476] Circ 23 July 2007
[477] Circulation 2006;113:1034-1044

- Soys main benefit is if and when it replaces junk food and then it improves BP and LDL in hypertensive women and BP in normotensive postmenopausal women[478]
- People who are able to produce equol -- a substance made by some types of "good" gut bacteria when they metabolize isoflavone micronutrients found in dietary soy, have lower levels of a risk factor for heart disease than their counterparts who cannot produce it. 50 to 60% of people in Asian countries produce it but only 20 to 30 percent of people in Western countries can. The daily intake of dietary isoflavones -- found in traditional soy foods such as tofu, miso and soymilk -- is 25 to 50 milligrams in China and Japan, while it is less than 2 milligrams in Western countries. It is thought that equol may have beneficial effects as equol-producers had 90-percent lower odds of coronary artery calcification, a predictor of heart disease, than the equol non-producers.[479]
- associations between intake of soy products and total and cause specific mortality in 42 750 men and 50 165 women aged 45-74 in a prospective study based in 11 of Japan's public health centre areas.7 During the 14.8 years of follow-up, the authors found that a higher intake of fermented soy (natto and miso) was associated with a significantly lower risk of all-cause mortality, but total soy product intake was not associated with all-cause mortality. Men and women who ate natto had a lower risk of cardiovascular mortality than those who did not eat natto.[480]

Smoked food[481]

The smoking process can cause carcinogens to form in foods. Not all smoked foods are dangerous, but most can contain low levels of these substances. Filters, made from zeolite, a porous aluminosilicate mineral used in car tailpipes, to reduce pollutants, removed as much as 93% of benzo[a]pyrene, a known carcinogen.

Smoke Point for Cooking Oils

If and when smoke is a problem (as it is in submarines and small apartments) then a high smoke point oil may be preferable. I have found such tables somewhat

---

[478] Arch Int Med 2007;167:1060-67

[479] Significant inverse association of equol-producer status with coronary artery calcification but not dietary isoflavones in healthy Japanese men. British Journal of Nutrition, 2017; 117 (02): 260 DOI: 10.1017/S000711451600458X

[480] BMJ doi:10.1136/bmj.m34

[481] American Chemical Society

contradictory and some only give the refined oil values when I very much recommend only cold pressed oils.

Spinach

Consuming the concentrated extract of thylakoids found in spinach can reduce hunger and sweet cravings.[482]

Spirulina or blue-green "pond" algae is cultivated as feedstock in Africa and Mexico. It became famous after it was used by NASA as a dietary supplement for astronauts on space missions. It does not, however, contain all nine essential amino acids. Despite the many claims there are no known medical uses for spirulina in humans.

Sperm

A supplement of vitamins C, E and D, selenium, l-carnitine, zinc, folic acid and lycopene did not help men with fertility problems.[483]

Statistics

Relative risk or **risk** ratio (RR) is the ratio of the probability of an event occurring (for example, developing a disease, being injured) in an exposed group to the probability of the event occurring in a comparison, non-exposed group.

In general: If the risk ratio is 1 (or close to 1), it suggests no difference or little difference in risk (incidence in each group is the same).

A risk ratio > 1 suggests an increased risk of that outcome in the exposed group. A risk ratio < 1 suggests a reduced risk.

Hazard Ratio and Relative Risk (risk ratio) are essentially the same: Hazard ratio s the instantaneous risk at a particular time while relative risk gives cumulative risk over a time span.

---

[482] Acute Effects of a Spinach Extrac Rich in Thylakoids on Satiety: A Randomized Controlled Crossover Trial. Journal of the American College of Nutrition, 2015; 1 DOI: 10.1080/07315724.2014.1003999

[483] Fertility and Sterility, Eunicen Kennedy Shriver (Institute NICHD) 2020

Sugar

- U.S. adult consumption of added sugars increased by more than 30% over three decades. Even more alarming is the fact that the top 20% of adult consumers are eating 721 calories from added sugar per day, on average. This is equally alarming for the top 20% of children who are consuming on average 673 calories from added sugar per day[484]
- These are essentially wasted calories, with no nutritional value other than energy. Weight gain is one obvious consequence. A cross sectional analysis of the survey data suggests that foods containing added sugars are also associated with adverse lipid profiles and increased risk of cardiovascular disease especially lower HDL. The link was independent of body mass index and other factors[485]
- Estimates of American sugar consumption vary between 77 to 152 pounds per year. An estimated 13% of Americans derive at least 25% of their total caloric intake from added sugars.
- In a study of more than 1000 US adolescents, more than half of their total caloric intake was derived from added sugars.
- The American Heart Association recommends no more than 6 teaspoons of added sugars per day among women and no more than 9 teaspoons for men. Current levels of average sugar consumption are 4 to 5 times higher than these limits.
- Added sugars in the diet promote obesity and insulin resistance. Insulin resistance is encountered in 25% of adults and up to 80% of persons with essential hypertension. Insulin resistance may be a greater factor than obesity in promoting hypertension.
- Compared with patients who consume less than 10% of their calories from added sugars, those for whom added sugars constitute 10% to 24.9% of total caloric intake experience a 30% higher risk for incident cardiovascular disease.
- Consumption of more than one 12-ounce sugar-sweetened beverage per day is associated with at least a 6% increase in the risk for incident hypertension.
- A meta-analysis of clinical trials found that higher sugar intake was associated with increases in systolic and diastolic blood pressure of 6.9 and 5.6 mm Hg, respectively.
- Fructose may particularly increase the risk for cardiovascular disease. Sucrose has an equal balance between fructose and glucose, but high-fructose corn syrup generally contains approximately 55% fructose.

---

[484] Obesity Society. "U.S. adult consumption of added sugars increased by more than 30% over three decades." ScienceDaily. ScienceDaily, 4 November 2014.

[485] JAMA 2010;303:1490-7

- In a randomized trial, consumption of a fructose solution was associated with an average 6.8 mm Hg increase in systolic blood pressure, whereas drinking a glucose solution did not significantly change blood pressure.
- Higher consumption of added sugars is associated with negative consequences on serum lipid levels, and fructose is also implicated in promoting the metabolic syndrome.
- Both fructose and glucose can increase blood pressure variability and myocardial oxygen demand[486]
- Sugar content in fruit drinks, juice and smoothies marketed to kids contained the entire recommended intake of 19g in nearly half those tested in the UK. Smoothies were worst @ 13g/100ml[487]

Sugar / High Fructose Corn Syrup

- The average American today consumes 53 teaspoons of sugar each day
- The average person in the UK eats 71.7 g of sugar a day in packaged foods
- A single can of soft drink has about 13 teaspoons of sugar in the form of High Fructose Corn Syrup
- Average American drinks about 55 gallons of soft drink a year
- 10% to 15% of all calories consumed by American teenage girls come from soft drinks
- Sugary drinks boost risk factors for heart disease
- The risk of death from cardiovascular disease -- the leading cause of death around the world -- increases as the amount of added sugar consumed increases. Beverages sweetened with low, medium and high amounts of high-fructose corn syrup significantly increase risk factors for cardiovascular disease, even when consumed for just two weeks by young, healthy men and women. Even the participants who consumed the 10-percent dose exhibited increased circulating concentrations of low-density lipoprotein cholesterol and triglyceride compared with their concentrations at the beginning of the study. Most of the increases in lipid/lipoprotein risk factors for cardiovascular disease were greater in men than in women and were independent of body weight gain[488]
- Sports drinks contain up to 13 teaspoons of sugar per bottle – more than a can of Coke

---

[486] Open Heart. 2014;1;e000167

[487] "How much sugar is hidden in drinks marketed to children? A survey of fruit juices, juice drinks and smoothies" BMJ Open 2016; DOI: 10.1136/bmjopen-2015-010330.

[488] A dose-response study of consuming high-fructose corn syrup–sweetened beverages on lipid/lipoprotein risk factors for cardiovascular disease in young adults. Am J Clin Nutr, April 2015 DOI: 10.3945/ajcn.114.100461

- Drinking sugar-sweetened beverages (more than 12 ounces per day) was associated with a 53% higher incidence of high triglycerides and a 98% higher incidence of low HDL cholesterol (the "good" cholesterol) compared to those who drank less than one serving per month.[489]

Supplements

U.S. and most Government laws does not oblige manufacturers or vendors of dietary supplements to prove the effectiveness of their product. Claims that the product is "all natural" or "naturally grown and harvested" should not be understood as a guarantee of safety. Often only 10% content is needed to claim "Natural". The FDA and other Governments don't require supplement makers to demonstrate that a product is safe or effective before it is sold. Nor to guarantee the contents of a supplement. Some products may have different amounts of ingredients than advertised or have contaminants or pesticides.

I Am Fit and Healthy: I'd Better Take a Supplement to make sure. Why Not? or, I'm Tired All The Time I'd Better Take A Supplement

Americans spend more than $30 billion a year on dietary supplements — vitamins, minerals and herbal products, among others — most of which are unnecessary or of doubtful benefit.

There are some 83,000 supplements sold in the USA.

The passage of the Dietary Supplement Health and Education Act of 1994 opened the floodgates to an industry that can bring these products to market without submitting any evidence to the Food and Drug Administration that they are safe and effective in people. The government can halt sales of an individual product *only after it is on the market and shown to be mislabeled or dangerous.* After 1994, sales of a very wide range of supplements skyrocketed, and because the law allowed it, many continued to be sold even after high-quality research showed they were no better than a placebo at supporting health. The law allows the products to be promoted as "supporting" the health of various parts of the body, but people translate this to mean to a proven benefit.

52% of adults used one or more supplements in 2012. In one study 45% of people said they took them to "improve" and 33% to "maintain" overall health. But what is bizarre is that these consumers were apparently among the healthiest members

[489] American Heart Association

of the population. They were more likely than non-users to report being in very good or excellent health, to use alcohol moderately, to refrain from cigarette smoking, to exercise frequently and to have health insurance. Other studies have shown that supplement use is also more frequent among those who are older, who weigh less and have higher levels of education and socioeconomic status.

Unlike the commercial food processed 'health' bars, a fruit-based micronutrient and fiber-dense supplement bar, the CHORI-bar is not just another nutrition bar but a serious intervention to improve health. Its complex composition required a number of years to develop and was shown in clinical trials to improve metabolism in overweight/obese otherwise healthy adults in ways that are consistent with reduced risk of type 2 diabetes and cardiovascular disease. Consumption of the bar for two months also reduced chronic inflammation and initiated a reduction in weight and waist circumference. The full potential of scientifically food-based supplements to do the work of some drug without their negative side effects is just beginning to be seriously investigated. .[490]

Fresh natural produce are the best source of most, if not all, of the human body needs. However, we do not live in a perfect world and the elderly or the economically distressed, often eat poorly and eat rubbish.

But so too are the affluent and busy who, time poor, "just grab a bite".

Supplements are then indicated, and multi-vitamins proven beneficial.

At the end of the day taking extra vitamins and minerals do more harm than good. While dietary supplements may be advertised to promote health, research shows a link between consumption of over-the-counter supplements and increased cancer risk, if the supplements are taken in excess of the recommended dietary amount.[491]

A study by the Department of Medical Physics and Applied Radiation Sciences, McMaster University, Canada found that in a mouse model of accelerated aging and severe cognitive decline, a combination of vitamins and minerals, as well as nutraceuticals, such as beta carotene, bioflavonoids, cod liver oil, flax seed, garlic, and green tea extract, not only maintained brain cell numbers and mass and cognitive function but also appeared to prevent deterioration of sight and smell. It

---

490 A multicomponent nutrient bar promotes weight loss and improves dyslipidemia and insulin resistance in the overweight/obese: chronic inflammation blunts these improvements. *The FASEB Journal*, 2015; DOI: 10.1096/fj.15-271833

491 University of Colorado Cancer Center. "Excessive use of dietary supplements linked to increase cancer risk." ScienceDaily. ScienceDaily, 20 April 2015. <www.sciencedaily.com/releases/2015/04/150420182403.htm>.

is optimistic that the effects of the supplement will translate into humans as the supplement works on fundamental mechanisms that are pretty much ubiquitous across any organism that breathes air, essentially. These mechanisms, which include oxidative stress, inflammation, and mitochondrial dysfunction, which happen in a multitude of species as they get older and are not something that is specifically a human phenomenon. Previous research showed that the supplement extended longevity and reduced cognitive and age-related physical deterioration in mice. The findings support the notion that nutraceuticals are more likely to be effective when taken in combination with other supplements rather than when taken alone as a single supplement. The supplement is not subject to intellectual property protection, owing to the fact that it is composed of nutraceuticals that are available in health food stores although a company has licensed the formulation from McMaster University to commercialize it should the supplement be shown to have similar effects in humans.[492]

Update 2020

Dietary supplements are wildly popular right now. Seventy-seven percent of Americans use them, according to a 2019 survey. And the industry will be worth an estimated $50 billion in the U.S. by the end of the year. People are consuming them in the hopes of improving their immunity, calming anxiety, and staving off diseases like cancer and Alzheimer's. Yet experts warn they're inadequately regulated and can even be dangerous.

In a large study published in 2019, researchers from Tufts University looked at the association between supplement use and premature death. They found that people who got adequate amounts of certain nutrients from their diet had a lower risk of death during the study period, wh ile those who took supplements to get their nutrients did not. It's preferable to get vitamins and minerals from food they are better absorbed, and you get the other health benefits, like fiber and antioxidants.

Future Hope?

A dietary supplement containing a blend of thirty vitamins and minerals—all-natural ingredients - has shown remarkable anti-aging properties that can prevent and even reverse massive brain cell loss, according to research in mice. It's a mixture that scientists from McMaster University believe could someday slow the

[492] Environ Mol Mutagen. Published May 20, 2016.

progress of catastrophic neurological diseases such as Alzheimer's, ALS and Parkinson's.[493]

Sweet Potatoes

Purple sweet potatoes (the darker the better) have high contents of anthocyanin which have been epidemiologically associated with a reduced cancer risk. The purple sweet potato had a much higher total phenolic content than the other regularly occurring sweet potatoes. Phenols are chemical compounds that have been found to have anti-aging and antioxidant components.[494]

Orange Sweet Potato is high in vitamin A and now grown extensively in parts of Africa to combat deficiencies.

Tea

- Also see Polyphenols
- Many claims have been made. As it does no harm then there's no harm in trying.
- May help prevent / slow bladder Ca
- Habitual green & oolong tea drinking in Taiwan significantly reduced risk of developing BP[495]
- Epithelial ovarian Ca risk seems reduced[496]
- Green tea may protect against diabetes 2[497]
- Following nearly 14,000 Japanese adults age 65 and older, they found that people who drank the most green-tea were the least likely to become functionally disabled over the next three years. People who drank at least five cups a day were one-third less likely to develop disabilities than those who had less than a cup a day. And people who averaged three or four cups a day had a 25% lower risk[498]

---

[493] A multi-ingredient dietary supplement abolishes large-scale brain cell loss, improves sensory function, and prevents neuronal atrophy in aging mice. Environmental and Molecular Mutagenesis, 2016; DOI: 10.1002/em.22019

[494] Kansas State University (2009, June 30). Purple Sweet Potato Means Increased Amount Of Anti-cancer Components. ScienceDaily. Retrieved July 1, 2009, from http://www.sciencedaily.com-/releases/2009/06/090629132250.htm

[495] Arch Int Med 2004;164:1534-40

[496] Arch Int Med 2005;165:2683-86

[497] Ann Int Med 206;144:554-62

[498] Am J Clin Nutr 2012.

- Green tea has the potential to help in the prevention and treatment of osteoporosis and other bone diseases.[499]
- Tea, 3 cups a day reduced CAD 27%, cardiac death 26%, stroke 18% total mortality 24%, intracerebral hemorrhage 21% and cerebral infarction 16%[500]
- Tea consumption was associated with reduced risks of atherosclerotic cardiovascular disease and all-cause mortality, especially among those consistent habitual tea drinkers. Compared with people who drank fewer than three cups of tea a week, those who drank more had a 20 percent reduced risk for a cardiovascular incident, a 22 percent reduced risk for cardiovascular death and a 15 percent reduced risk for all-cause premature death.[501]

Telomere Protection

Telomeres are repetitive DNA sequences at the ends of chromosomes that progressively shorten with age. Shorter telomeres are associated with shorter life expectancy and greater risk for age-related diseases. Obesity, cigarette smoking, and other lifestyle factors have been linked to shorter telomere length. Oxidative stress and inflammation speed up telomere shortening.

Tofu

Consuming tofu, which is high in isoflavones, more than once a week was associated with a 18% lower risk of heart disease, compared to a 12% lower risk for those who ate tofu less than once a month.

Tomatoes

It was thought that the Lycopene in tomatoes protected against prostate cancer, but a later bigger trial has thrown doubt on this effect. However, it seems to slow down development of enlarged prostate[502]

- tomatoes may reduce platelet activation (clotting) and therefore be cardioprotective[503] The yellow fluid around tomato seeds appears to suppress platelet activation without affecting blood clotting[504]

---

[499] Effects of Tea Catechins, Epigallocatechin, Gallocatechin, and Gallocatechin Gallate, on Bone Metabolism. Journal of Agricultural and Food Chemistry, 2009; 57 (16): 7293 DOI: 10.1021/jf901545u

[500] European Journal of Epidemology Feb 2015, Vol 30 issue 2. pp 103-113

[501] European Journal of Preventive Cardiology,Jan 8th 2020, https://doi.org/10.1177/2047487319894685

[502] Oncology and Cancer Case reports May 2016 online

[503] Am J Clin Nutr September 2006 vol. 84 no. 3 570-579

[504] Adv Food Nutr Res. 2013;68:273-82.

- Lycopene in tomatoes is fat soluble-use oil

Trans-fats

- TFs are 'metabolic poison' and are more harmful than any other fat.
- Usually occur when vegetable oil is hydrogenated to make it solid at room temperature. The 'pure' white solid cooking 'oil' that most restaurants and fast-food outlets used was mostly saturated and hydrogenated Palm Oil which was then made even worse by heating causing Trans Fats to develop. The amount of Trans Fats varied widely in the same foods e.g. KFC, McDonalds around the world and even from town to town by according to what they had been cooked in[505]
- Liquid vegetable oils e.g. soy, canola or olive oil eliminates TFs
- Most Fast Foods have switched but many processed have not

Ubiquinone, also known as Coenzyme Q10

Widely believed to function as an antioxidant, protecting cells against damage from free radicals but a study finds that it is not a crucial antioxidant -- and that consuming it is unlikely to provide any benefit.[506]

Vitamins & Minerals

Let me be quite clear here: Vitamins are essential - all I advocate is how we get them. It is my opinion that fresh food, especially a wide variety of vegetables and fruit, not only supply all the vitamins and minerals but also in the correct dose and in a form that the body can best absorb and utilize. But further, natural foods also contain thousands of micronutrients that also contribute to our metabolic pathways. If you eat the Newtrition recommended foods, you should not need supplements. Any of the benefits, as below, probably occurred in people who were deficient from a poor diet - often found even in affluent societies eating processed foods.

Researchers and Vitamin Companies will make claims that may well be premature if they improve their chances of a research grant or sales e.g. observational studies on vitamin D make claims not supported by randomised trials.

[505] NEMJ 150406

[506] Mitochondrial function and lifespan of mice with controlled ubiquinone biosynthesis. Nature Communications, 2015; 6: 6393 DOI: 10.1038/ncomms7393

In the overall picture of life, it is patently absurd to remove the vitamins from natural food, as in de-husking grains, only to then add them back in the form of synthetic vitamins into our bread. Crazy no?

Many synthetic vitamins are made from coal tar derivatives, chemically processed sugar, acids and industrial chemicals with the word 'natural' used when only some 10% of their content need be natural or, when analyzed, e.g. fish oil capsules, don't contain amounts they claimed.

The claims and counter claims are confusing. The highly respected Annals of Internal medicine reported, as below in 2003, how vitamin C, admittedly as a multivitamin combination, did not reduce cardiovascular disease (CVD). However, in 2015, a Danish study found, when sourced from fruit and vegetables, it did.

In the large-scale randomized trial of 14,641 middle-aged and older USA Physicians, a daily multivitamin supplement significantly but modestly reduced the risk of total cancer during a mean of 11 years of treatment and follow-up. Although the main reason to take multivitamins is to prevent nutritional deficiency, these data provide support for the potential use of multivitamin supplements in the prevention of cancer in middle-aged and older men.[507] The later 2016 study suggests that Vitamin D can prevent some 67% of cancers.[508]

However, the best advice, in my opinion, is to source your vitamins from a good varied diet. In other words, if you benefit from or need a multi-vitamin you are not eating correctly.

Most vitamin deficiencies are usually associated with the elderly who cannot care for themselves, are indoors and eat a poor diet. Some trials, however, have shown how vitamins are not only not necessary with a good diet and exercise, but may well be harmful.

- Vit A, C or E, Multivitamins with Folic A or combinations did not prevent CVD or cancer and are not recommended. Cancer incidence increased in smokers taking Beta-carotene[509]
- Although findings that a healthy diet is good for the heart aren't really a surprise anymore, this research suggests that this may be because of the

---

[507] Multivitamins in the Prevention of Cancer in Men: The Physicians' Health Study II Randomized Controlled Trial JAMA. 2012;308(18):1871-1880. doi:10.1001/jama.2012.14641.

[508] PLoS One. 2016;11:e0152441.

[509] Ann Int Med 2003;139:51-55 & 56-70

increase in vitamin-C levels that come from a high intake of fruit and vegetables· Evaluation of almost 100,000 individuals from the Copenhagen General Population Study (CGPS) and Copenhagen City Heart Study showed that those who ate the most fruit and vegetables had a 13% lower risk of CVD and a 20% lower risk of all-cause mortality compared with the subgroup that ate these foods only rarely[510]

- Beta-carotene, vitamins A and E may increase mortality[511]
- Higher dietary intake of vitamin C has been found to have a potentially preventative effect on cataract progression. The human body cannot manufacture vitamin C, so we depend on vitamins in the food we eat.
- Overweight and obese adults are advised to exercise to improve their health but taking vitamin C supplements daily can have similar cardiovascular benefits as regular exercise in these adults. The blood vessels of overweight and obese adults have elevated activity of the small vessel-constricting protein endothelin (ET)-1. Exercise has been shown to reduce ET-1 activity but incorporating an exercise regimen into a daily routine can be challenging. Daily supplementation of vitamin C (500 mg/day, time-released) reduced ET-1-related vessel constriction as much as walking for exercise did[512]
- 6 g/day dose vitamin C shortened colds by 17%, twice as much as the 3g/day doses did. 8g/day dose shortened colds by 19%, Self-dosing of vitamin C must be started as soon as possible after the onset of common cold symptoms to be most effective.[513]
- Supplements may interfere with statins
- **Vit E does not prevent atherosclerosis[514]**
- Vit E, C & Beta-carotene supplements gave no reduction in mortality, CVD, Ca or anything[515] including stroke[516]
- Vit E does nothing to reduce incidence of diabetes[517]
- When testing mice whose immune cells lacked the repair enzyme, the immune cells were saved from cell death by mixing a high dose of vitamin E into the animals' food. That was enough antioxidant to protect the T cells' cell membranes from damage, so they could multiply and successfully fend off

---

[510] Genetically high plasma vitamin C, intake of fruit and vegetables, and risk of ischemic heart disease and all-cause mortality: a Mendelian randomization study. Am J Clin Nutr 2015; 101:1135-1143

[511] Cardiosource 27 Mar 2007

[512] American Physiological Society (APS). "Vitamin C: The exercise replacement?." ScienceDaily. ScienceDaily, 4 September 2015. <www.sciencedaily.com/releases/2015/09/150904144604.htm>.

513 Vitamin C and Infections. Nutrients, 2017; 9 (4): 339 DOI: 10.3390/nu9040339

514 Lancet 2003;361:2017-23

515 Lancet 2002;360:23-33

516 Ann Int Med 1999;130:963-970

517 Diabetes 2006;55:2856-62

the viral infection. At 500 milligrams per kilogram of mouse feed, this quantity of vitamin E was ten times higher than was present in the standardized normal food.[518] May be worth a try with your next cold sore?

- Multivitamin & mineral supplement seemed to reduce infections esp. in Type 2 Diabetics[519]
- 22% of Kids in UK were consuming less than the minimum safe amounts of vitamins and 50% girls were consuming less than safe amounts of minerals (Fe, Mg)[520]
- B6 and B12 vitamin pills & Folate failed to keep elderly people's brains and memories sharp[521]
- Folate, Vit C and E proved useless in preventing pre-eclampsia in pregnancy
- 57% women and 47% men take supplements[522]
- 31.8% of USA Children take supplements. Highest use 48.5% ages 4 to 8 years.
- Most taken: Vit C (28.6%), retinol (25.8%), Vit D (25.6%), calcium (21.1%) and iron (19.3%)
- Bioflavenoids, ginseng, Echinacea, gingko, grape seed extract
- Supplement use was associated with higher family income, a smoke free environment, lower BMI, less daily recreational TV/computer) time[523]
- In those who are otherwise healthy, there is no evidence that supplements have any benefits with respect to cancer or heart disease. Vitamin A and E supplements not only provide no health benefits for generally healthy individuals, but they may increase mortality, though the two large studies that support this conclusion included smokers for whom it was already known that beta-carotene supplements can be harmful. Other findings suggest that vitamin E toxicity is limited to only a specific form when taken in excess[524]
- It was found that many common store-brand herbal supplements did not contain the ingredient listed on the product's label or contained contaminants or fillers not included on the label. Only 21% of the test results from store-

---

518 M. Matsushita, S. Freigang, C. Schneider, M. Conrad, G. W. Bornkamm, M. Kopf. T cell lipid peroxidation induces ferroptosis and prevents immunity to infection. *Journal of Experimental Medicine*, 2015; 212 (4): 555 DOI: 10.1084/jem.20140857

519 Ann Int Med 2003;138;365-371

520 Prof Lean Uni Glasgow 2003

521 University of Otago study 2006.

522 NHANES- National Health & Nutrition Examination Survey USA 2007

523 Arch Paedtr Adolesc Med 2007;161: 978-985

524 "Vitamin, Mineral, and Multivitamin Supplements for the Primary Prevention of Cardiovascular [185] Disease and Cancer: U.S. Preventive Services Task Force Recommendation Statement.". Mortality in Randomized Trials of Antioxidant Supplements for Primary and Secondary Prevention: Systematic Review and Meta-analysis". *JAMA* 297 (8): 842–57. doi:10.1001/jama.297.8.842. PMID 17327526.

[186] "Tocotrienols: Vitamin E beyond tocopherols". *Life Sciences* 78 (18): 2088–98.

brand herbal supplements indicated that the supplements had DNA from the plants listed on the labels. The worst had only 4% of the advertised content. Also see Fish Oils[525]

- Vitamin K2: May be important in preventing osteoporosis and coronary artery calcification: A large volume of alternative literature has been hyping vitamin K2 as active in preventing or treating arterial calcification for years. But serious science now seems to be backing that up. The relationship of vitamin D, vitamin K2, and calcium may hold a real key to a better understanding of harmful arterial calcification. But which came first: the chicken or the egg? Was the vascular wall calcium an instigating progenitor, a fellow traveler as simple dystrophy, a part of the inflammatory pathogenesis, or a culminating bony add-on for advanced atherosclerosis? Watch this space.
- Boiling vegetables often loses their vitamins especially vitamin C, so does using baking soda (although it helps maintain color).
- Microwaving / Steaming is one of the best cooking methods for preserving nutrients, including water-soluble vitamins or use as little water as possible when poaching or boiling.
- Don't peel vegetables to maximize their fiber and nutrient content.

Vitamin D

Vitamin D offers some protection against Covid-19 see front pages

Vitamin D *may* play a vital role in the prevention and treatments of chronic diseases associated with aging such as cognitive decline, depression, osteoporosis, cardiovascular disease, high blood pressure, Type 2 diabetes and cancer.[526]

But see start of this section. The above may be true for the elderly nutritionally deprived but research often makes claims which are premature. A good diet and exercise is what is recommended. Further the measurement of vitamin D which has an inactive and several active forms is far from clear. Get out, get exercise and eat well.

A review of the major studies and research published in the BMJ November 2016 found little or no benefit is supplementation for almost any health outcome, disease or illness and doubts that any further research or studies will find otherwise and any improvements from supplementation are too small as to be non-

---

[525] *New York Times 2015* story

[526] The Role of Vitamin D in the Aging. Journal of Aging and Gerontology, 2014; 2 (2): 60 DOI: 10.12974/2309-6128.2014.02.02.1

beneficial and that benefit are most likely to be seen in populations with severe vitamin D deficiency.[527]

It should be noted in the following that many of these "improvements" were in the severely mal-nourished and vitamin deficient.

- Our skin makes most of the vitamin D in our bodies after exposure to sunlight. Because most of us are indoors most of the 24-hour day, many of us have relatively low blood levels of vitamin D.
- Studies have found that people with low blood levels of vitamin D are at greater risk for several important diseases, including heart disease, some kinds of cancer, and autoimmune diseases, than people with higher levels of vitamin D. So it seems logical that taking a vitamin D pill that will raise your blood levels of the vitamin would be a good thing. But the only way to prove that such higher levels bring health benefits is to perform a large randomized study in which some people take vitamin D every day and some take an identical-looking sugar pill (placebo). As at 2016 such a study is under way, and preliminary results are expected within two to three years.

Vitamin D and Colorectal Cancer

Higher blood vitamin D concentration showed a strong dose—response inverse association with colorectal cancer risk (men and women). Subjects in the highest fifth of blood vitamin D levels showed a 40% reduced risk compared with those in the lowest fifth. Subjects with very low levels showed a significantly higher risk of colorectal cancer.[528]

Reduction in Colds and Influenza

Vitamin D supplementation does cut respiratory infections but the absolute risk reduction of 2% found in the study would not be a sufficient justification for most of the general population to take supplements but it was safe, and it protected against acute respiratory tract infection overall.

---

[527] BMJ 2016;355:i6201

[528] Association between pre-diagnostic circulating vitamin D concentration and risk of colorectal cancer in European populations: a nested case-control study. BMJ. 2010 Jan 21;340:b5500. PMID: 20093284

Prediagnostic 25-hydroxyvitamin D, VDR and CASR polymorphisms, and survival in patients with colorectal cancer in western European populations. Cancer Epidemiol Biomarkers Prev. 2012 Apr;21(4):582-93. PMID: 22278364

Vitamin and Mineral Supplements for Primary Prevention of Cardiovascular Disease and Cancer

The U.S. Preventive Services Task Force recommends against vitamin E supplements and notes that evidence is insufficient to support multivitamin use.[529]

Increased All-Cause Mortality from Vitamins

The long-term impact of supplementation is unknown, and some studies suggested a relationship between supplements and increased mortality. In light of this uncertainty the use of vitamin and mineral supplements among 38,772 postmenopausal women participating in the Iowa Women's Health Study was studied. The mean age of the women at baseline in 1986 was 61.6. After adjustment for demographics, dietary and lifestyle factors, comorbidities, and use of hormone replacement therapy, the following supplements were associated with a greater risk of death during follow-up:

Multivitamins, Magnesium, Zinc, Iron, Vitamin B6, Folic acid, Copper. Absolute increases in risk ranged from 2.4% with multivitamins to 18% with copper. In contrast calcium supplementation was associated with a lower risk of death. The absolute risk reduction was 3.8%. It was concluded that "a better investment in health would be eating more fruits and vegetables because commonly used vitamin and mineral supplements have no known benefit on mortality rate and have been shown to confer risk"[530]

- Up to 50% of U.S. adults regularly take mineral- vitamin supplements.
- Vitamin E was associated with a higher rate of prostate cancer and hemorrhagic strokes[531]
- Large, hard multivitamin and calcium supplements are a frequent cause of choking in seniors.[532]

Walnuts

A study showed walnuts have a beneficial effect on serum lipid levels and blood pressure, coronary heart disease, and cardiovascular disease but not on age-related cognitive decline.[533]

---

529 Ann Intern Med 2014 Apr 15

530 "Dietary supplements and mortality rate in older women: the Iowa Women's Health Study" *Arch Intern Med* 2011; 171: 1625-1633.

531 The Selenium and Vitamin E Cancer Prevention Trial (SELECT)" *JAMA* 2011; 306: 1549-1556.

532 August 19 in *Annals of Internal Medicine*.

533 *Am J Clin Nutr*. Published online January 7, 2020

Wheatgrass

There is no sound evidence to support the claim that wheatgrass is better than other fruits and vegetables in terms of nutrition. It cannot be recommended above any other choices in this food group.

Xantham gum

Is a polysaccharide, a type of carbohydrate created when sugar is fermented by the bacteria Xanthomonas campestris. It's often used in processed foods, medicines, and toothpastes as a thickener and stabilizing agent to improve consistency and texture and extend the shelf life. The body is unable to digest xanthan gum and it doesn't provide any calories or nutrients, so it's neither healthy or unhealthy but it should alert that this is probably processed food that it is in.

Yeast

See Nooch

Yoghurt

Beneficial if natural with plenty of microbes (1 billion colony-forming-units CFUs). Avoid low-fat with concentrated fruit and sugar or sweeteners.

Zinc

The trace element zinc has an impact on the essential metabolic functions of most living organisms. Even minimal zinc deficiency impairs digestion, albeit without any typical symptoms such as skin problems or fatigue. Hence, short-term zinc deficiency in the diet should be avoided. Vegans, vegetarians and older people should monitor their zinc intake. Among other things, a subclinical zinc deficiency in humans has been attributed to increased levels of inflammation markers and reduced immuno-competence.[534]

---

534 Subclinical zinc deficiency impairs pancreatic digestive enzyme activity and digestive capacity of weaned piglets. *British Journal of Nutrition*, 2016; 1 DOI: 10.1017/S0007114516002105

PART D

FOOD ANALYSIS

and

The MICRO-NUTRIENT

REVOLUTION

CHAPTER 15

FOOD GROUPS

The macronutrients are the **Proteins, Carbohydrates and Fats** which we all know, but their discoveries, let alone nutritional science, is surprisingly recent.

FOOD COMPOSITION

A: MACRONUTRIENT GROUPS

1. **Protein e.g. meats, beans**
2. **Carbohydrates + Fiber e.g. plants**
3. **Fats**
    - **Saturated** – solid at room temperature: Butter, lard, palm oil
    - **Unsaturated** = Omega **or** ω **(ω Greek letter omega) or** n
        - 9 = Mono – **Olive oil, canola, avocado, peanut**
        - 6 = Poly -- **Vegetable oils**
        - 3 = 'Super' – **Fish, linseed (flax), walnuts, soy**

Note: 'Super' is my terminology as these omega 3s are super-unsaturated.

B: MICRONUTRIENTS: Chemical elements required in trace amounts for the normal growth and development. Some are "essential" for life.

4. **Vitamins**
5. **Minerals**
    - Major
    - Trace
    - Ultra Trace Elements
6. **Phytochemicals or nutrients**
    - Amino Acids
    - Phytochemicals

Most natural foods are a combination of all three macro-nutrients.

Only a few foods, such as some oils and sugars, are made up of a single nutrient

Most foods contain a mixture of protein, carbohydrate and fat e.g:

Food (g)	Water	Protein	Fat	Carbohy-drate	Alcohol
Wheat flour	15	13.6	2.5	69.1	
White bread	38.3	7.8	1.4	52.7	
Rice, raw	11.7	6.2	1.0	86.8	
Milk whole	87	3.4	3.7	4.8	
Butter	13.9	0.4	85.1	trace	
Cheddar cheese	37	25.4	34.5	trace	
Beef, fried	56.9	20.4	20.4	0	
Haddock, fried	65.1	20.4	8.3	3.6	
Potatoes raw	80	2.5	Trace	15.9	
Peas, canned	72.7	5.9	Trace	16.5	
Cabbage boiled	95.7	1.3	Trace	1.1	
Orange, w peel	64.8	0.6	Trace	12.2	
Apple	47	84.1	0.3 trace	12.2	
Sugar white	Trace	Trace	0	105	
Beer	96.7	0.2	Trace	2.2	3.1
Spirits 70%	63.5	Trace	0	Trace	31.5

CHAPTER 16.

PROTEINS

Proteins are formed from 20 amino acids (see) and are mostly intra-cellular.

Functions:

1. Growth and Maintenance

Body protein needs are dependent upon age, health and activity levels.

Our bodies need protein for growth and maintenance of tissues. We grow rapidly until age 17 – 27 years and are then in a protein deficit or 'negative nitrogen balance'. But then our body's proteins are in a constant state of turnover, breaking down the same amount of protein that it uses to build and repair tissues.

Other times, it breaks down more protein than it can create, thus increasing needs. This typically happens in periods of illness, during pregnancy and while breastfeeding, when recovering from an injury or surgery. The elderly and athletes require more protein as well.

2. Provides Structure

Some proteins help form the body's connective tissue framework. They are fibrous and provide cells and tissues with stiffness and rigidity.

Keratin is a structural protein that is found in skin, hair and nails.

Collagen is the most abundant protein in the body and is the structural protein of bones, tendons, ligaments and skin.

Elastin is several hundred times more flexible than collagen. Its high elasticity allows many tissues in your body to return to their original shape after stretching or contracting, such as lungs, arteries and the uterus.

3. Biochemical Reactions

Enzymes are proteins that aid the thousands of biochemical reactions that take place within and outside cells. The structure of enzymes allows them to combine with other molecules inside the cell called substrates, which catalyze reactions that are essential to metabolism. Enzymes may also function outside the cell, such as digestive enzymes like lactase and sucrase, which help digest sugar. Some enzymes require other molecules, such as vitamins or minerals, for a reaction to take place. Bodily functions that depend on enzymes include

- Digestion
- Energy production
- Blood clotting
- Muscle contraction

4. Hormones

Hormones transmit information between cells, tissues and organs as chemical messengers. They are made and secreted by endocrine tissues or glands and then transported in the blood to their target tissues or organs where they bind to protein receptors on the cell surface. Protein and polypeptides make up most hormones.

Hormones can be grouped into three main categories:

1. Protein and peptides: These are made from chains of amino acids, ranging from a few to several hundred.

2. Steroids: These are made from the fat cholesterol. The sex hormones, testosterone and estrogen, are steroid-based.

3. Amines: These are made from the individual amino acids tryptophan or tyrosine, which help make hormones related to sleep and metabolism.

Some protein hormone examples include:

- *Insulin*: Signals the uptake of glucose or sugar into the cell.
- *Glucagon*: Signals the breakdown of stored glucose in the liver.
- *HGH* (human growth hormone): Stimulates the growth of various tissues, including bone.
- *ADH* (antidiuretic hormone): Signals the kidneys to reabsorb water.
- *ACTH* (adrenocorticotropic hormone): Stimulates the release of cortisol, a key factor in metabolism.

5. Maintain pH

The pH is a measure of whether a substance is acid or alkali. Proteins plays a vital role in regulating the concentrations of acids and bases in the blood and interstitial fluid and other body fluids via a variety of buffering systems.

An example is hemoglobin, a protein in red blood cells which binds small amounts of acid, helping to maintain the normal pH value of the blood. Another major buffer system is the acid-base balance with phosphate and bicarbonate.

6. Fluid Balance

The proteins albumin and globulin in the blood that help maintain the body's fluid balance by attracting and retaining water. Without enough protein, levels of albumin and globulin eventually fall and can no longer keep blood in the blood vessels, and the fluid is forced into the (Interstitial) spaces between cells leading to swelling or oedema. Severe protein malnutrition, as with starving, can be seen in the swollen abdomens of those natives in Africa.

7. Bolsters Immune Health

Proteins help form immunoglobulins, or antibodies, to fight infection. When bacteria or viruses enter cells, the body produces antibodies that tag them for elimination. Without these antibodies, bacteria and viruses would be free to multiply and overwhelm with the disease they cause. Once a person has produced antibodies against a particular bacteria or virus, their cells never forget how to make them which allows the antibodies to respond quickly the next time a particular disease agent invades and immunity against the diseases to which it is exposed is developed.

8. Transports and Stores Nutrients

Transport proteins carry nutrients like vitamins or minerals, blood sugar, cholesterol and oxygen.

- *Hemoglobin* carries oxygen from your lungs to body tissues.
- *Glucose transporters (GLUT)* move glucose to the cells, while lipoproteins transport cholesterol and other fats in the blood.

Protein transporters are specific and will only bind to specific substances.

Storage

- *Ferritin* is a storage protein that stores iron
- *Casein* is the principal protein in milk that helps babies grow.

9. Emergency Energy Supply

Protein can supply energy but as a last resort as this valuable nutrient is widely used throughout your body and carbs and fats are much better suited, metabolizing more efficiently compared to protein.

However, in a state of fasting (18–48 hours of no food intake), your body breaks down skeletal muscle so that the amino acids can supply you with energy. The body also uses amino acids from broken-down skeletal muscle if carbohydrate storage is low. This can occur after exhaustive exercise or if you don't consume enough calories in general.

CHAPTER 17.

CARBOHYDRATES (CARBS / CHOs)

Carbohydrates, "Carbs", are the sugars, starches and fibers found in fruits, grains, vegetables and milk products. They are important to a healthy diet, their primarily function is for fast / instant energy releasing 4 Cal/g and response and their metabolism appears to depend largely on individual response.

The progressive introduction of fast foods has seen *whole-natural-complex* carbs processed to *simple-refined* carbs, and this would seem to be the main problem. They are maligned in fad diets but this is due to these simple processed carbs.

Numerous studies show that eating refined simple processed carbohydrates is associated with health problems like obesity and type 2 diabetes. They tend to cause major spikes in blood sugar levels, which leads to a subsequent crash that can trigger hunger and cravings for more high-carb foods - the "blood sugar roller coaster".

But many studies on high-fiber carbohydrates, including vegetables, fruits, legumes and whole grains revealed improved health.

Many studies have shown that low-carb diets can cause more weight loss and greater improvement in various health markers, including HDL (the "good") cholesterol. For people who are obese or have metabolic syndrome and/or type 2 diabetes, low-carb diets can have life-saving benefits for people with the Metabolic Syndrome and Type 2 Diabetes but they are not the answer for everyone.

Many populations have lived longer and in excellent health on a high-carb diet, such as the Okinawans and Asian rice eaters. Once again it is to be emphasised that these 'primitive' diets were natural complex foods and not fast-processed junk.

Good Carbs: As per Newtrition

Fruits: Eat the whole fruit as its (good) fiber drags through its fructose
Vegetables: Eat a variety of vegetables every day.
Legumes: Lentils-pulses, beans, peas
Nuts: All – a hand-full every day
Seeds: Variety – Chia, pumpkin
Whole grains: Raw oats, quinoa, brown rice, multi-grain bread
Tubers: Sweet potatoes esp. purple, potatoes (cold best)

Bad Carbs:

Sugary drinks: Sugar Sweetened Beverages (SSB): Coca cola, Pepsi etc
Fruit juices: Unfortunately, fruit juices may have similar metabolic effects as sugar-sweetened beverages. Most only contain 2% actual fruit.
White bread:
Pastries, cookies and cakes:
Ice cream: A 50/50 ratio of fat and sugar that does not occur in nature
Candies and chocolates: Dark chocolate >70% cocoa is good. Rest bad.
French fries and potato chips:
Most carbs get broken down or transformed into glucose, which can be used as energy. Carbs can also be turned into fat (stored energy) for later use.

Classification: is by the number of forming units:

- monosaccharides
- oligosaccharides
- polysaccharides

Dietary carbohydrates can be split into three main categories:

1. Sugars: Sweet, short-chain carbohydrates found in foods. Examples are glucose, fructose, galactose and sucrose.
2. Starches: Long chains of glucose molecules, which eventually get broken down into glucose in the digestive system.
3. Fiber: Humans cannot digest fiber, although the bacteria in the digestive system can make use of some of them.

Storage Reservoirs

* Glycogen is the storage form of carbohydrates in mammals in two forms of energy reserves,
    1. glycogen being for short-term stored primarily skeletal muscle and the liver
    2. Triglycerides for long-term stored in body fat
* 70kg Reference Man stores 18 hrs of fuel supply as glycogen
* And 2 months supply as fat
* Glucagon raises Blood Glucose: Insulin lowers it
* Non-digestible part = Fiber (soluble & insoluble)
* Glycaemic Index is how much 50g of carbohydrate raises the BG
* Glycaemic Load is the amount of food needed to contribute 50g

Big human brains needed carbs: Importance of dietary carbohydrate

The Paleo is a diet based on the types of foods presumed to have been eaten by early humans, but it eschews grains and dairy. It is a Low-carbohydrate, high-fat (LCHF) diet. Why humans evolved such large brains is one of the most puzzling issues in the study of human evolution and it is argued that carbohydrate consumption, particularly in the form of starch, was critical for the accelerated expansion of the human brain over the last million years. Eating meat may have kick-started the evolution of bigger brains, but cooked starchy foods together with more salivary amylase genes made us smarter still and the importance of carbohydrate had been largely overlooked.

The following observations build the case for dietary carbohydrate being essential for the evolution of modern big-brained humans:

1. The human brain uses up to 25% of the body's energy budget and up to 60% of blood glucose. While synthesis of glucose from other sources is possible, it is not the most efficient way, and these high glucose demands are unlikely to have been met on a low carbohydrate diet
2. Human pregnancy and lactation place additional demands on the body's glucose budget and low maternal blood glucose levels compromise the health of both the mother and her offspring
3. Starches would have been readily available to ancestral human populations in the form of tubers, seeds and some fruits and nuts
4. While raw starches are often only poorly digested in humans, when cooked they become far more easily digested
5. Salivary amylase genes are usually present in many copies (average 6 in humans, but in only 2 copies in other primates). This increases the amount of

salivary amylase produced and so increases the ability to digest starch. The exact date when salivary amylase genes multiplied remains uncertain, but genetic evidence suggests it was at some point in the last 1 million years

After cooking became widespread, the co-evolution of cooking and higher copy number of the salivary amylase (and possibly pancreatic amylase) genes increased the availability of pre-formed dietary glucose to the brain and fetus, which in turn, permitted the acceleration in brain size increase which occurred from around 800,000 years ago onwards. The better absorption facilitated by cooking also allowed the human gut to shorten dramatically, by a third, without the need to graze and eat all day like the lower primates and animals. Eating meat may have kick-started the evolution of bigger brains, but cooked starchy foods together with more salivary amylase genes made us smarter still.[535]

FIBER OR ROUGHAGE

- Fiber is the skeletal remains of plants that resist digestion (No fiber in meat or fats)
- Fiber consumption reduced by > 55% between 1909 and 1975.
- Daily need = 25 – 35g Maybe up to 50g.
- Present consumption <20g. It is thought we need to eat more
- It is essential for normal gut function with three primary mechanisms: bulking, viscosity and fermentation.
- We need to increase fiber intake; it reduces cholesterol, heart and diverticular disease, diabetes 2, constipation and may reduce risk of the metabolic syndrome and Colorectal Cancer.

* Eat whole fruits instead of juices
* Replace white rice, bread, pasta with brown rice and whole grain
* Choose whole grain cereals if you eat breakfast
* Use raw vegetables for snacks
* Substitute pulses (legumes) for meat two to three times a week

[535] The Importance of Dietary Carbohydrate in Human Evolution. The Quarterly Review of Biology, 2015; 90 (3): 251 DOI: 10.1086/682587

Benefits Overall

* Reduces heart disease, diabetes, diverticulitis, constipation, metabolic syndrome and maybe Colon Cancer
* A study indicated that a radically simple diet that focused solely on increasing fiber intake to at least 30g/day might be nearly as beneficial as a more traditional, complex diet. Americans now average only 16g/day of fiber, and just 7% of adults between ages 40 and 59 consume 30 g/day or more. 240 adults with metabolic syndrome were randomized to the multicomponent American Heart Association (AHA) diet or this Higher Fiber diet and the results were essentially the same.[536]
* Diet rich in fiber, esp. water soluble, reduces risk of CVD
* A high fiber diet cf low had a 40% lower risk of coronary heart disease in a 40,000 study of men[537]
* Cereal fiber seemed more beneficial and lowered women's risk of CHD[538]
* Consumption of fiber from cereals & fruit is inversely related to risk of CHD[539]
* Delays absorption of CHO and lowers total & LDL cholesterol[540]

Classification

1. Insoluble Fiber: Best source are 1. Vegetables 45%, cereals 35%, fruit 20% Bran (wheat, corn, rice) skins of fruit & veg, nuts, seeds, dried beans, whole grains or whole wheat, wheat bran, corn bran, seeds, nuts, barley, couscous, brown rice, bulgur, zucchini, celery, broccoli, cabbage, onions, tomatoes, carrots, cucumbers, green beans, dark leafy vegetables, raisins, grapes, fruit, and root vegetable skins. Insoluble fiber is associated with reduced diabetes risk. One type of insoluble dietary fiber, resistant starch has been shown to directly increase insulin sensitivity in healthy people, in type 2 diabetics and in individuals with insulin resistance, possibly contributing to reduced risk of type 2 diabetes

2. Soluble Fiber: Fruits, veg, oat bran, barley, husks, flaxseed, psyllium, dried beans, peas, soy, nuts, seeds, lentils, citrus fruits, apples, strawberries, and carrots or oatmeal, oat cereal, oranges, pears, flaxseeds, beans, dried peas, blueberries, cucumbers, celery. Soluble fiber causes increased production of an

---

536 *Ann Intern Med.* 2015;162(4):248-257. doi:10.7326/M14-0611

537 Rimm EB et al, Vegetable, fruit and cereal fiber intake and risk of coronary heart disease among men. JAMA, 1996; 275:447-51

538 Brown L, et al, Cholesterol-lowering effects of dietary fiber: a meta-analysis. AmJ Clin nutr. 1999;69:30-42

539 Arch Int Med 2004;164:370-76

540 Arch Int Med 2003;163:1897-1904

anti-inflammatory protein interleukin-4, that helps us recover faster from infection with positive changes in the immune system.

Some soluble fibers bind to bile acids making them less likely to re-enter the body, which in turn lowers cholesterol levels. Viscous soluble fibers may also attenuate the absorption of sugar, reduce sugar response after eating, normalize blood lipid levels and, once fermented in the colon, produce short-chain fatty acids with wide-ranging physiological activities.

3. *Resistant starch* is readily fermented by gut microbes to produce beneficial molecules called short-chain fatty acids, such as butyrate. Good examples of natural sources of resistant starch include bananas that are still slightly green, cooked and cooled potatoes (such as potato salad), whole grains, beans, chickpeas, and lentils. Consumption of resistant starch that acts like fiber may help reduce colorectal cancer risk associated with a high red meat diet.[541]

A fiber-rich diet may reduce the risk of developing type 2 diabetes by 18%. Cereal fiber emerged as the strongest protector against diabetes, compared with vegetable fiber and fruit fiber.[542]

When I was a medical student Dr Denis Burkitt, an Irish Surgeon, was collecting and weighing the faeces of natives in Africa and while this led to some raised eyebrows, he pointed out in one study that people back in England who ate very low levels of fiber—less than 10 grams per day—had an 18% higher risk of colorectal cancer (CaC). There have been considerable studies done subsequently. Some studies have shown an association of higher fiber intake with a reduction in colon cancer. Others have not. Unfortunately, most of these studies both for and against seem to have been well-designed and provide valid trials. I will only list two of the many. As you can see the gut microbiome may be the key. Be that as it may I feel gut transit time is also important - see next section. In any event a high fiber intake is certainly of more benefit than a low intake.

---

[541] Dietary Manipulation of Oncogenic MicroRNA Expression in Human Rectal Mucosa: A Randomized Trial. Cancer Prevention Research, 2014; 7 (8): 786 DOI: 10.1158/1940-6207.CAPR-14-0053

[542] Diabetologia Source Reference: The InterAct Consortium "Dietary fiber and incidence of type 2 diabetes in eight European countries: the EPIC-InterAct Study and a meta-analysis of prospective studies" Diabetologia 2015; DOI: 10.1007/s00125-015-3585-9.

- A meta-analysis found there was a 10% reduction in risk of colorectal cancer for each 10 g/day intake of total dietary fiber and cereal fiber and about a 20% reduction for each three servings (90 g/day) of whole grain daily, and further reductions with higher intake. It was also suggested that there was a particular benefit of increasing cereal fiber and whole grain intake. Increasing the intake of dietary fiber and whole grains is also likely to reduce the risk of cardiovascular disease, type 2 diabetes, overweight and obesity, and possibly overall mortality, thus there are several health benefits by increasing fiber intake and replacing refined grains with whole grains.[543]
- A high-fiber diet, however, does not seem to protect against colon cancer, unless you have the right gut bacteria, a study in mice suggests. In the study, mice were fed a high-fiber diet and some had a type of bacteria in their gut that ferments fiber into a chemical called butyrate and they had 75% less tumors. However, the high-fiber diet by itself, without the butyrate-producing bacteria, did not protect against colon cancer; nor did a low-fiber diet with butyrate-producing bacteria[544].

Food gut transit time: A key factor in digestive health

Early in writing this series I expressed the simplistic opinion that the longer any foreign object is in contact with human tissue, the greater the chance for irritation and, in the case of the gut, I suggested that the longer the transit time the greater the chance for irritation then inflammation and gut reaction and thus cancer. From the above it can be seen the many articles that refute my simplistic but clinical observations. Now a study from Denmark supports my contention:

"We find that a long colonic transit time associates with high microbial richness and is accompanied by a shift in colonic metabolism from carbohydrate fermentation to protein catabolism as reflected by higher urinary levels of potentially deleterious protein-derived metabolites. Additionally, shorter colonic transit time correlates with metabolites possibly reflecting increased renewal of the colonic mucosa. Together, this suggests that a high gut microbial richness does not *per se* imply a healthy gut microbial ecosystem."[545]

The more complete explanation follows but this study which concurs with my own I suggest, is only a matter of common sense.

"In short, the longer food takes to pass through the colon, the more harmful

543 BMJ 2011;343:d6617 doi: 10.1136/bmj.d6617
544 Why a High-Fiber Diet Prevents Cancer. Sci. Signal. 8, ec8 (2015)
545 *Nature Microbiology* 1, Article number: 16093 (2016) doi:10.1038/nmicrobiol.2016.93

bacterial degradation products are produced. Conversely, when the transit time is shorter, we find a higher amount of the substances that are produced when the colon renews its inner surface, which may be a sign of a healthier intestinal wall".

The time it takes for ingested food to travel through the human gut – also called transit time – affects the amount of harmful degradation products produced along the way. This means that transit time is a key factor in a healthy digestive system. Food has to travel through eight meters of intestine from the time it enters the mouth of an adult until it comes out the other end. Recent research has focused mainly on the influence of the bacterial composition of the gut on the health of people's digestive system.

The effect of food's transit time

Intestinal bacteria prefer to digest dietary carbohydrates, but when these are depleted, the bacteria start to break down other nutrients such as proteins and the resultant degradation products have been associated with the development of various diseases including colorectal cancer, chronic renal disease and autism.

Better understanding of constipation as a risk factor

The study shows that transit time is a key factor in the activity of the intestinal bacteria, and this emphasizes the importance of preventing constipation, which may have an impact on health. This is highly relevant in Denmark where up to as much as 20% of the population suffers from constipation from time to time and where constipation is considered a risk factor, such as colorectal cancer and Parkinson's disease as well as afflictions where constipation often occurs such as ADHD and autism.

Influencing food's transit time

People's dietary habits can influence transit time:

You can help food pass through the colon by eating a diet rich in fiber and drinking plenty of water. It may also be worth trying to limit the intake of for example meat, which slows down the transit time and provides the gut bacteria with lots of protein to digest. Physical activity can also reduce the time it takes for food to travel through the colon.[546]

---

[546] Colonic transit time is related to bacterial metabolism and mucosal turnover in the gut. *Nature Microbiology*, 2016; 1: 16093 DOI: 10.1038/nmicrobiol.2016.93

The importance of the "quality of the intestinal bacteria" and the impact that this has on the fermentation of malabsorbed carbohydrates has now been recognized. A new hypothesis is that it is early priming that gives the African a more robust gut microflora, better able to withstand the insults in adult life. The corollary is also that if we expect fiber and oligosaccharides that are promoted as prebiotics to enhance the proliferation of 'good bacteria', we have to start feeding these substrates to our gut in the early years of life.

CHAPTER 18.

FATS and OILS

Fatty acids are the chemical compounds that make up fats. They are abundant in animal tissues, as they are the major component of cellular membranes and have vital functions in nearly every metabolic action within the body. Fats can be solid or oils.

- Most commonly they are found in carbon chains of 16-18 carbons (C) with several double bonds making them polyunsaturated.
- What we all understand as 'fats' are Fatty Acids which are derived from triglycerides or phospholipids
- Energy rich 9 Cal / g for long-term storage
- Stored as adipose tissue for energy, as protection for organs & subcutaneous for insulation
- Famine quality. Fat deposits allowed weeks / months survival
- Humans don't recognize excess so keep eating it.
- Food manufacturers use fat to impart textural enhancement
- Low-fat diets did not seem to confer any CVS or anti-cancer (breast/colon) benefits[547]
- New diet recommendations do not restrict eating fat
- Fat is stored in our bodies as adipose tissue under the skin (sub-cutaneous) and around our organs (visceral and brown fat) and as triglycerides within skeletal muscle fibers.

Classification

Classification is according to the presence and number of double bonds in their carbon chain.

1. **Saturated (SFA)** : no double bonds
2. **Monosaturated (MUFA) or 9:** one double bond
3. **Polyunsaturated (PUFA) or 6:** more than one double bond

---

547 JAMA 2006;295:629-42

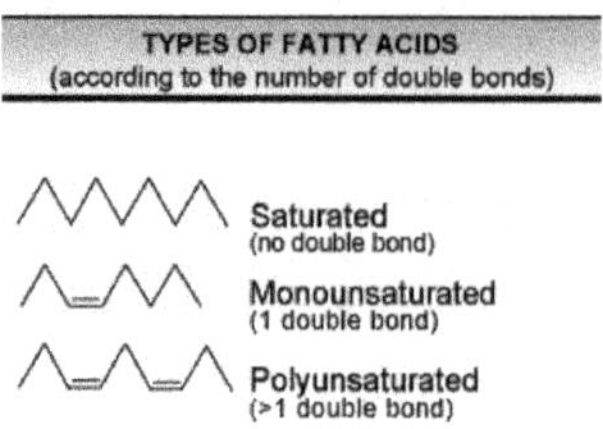

Unsaturated can also be classified as "*cis*" (bent) or "*trans*" (straight).

The further classification of fats is complicated, to say the least.

Essentially what we all have to know for our health is what fats are good and what are bad.

Fat is perhaps the most diverse class of dietary macronutrients in regards to nutritional value and physiological effects. It used to be thought that Unsaturated fat was good and Saturated fat was bad and Trans-fat very bad. Now there has been more research such that some fatty acids in saturated fats may be beneficial while some in unsaturated fats may be harmful.

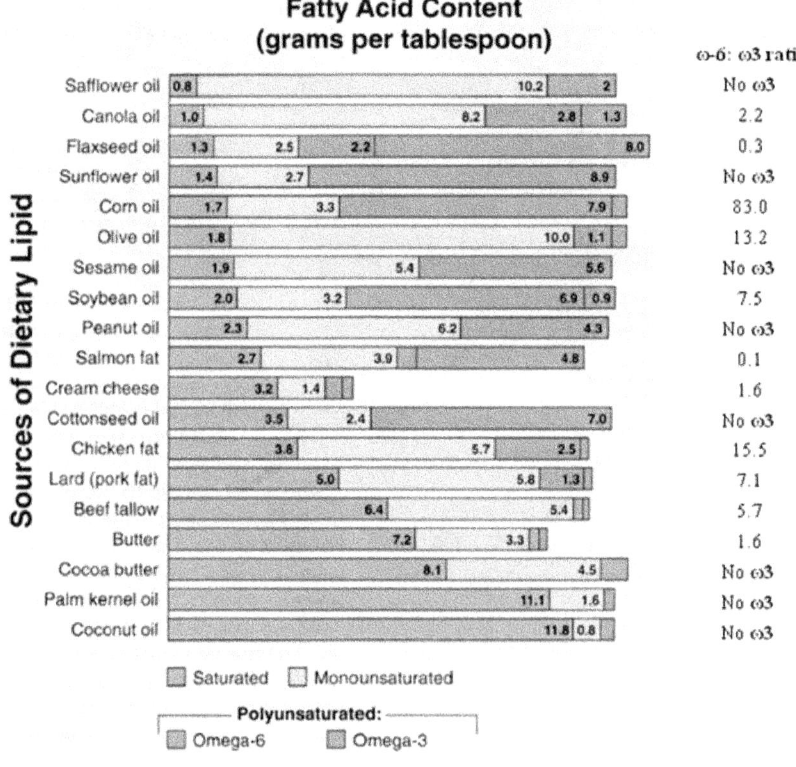

Saturated (SFA) = no double bonds
solid at room temperature
butter, lard, palm oil, the fat in meats

Unsaturated Also identified by the Greek letter **Omega** or Ω or **ω**

Mono-saturated = **Omega-9** (or n-9) fatty acids
first double bond at the ninth carbon atom mainly oleic acid (Olive oil), canola, avocado, peanut

Polyunsaturated = **Omega-6** (or n-6) fatty acids

first double bond at the sixth carbon atom Vegetable oils linoleic acid (LA) and its derivative arachidonic acid (AA).

Omega-3 (or n-3) fatty acids
first double bond at the third carbon atom alpha-linolenic acid (ALA) and its derivatives eicosapentaenoic acid (EPA) and docosahexaenoic acid (DHA).

There are two dietary sources:
1.EPA and DHA are primarily found in fish, such as salmon, tuna, and anchovies.
2.Alpha-linolenic acid (ALA) is plant-based and an essential omega-3 fatty acid that must be obtained through the diet.
Canola, flaxseeds, nuts, soya, meat, dairy.

Fatty acids are often described based on the length (number of carbon atoms), the number of double bonds and the omega class to which they belong e.g:

1. Linoleic acid (LA): C18:2 n-6, indicating that it has 18 carbon atoms, 2 double bonds and belongs to the omega-6 fatty acid family.

2. Alpha linolenic acid (ALA): C18:3 n-3, has 18 carbon atoms, 3 double bonds and belongs to the omega-3 fatty acid family.

Common name	Symbol (*)	Typical dietary source
SATURATED FATTY ACIDS		
Butyric	C4:0	Butterfat
Caprylic	C8:0	Palm kernel oil
Capric	C10:0	Coconut oil
Lauric	C12:0	Coconut oil
Myristic	C14:0	Butterfat, coconut oil
Palmitic	C16:0	Most fats and oils
Stearic	C18:0	Most fats and oils
Arachidic	C20:0	Lard, peanut oil
MONOUNSATURATED FATTY ACIDS		
Palmitoleic	C16:1 n-7	Most fats and oils
Oleic	C18:1 n-9 (cis)	Most fats and oils
Elaidic	C18:1 n-9 (trans)	Hydrogenated vegetable oils, butterfat, beef fat
POLYUNSATURATES PUFA		
Linoleic	C18:2 n-6 (all cis)	Most vegetable oils
Alpha-linolenic	C18:3 n-3 (all cis)	Soybean oil, canola/rapeseed oil
Gamma-linolenic	C18:3 n-6	Blackcurrant seed oil, borage oil, evening primrose oil
Arachidonic	C20:4 n-6 (all cis)	Pork fat, poultry fat
Eicosapentaenoic	C20:5 n-3 (all cis)	Fish oils
Docosahexaenoic	C22:6 n-3 (all cis)	Fish oils

Most natural fats are a combination of all of these, saturated and unsaturated.

	Saturated	Mono-unsaturated	Poly-unsaturated	Cholesterol
	g/100g	g/100g	g/100g	mg/100g
Animal fats				
Lard	40.8	43.8	9.6	93
Duck fat	33.2	49.3	12.9	100
Butter	54.0	19.8	2.6	230
Vegetable fats				
Coconut oil	85.2	6.6	1.7	0
Cocoa butter	60.0	32.9	3.0	0
Palm kernel oil	81.5	11.4	1.6	0
Palm oil	45.3	41.6	8.3	0
Cottonseed oil	25.5	21.3	48.1	0
Wheat germ oil	18.8	15.9	60.7	0
Soybean oil	14.5	23.2	56.5	0
Olive oil	14.0	69.7	11.2	0
Corn oil	12.7	24.7	57.8	0
Sunflower oil	11.9	20.2	63.0	0
Safflower oil	10.2	12.6	72.1	0
Hemp oil	10	15	75	0
Canola/Rapeseed oil	5.3	64.3	24.8	0

It can be seen that olive oil has the greatest amount of monosaturates. It was thought that canola / rape oil also high in monosaturates would also improve cardiovascular disease but in one study it did not.

Overall, canola oil would appear to have the most balanced fatty acid composition, but there are reservations:

It was originally Rape Seed used as a ship's lubricant in WW2. After that the Canadians were desperate to find another market and rapeseed oil extracts were first put on the market in 1956–1957 as food products, but these suffered from several unacceptable characteristics, a distinctive taste and a disagreeable greenish color, due to the presence of chlorophyll. So, they modified the chemical composition by reducing the erucic acid and this new oil was called "Canola", a condensation of "Can" from Canada and "OLA " meaning "Oil, low acid" has been tested as safe for human use.

However, almost all Canola is chemically extracted with hexane and, if you want to use it, make sure you get some that is guaranteed "cold-pressed".

Olive oil, although moderately high in the omega-6 : omega-3 ratio, also contains a high percentage of monounsaturated fat. Most importantly, olive oil also contains a high amount of antioxidants and the substance squalene that has been shown to have anti-cancer effects. The PREDIMED Study also found it was beneficial for the heart.

Fatty fish such as salmon are excellent sources of omega-3. Flaxseed oil is also a rich source of omega-3 but not for EPA and DHA.

While the use of omega 6 PUFAs is credited with lowering the epidemic of heart disease, beware, Western societies get almost 70% of their omega-6 from packaged biscuits and pastries (made with shortening which is any fat that is a solid at room temperature i.e. saturated, and used to make crumbly pastry), margarine, French fries (cooked in vegetable oil), and processed, high-sugar, high-vegetable oil junk food and just 6% from beans, seeds, and nuts, 1% from eggs and 13% from meat.

And much of this oil, especially in restaurants, fast food outlets and industries, and not just in Western societies, is reheated and used a number of times with increasing detrimental by-products.

Oils Ain't Oils

The Italian olive oil industry was making more money, from adulterating olive oil and re-labeling it as "pure" "Extra-Virgin Olive Oil", than from dealing cocaine. That was a couple of decades ago and I don't know if it has changed.

But the latest scam is "Fish Oil" and its many manifestation such as "Krill" and such. Firstly, even if they contained the actual fish oil they claimed, it doesn't do much good, if any, whereas actual oily fish do donate benefits. Secondly, most comes from fish caught off Peru and Chile and then sent in tankers, progressively being oxidized and becoming rancid on the way, to China, where samples of the capsules reveal most don't even contain the amounts their labels state let alone the dubious state of the oxidized-rancid contents.

Don't take fish-oil supplements and research the supplier of any olive oil.

Higher Consumption of Saturated Linked with Higher Mortality

The health effects of specific types of fats depend on what people were replacing them with. People who replaced saturated fats with unsaturated fats -- especially polyunsaturated fats--had significantly lower risk of death overall, as well as lower risk of death from CVD, cancer, neurodegenerative disease, and respiratory disease, compared with those who maintained high intakes of saturated fats. The findings for cardiovascular disease are consistent with many earlier studies showing reduced total and LDL ("bad") cholesterol when unsaturated fats replace trans or saturated fats.

A recent American Heart Association advisory, written by Lichtenstein and colleagues and published in the journal Circulation, analyzed a number of studies examining what happens when people replace saturated fat with unsaturated fat. Several studies, including the Oslo Diet-Heart Study and studies conducted at the Veterans Administration center in Los Angeles, provided evidence that replacing saturated fat with polyunsaturated fat lowers the risk of heart attack, stroke, and angina. The authors of the advisory concluded that replacing foods high in saturated fat like butter, meat, and coconut oil with polyunsaturated fat-rich vegetable oils such as soybean and corn oils* could lower rates of CVD by about 30 percent. Replacing foods high in saturated fat with monounsaturated-rich vegetable oils such as canola and olive oils was found to be associated with a 15 percent lower rate of CVD.

*As noted, Newtrition recommends replace with EVOO

People who replaced saturated fats with refined carbohydrates had only slightly lower mortality risk. In addition, replacing total fat with carbohydrates was associated with modestly higher mortality. This was not surprising because refined starch and sugar, have a similar influence on mortality risk as saturated fats. The study included 126,233 participants from two large long-term studies -- the Nurses' Health Study and the Health Professionals Follow-Up Study -- who answered survey questions every 2-4 years about their diet, lifestyle, and health for up to 32 years. The study is the most detailed and powerful examination to date on how dietary fats impact health.

Replacing saturated fats like butter, lard, and fat in red meat with unsaturated fats from plant-based foods -- like cold pressed olive oil -- can confer substantial health benefits.[548]

Since 1950 or thereabouts, certainly for the last 40 years, the advice has been to reduce saturated fat while boosting unsaturated fats, usually with plant or fish oils. This has recently been challenged in that eating high saturated fat or cholesterol foods does not seem to raise our blood cholesterol, which has been shown to be associated with CVD and heart attacks. Nevertheless, by reducing ingestion of saturated fat and changing to polyunsaturated oils, heart disease has dropped dramatically. This may be due to better diagnosis and the use of statins but, as above, there are good, bad and ugly fats. All fats and oils contain saturated,

[548] Specific Dietary Fats in Relation to Total and Cause-Specific Mortality. JAMA Internal Medicine, July 5, 2016 DOI: 10.1001/jamainternmed.2016.2417

polyunsaturated and monosaturated fats in various ratios and different types of the many 16 or so different fatty acids in our diets. It is unknown which fatty acids, or which ratios or which combinations are good for us or bad for us but in an impressive study Olive Oil lowered the risk of cardiovascular disease whereas in another Canola / Rape Oil, considered a viable alternative, did not.[549]

New research has found there are striking differences in the accumulation of saturated and unsaturated fatty acids in cardiac muscle cells (cardiomyocytes). Saturated fatty acids are toxic to cardiomyocytes and induce the death of these cells through endoplasmic reticulum stress (ER stress), a cellular process known to be involved in the development of many diseases and this validates a critical role for saturated fatty acids in the development of heart diseases. In stark contrast, unsaturated fatty acids are not only harmless but also provide protection against the damage done by saturated fatty acids.[550]

Essential Fatty Acids (EFAs)

These two are critical as humans cannot make them and they must be obtained from food.

1. Alpha-Lenolenic (ALA) - omega 3

   ALA, the most common omega-3 fat, is not biologically active until it's converted into EPA or DHA. This conversion is inefficient from plants and obtaining EPA and DHA is best from fatty fish and other seafoods.
2. Lenoleic (omega 6)

Increasing the amount of omega-3s in your diet, whether from fish or flax, will likely decrease your risk of getting heart disease. A substantial amount of evidence exists supporting the heart-health benefits of eicosapentaenoic acid (EPA) and docosahexaenoic acid (DHA), marine-derived omega-3 fatty acids, but alpha-linolenic acid (ALA), a plant-based omega-3 fatty acid is likely just as effective as EPA and DHA have proven to be. ALA is found in flaxseed, chia,

---

[549] Impact of a 6-wk olive oil supplementation in healthy adults on urinary proteomic biomarkers of coronary artery disease, chronic kidney disease, and diabetes (types 1 and 2): a randomized, parallel, controlled, double-blind study. First published November 19, 2014, doi: 10.3945/ ajcn.114.094219 Am J Clin Nutr ajcn.094219

[550] Saturated fatty acids induce endoplasmic reticulum stress in primary cardiomyocytes, Endoplasmic Reticulum Stress in Diseases. Endoplasmic Reticulum Stress in Diseases, Volume 2, Issue 1, 2015 DOI: 10.1515/ersc-2015-0004

walnuts, canola, soya and is now available in supplement form and fortified foods.[551]

Recent analyses of fish oil capsules in both New Zealand and USA have found these do not contain the amount of fish oils advertised and most is oxidized and rancid. Obtaining Omega-3s from plant foods is advised.

TYPE	SHORT	FULL NAME	DIET SOURCE
Omega-3	ALA	a-Linolenic	Flax, Olive, Canola Oils
	EPA	Eicosapentaenoic	Fish, algae
	DHA	Docosahexaenoic	Fish, algae
Omega-6	LA	Linoleic	Corn, safflower, Sunflower, Soya, Peanut oils
	AA	Arachidonic	Meat, dairy, Eggs

The most common omega-3 fatty acids in the human diet are ALA, EPA, and DHA while the most common omega-6 fatty acids are LA and AA.

Adequate amounts of omega-6 fatty acids are beneficial to human health since many bioactive signaling molecules, especially ones involved in immune response and cardiomyocyte (muscle cells) contraction, are derived from them. However, omega-6 fatty acids tend to be over-supplied while omega-3 fatty acids are under-supplied in Western diets due to industrialized food oil production. This overwhelming intake of omega-6 leads to hyperimmune responses and interferes with the proper function of omega-3 fatty acids, causing detrimental effects associated with chronic cardiovascular diseases and inflammatory responses.

High omega-6 levels can protect against premature death552

Linoleic acid (LA) is the most common polyunsaturated omega-6 fatty acid and the higher the blood linoleic acid level, the smaller the risk of premature death.

Although omega-6 polyunsaturated fatty acids are known for their beneficial effect on blood cholesterol levels, it has been speculated that they may increase the risk of several chronic diseases by promoting low-grade inflammation, among other things. The reasoning behind this speculation is that in the human body,

[551] The Evidence for -Linolenic Acid and Cardiovascular Disease Benefits: Comparisons with Eicosapentaenoic Acid and Docosahexaenoic Acid. Advances in Nutrition: An International Review Journal, 2014; 5 (6): 863S DOI: 10.3945/an.114.005850
[552] American Journal of Clinical Nutrition, julkaistu internetissä 16.3.2018
Linkki artikkeliin: https://academic.oup.com/ajcn/article-abstract/107/3/427/4939343
DOI: https://doi.org/10.1093/ajcn/nqx063

linoleic acid is converted into arachidonic acid (also an omega-6 fatty acid) which, in turn, is converted into various inflammation-promoting compounds. However, omega-6 fatty acids also increase the production of anti-inflammatory compounds.

The risk of premature death was 43% lower in the group with the highest level, when compared to the group with the lowest level. A more detailed analysis of the causes of death showed that a similar association exists for death due to cardiovascular diseases, as well as for death due to some other reason than cardiovascular diseases or cancer. However, no association was observed for death due to cancer. Similar, although slightly weaker, associations were also observed for the blood arachidonic acid level.

Another significant finding of the study is that the outcome is very similar regardless of whether the study participants suffered from cardiovascular diseases, cancer or diabetes at the onset of the study.

A higher dietary intake of linoleic acid and a higher blood linoleic acid level results in a smaller risk of cardiovascular diseases and type 2 diabetes, without increasing the risk of cancer. The observed association of arachidonic acid with a reduced risk of death is a new finding.

The blood linoleic acid level is determined by a person's diet, and the main sources of linoleic acid are vegetable oils, plant-based spreads, nuts and seeds. However, a person's diet will affect his or her blood arachidonic acid level only a little.

The 'Linoleic acid theory of coronary heart disease'[553]

Dietary linoleic acid, especially when consumed from refined omega-6 vegetable oils, gets incorporated into all blood lipoproteins (such as LDL, VLDL and HDL) increasing the susceptibility of all lipoproteins to oxidise and hence increases cardiovascular risk. The most prevalent fatty acid in LDL is linoleic acid.

The intake of omega-6 vegetable oils, particularly soybean oil, began to increase in the USA starting in the early 1900s at a time when the consumption of butter and lard was on the decline. This caused a more than two-fold increase in the intake of linoleic acid, the main omega-6 polyunsaturated fat found in vegetable oils, which now makes up around 8% to 10% of total energy intake in the Western

---

[553] BMJ Open Heart. 2018:5(2): e000898.

world. Linoleic acid concentration in subcutaneous adipose tissue in the USA revealed an approximate 2.5-fold increase.

The amount of linoleic acid in adipose tissue, but also in platelets, is positively associated with coronary artery disease (CAD), whereas long-chain omega-3 (eicosapentaenoic acid (EPA) and docosahexaenoic acid (DHA)) levels in platelets are inversely related to CAD. This provides rather compelling evidence that omega-3s protect whereas omega-6 linoleic acid promotes heart disease.

Authors comment:

Despite this 'compelling evidence' (that "omega-6 linoleic acid promotes heart disease") the increased use of vegetable oils saw heart disease drop. But this Linoleic Acid Theory is interesting. My take on it is that soya bean oil, the most used oil in the USA, has, as below, more polyunsaturated F.A. than any other. Furthermore, as it was and is mostly used in commercial foods it is most likely *not cold pressed* and thus more likely to have the bad oxidized form of Linoleic Acid.

From the graph below, it can be seen Olive Oil has the least polyunsaturated content (and the highest monosaturate) and, hedging my bets, I always use Extra Virgin Olive Oil (EVOO) which is cold-pressed.

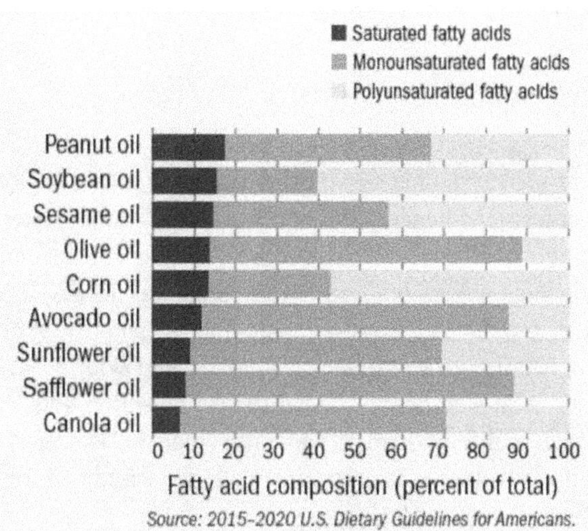

Source: 2015-2020 U.S. Dietary Guidelines for Americans.

The Effects of Omega 3 & 6s on Chronic Diseases

Chronic Disease	Risk factors	Comments	Omega-3	Omega-6
Cardiovasc. Disease	Arrhythmias	Sudden death	Reduces	Increases
	Thrombosis	Heart attack Stroke	Reduces	Increases
	Atheroma	Plaque	Reduces	Increases
	HDL	Good	Increases	Lowers
	LDL	Bad	Lowers	Increases
	Triglycerides		Lowers	Increases
Inflammatory Response	Interlukin IL-1	Inflammatory	Lowers	Increases
	Interlukin IL-6	Inflammatory	Lowers	Increases
	CRP	Inflammatory	Lowers	Increases

Omega 3[554]

Taking supplements of Omega 3s was not associated with significantly reduced risk of:

* Death from coronary heart disease
* Nonfatal myocardial infarction
* Any coronary heart disease events
* Major vascular events

Benefits also weren't seen in subgroups with prior coronary heart disease, diabetes, elevated lipid levels, or statin use.

The Omega-6:Omega-3 Ratio Theory[555]

Due to the opposing effects of omega-3 and omega-6 fatty acids, a healthy diet should contain a balanced omega-6: omega-3 ratio. Human beings evolved eating a diet with an omega-6: omega-3 ratio of about 1:1. Modern Western diets exhibit ratios ranging between 15:1 to 20:1, or more. Studies have concluded that while an exceptionally high omega-6:omega-3 ratio promotes the development of many chronic diseases, a reduced omega-6:omega-3 ratio can prevent or reverse these diseases. For example, a ratio of 4:1 was associated with a 70% reduction in mortality in secondary coronary heart disease prevention and a ratio of 2.5:1 reduced rectal cell proliferation in patients with colorectal cancer. A lower omega-6: omega-3 ratio in women was associated with decreased risk for breast cancer.

---

554 "Associations of omega-3 fatty acid supplement use with cardiovascular disease risks: Meta-analysis of 10 trials involving 77,917 individuals" JAMA Cardiol 2018; DOI:10.1001/jamacardio.2017.5205.

555 GB Health Watch

A ratio of 2:1–3:1 suppressed inflammation in patients with rheumatoid arthritis, and a ratio of 5:1 had a beneficial effect on patients with asthma, whereas a ratio of 10:1 had adverse consequences.

People in the U.S. and Western societies generally eat loads of corn oil and other vegetable oils high in omega-6. Soy and corn oils alone make up almost a third of USA calories. In centuries past, the amount of omega-6 we ate was much lower, with a ratio of around 4:1 omega-6 to omega-3 but as cheap vegetable oils became prominent in the middle of the 20th century, the ratio has increased, all the way up to the current ratio of around 15:1. While people occasionally make a tiny dent in their omega 6:3 ratio by eating fish, the main driver of this skewed ratio is ubiquitous and cheap vegetable oils.

One of the strongest predictors of heart disease is tissue omega-6 to omega-3 ratio, which can be estimated by a blood test. Western Societies typically have three times more omega-6 than omega-3 in their tissues, which is the reverse of what is optimal. Japanese and Mediterranean populations have far lower ratios, and also happen to have lower heart disease rates and longer lifespans. While this cannot prove causation, it's clear that eating high-PUFA oils such as corn oil is not necessary for optimal health and may very well be detrimental. Too much omega-6 compared to omega-3 is linked to a variety of chronic conditions. Some of that may be due to inflammation, but the exact mechanisms aren't fully understood. Studies have shown that a reduction in omega-6 fats is a primary factor in reaching a healthy omega-3 intake that can curb chronic disease. Coupled with the findings showing that PUFA is easily oxidized, along with the fact that omega-6 competes with omega-3s within our bodies, there does not seem to be much reason to purposely choose corn or vegetable PUFA-6 oils as a kitchen staple.

Certain plant foods contain fat, such as olives and avocado. You can taste the fat and quite easily press it out of the plant. Other plants aren't so high in fat, like corn. To get the fat out of corn, you have to bathe it in a hexane bath and chemically extract the fat, bleach and deodorize it. It turns out that processing corn for fat can make it a bit rancid. This is because corn oil is high in PUFAs, which are easily oxidized due to their chemical structures containing multiple double bonds. After purchasing it, cooking with corn oil can make it even more rancid. Oxidized PUFA can be dangerous when in our bodies, especially since oxidative damage to fat-containing LDL particles is a primary factor in the development of heart disease. And an omega-6 rich diet greatly increases oxidized LDL levels. The more PUFA we eat, the more that accumulates in our bodies' adipose tissue. Hence, we have more than double the linoleic acid in our body fat as do our parents' generation, and fatty acid turnover in adipose tissue can take years. So you may feel the health effects of your diet from the past year or two, even if you switch to a healthier diet.[556]

Omega-3 and omega-6 fatty acids compete for the same enzymes to produce eicosanoids and DHA-derived signaling molecules with opposing physiological functions. While omega-6 derived signaling molecules are pro-inflammatory, omega-3 derived are anti-inflammatory. Moreover, omega-3 and omega-6 fatty acids also compete to incorporate into cell membranes, directly impacting the function of the membrane. The opposing effects of omega-3 and omega-6 fatty acids lead to the omega-6: omega-3 ratio theory.

Summary

Based on evidence from studies on the evolutionary aspects of diet, modern day hunter-gatherers, and traditional diets, the omega-6:omega-3 ratio theory proposes that the genetic makeup of human beings is adapted to a diet in which the ratio of omega-6:omega-3 was about 1:1. In today's Western diets the ratio is 15:1 to 17:1. Many of the chronic conditions—cardiovascular disease, diabetes, cancer, obesity, autoimmune diseases, rheumatoid arthritis, asthma and depression—are associated with increased production of factors (thromboxane A2 (TXA2), leukotriene B4 (LTB4), IL-1β, IL-6, TNF and CRP) due to the high ratio of omega-6:omega-3 in dietary fat that is incompatible to our genetic makeup.

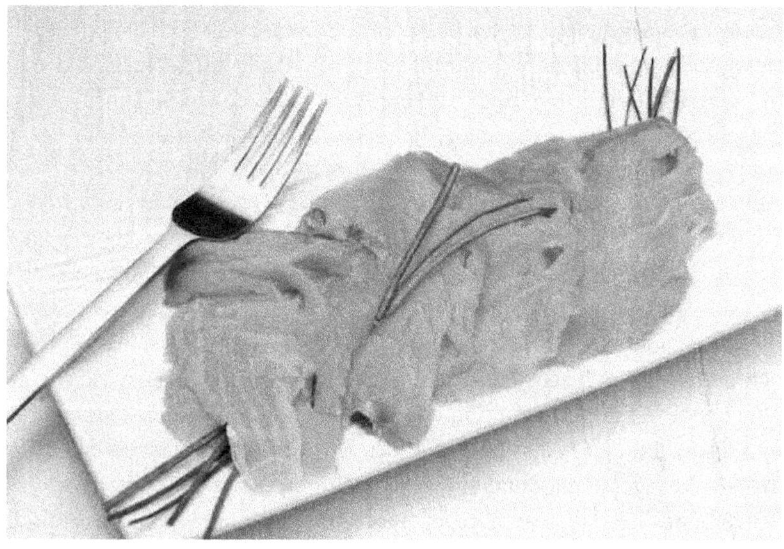

[556] MEDPAGE TODAY Wednesday, April 15, 2015 vascular function but does not affect oxidative stress markers or lipid levels. *Free Radical Research*, 2014; 48 (5): 599 DOI: 10.3109/10715762.2014.896458

Therefore, reducing your omega-6:omega-3 ratio to roughly 1:1 by including healthy oils or an omega-3 dietary supplement in your diet can help promote optimal health.

Oily fish, such as Salmon is excellent.

Further Information

Healthy ratios of omega-6: omega-3, according to some authors, range from 1:1 to 1:4. Others believe that ratio 4:1 (omega-6 is 4 times more than omega-3) is already healthy. Studies suggest the evolutionary human diet, rich in game animals, seafood, and other sources of omega-3, may have provided such a ratio.

Typical Western diets provide ratios in the range of 10:1 to 30:1 (i.e., dramatically higher levels of omega-6 than omega-3). The ratios of omega-6 to omega-3 fatty acids in some common vegetable oils are: canola 2:1, hemp 2-3:1, soybean 7:1, olive 3–13:1, sunflower (no omega-3), flax 1:3, cottonseed (almost no omega-3), peanut (no omega-3), grape seed oil (almost no omega-3) and corn oil 46:1 ratio of omega-6 to omega-3.

Polyunsaturated Vegetable Oils vs 'Super'-unsaturated Fish Oils

- Our modern diet usually has 8 to 14 times more Omega 6 (Vegetable Oils) than Omega 3 ('Fish' Oils) by some 14:1
- Our Omega 3 (fish/soy) consumption has decreased to 1/6th of what was in our food in 1850 while our Omega 6 (safflower, corn oils) consumption has doubled
- It is thought the early Palaeolithic / Hunter Gatherer Diet ratio was more 1:1

What is healthy **Veg : Fish Oil Ratio**

- The Inuit (Eskimo) =1 : 1.25 very low rate of heart attacks
- Traditional = 6 : 1
- Today = 20 : 1 present day vegetable oil diets
- Best estimate for health = 3 : 1
- We should try and reduce our PUFA 6 : SUFA 3 ratio from the current 20:1 to 3:1

This 3:1 ratio is found naturally in Hemp oil. It is said to taste 'nutty and good and free from the objectionable undertones of flax (linseed) oil'. Cannabis / Marijuana is a strain of hemp but there is no psycho-activity in nutritional hemp oil which is legal to use. Linseed (flax) does not taste good and needs to be super-fresh.

However

The evidence for a high omega 3 to 6 level is weak and a large study of many countries found high omega 6 of more benefit than omega 3.[557]

Omega 3 supplements (fish oil capsules etc) cannot be recommended especially as most have been found not to contain the amounts of omega-3 they claim on their labels.[558]

Get Cold Pressed

Most vegetable oils are "refined". This means they are chemically extracted using a solvent called hexane, then go through stages — such as bleaching and deodorizing — that involve chemical treatment and heat is often applied which can affect the stability of the oil's molecules, turn it rancid, destroy theomega-3s in it, and can even create trans fats.

Cold-pressed i.e. pure untampered-with oils just pressed or squeezed out, are available including canola, soy, corn, peanut, avocado palm oils – probably all – are available, but more expensive, and hard to find.

Nevertheless, it's your health and cold-pressed are highly to be recommended.

Extra Virgin Olive Oil covers most needs but read the notes in Part Cas some brands, especially Italian, have been highly adulterated. The book *"Extra Virginity: The sublime and scandalous world of olive oil"* by Tom Mueller, is to be recommended.

What to do

- Reduce vegetable oils if you are using them exclusively.
- Use cold-pressed olive oil, canola (rape), peanut for cooking
- Increase fish, flax, nuts (walnuts) and soy
- It seems that the reduction of saturated fats from the diet does not reduce the risk of cardiovascular diseases. What is added to the plate in place of saturated fat seems to be more important. The risk of cardiovascular diseases reduces when saturated fats are replaced with polyunsaturated fats. However,

---

557 Metabolic Profiling and cardiovascular event risk: A prospective study of three population-based cohorts. Circulation pii:114.013116 (8 Jan 2015)

558 Fish Oil Supplements in New Zealan are highly oxidized and do not meet label content of n-3 PUFA. Sci Rep;5:7928. Doi:10.1038/srep07928 (21 Jan 2015.

this has not been observed when replacing saturated fats with carbohydrates.[559]

Omega 3 Anti-Cancer[560]

Marine-based omega-3s are eight times more effective at inhibiting tumor development and growth when comparing the cancer-fighting potency of plant-versus marine-derived omega-3s on breast tumor development.

There are three types of omega-3 fatty acids: a-linolenic acid (ALA), eicosapentaenoic acid (EPA) and docosahexaenoic acid (DHA). ALA is plant-based and found in such edible seeds as flaxseed and in oils, such as soy, canola and hemp oil. EPA and DHA are found in marine life, such as fish, algae and phytoplankton.

Omega-3s prevent and fight cancer by turning on genes associated with the immune system and blocking tumor growth pathways Exposure to marine-based omega-3s reduced the size of the tumors by 60 to 70 per cent and the number of tumors by 30 per cent.

Based on the doses given in the study, humans should consume two to three servings of fish a week to have the same effect.

Omega-3 side effects

No side effect has been associated with omega-3 rich food. However, high intake of omega-3 supplements, such as more than 3 grams of fish oil daily, may increase the risk of bleeding. Higher doses of omega-3 dietary supplements may also compromise our immune function. Most of the side effects and precautions for fish oil also pertain to cod liver oil with a few exceptions. Cod liver oil contains both vitamin A and D. Consuming excessive amounts of these two vitamins can cause toxicity and dangerous side effects. Moreover, certain medications and mineral oil may interfere with the absorption of vitamin A. In addition, using vitamin A at higher dosages in conjunction with synthetic vitamin A derivatives can result in an increased risk of toxicity.

---

559 Dietary Fatty Acids and Risk of Coronary Heart Disease in Men: The Kuopio Ischemic Heart Disease Risk Factor Study. *Arteriosclerosis, Thrombosis, and Vascular Biology*, 2014; DOI: 10.1161/ATVBAHA.114.304082

560 Marine fish oil is more potent than plant based n-3 polyunsaturated fatty acids in the prevention of mammary tumors. *The Journal of Nutritional Biochemistry*, 2017; DOI: 10.1016/j.jnutbio.2017.12.011

Other Fats and Fat Like Substances: Triglycerides and Cholesterol

Lipids are organic compounds that are fatty acids or their derivatives. They include many natural oils, waxes, and steroids. Fats are made from lipid molecules.

Cholesterol and Triglycerides make up our Blood Lipids.

Cholesterol is a fat-like substance in the body and is used to build cell walls and produce some hormones. About three quarters of the cholesterol is produced by your liver; the rest comes from the food. Cholesterol is carried in the blood by lipoproteins. The main types of lipoproteins are high-density lipoprotein (HDL) and low-density lipoprotein (LDL).

HDL cholesterol is known as 'good' cholesterol. This is because HDL helps to remove cholesterol from your arteries by carrying cholesterol back to your liver for disposal.

LDL cholesterol is known as 'bad' cholesterol. This is because LDL leaves cholesterol in your arteries.

The total cholesterol test is a blood test that measures both HDL and LDL cholesterol.

Triglycerides are a type of fat in your blood that can also increase your risk of heart disease.

Lipid Profile

Triglycerides are usually tested along with cholesterol when you have a cholesterol blood test. The tests for total cholesterol, HDL cholesterol, LDL cholesterol and triglycerides are known as a lipid profile.

Elevation of both of these has been shown to increase the risk of cardiovascular problems especially heart attacks

Recently the eating of high fat, high cholesterol foods has been shown not to elevate our blood levels. Be that as it may, if you have high cholesterol or triglycerides a diet low in these will obviously help, after all a 20% drop would fix most.

Low-density lipoprotein (LDL) cholesterol was identified as a causal risk factor for coronary heart disease[561] and the intake of different types of fats was found to affect its concentration. A meta-analysis of 60 controlled dietary experiments carried out since 1970, showed that substituting saturated fats for carbohydrates as the source of 1% of energy intake increased LDL cholesterol by 0.032 mmol/L.

Substitution with monounsaturated fats decreased LDL cholesterol by 0.009 mmol/L and substitution with polyunsaturated fats decreased it by 0.019 mmol/L.[562] The strongest reductions in LDL cholesterol occurred when saturated fats were replaced by mono or polyunsaturated fats; monounsaturated fats reduced LDL cholesterol by 0.041 mmol/L and polyunsaturated fat by 0.051 mmol/L. Replacement of carbohydrates by all three types of fats increased high-density lipoprotein (HDL) cholesterol (the "good" cholesterol) and decreased triglycerides levels.

High-cholesterol diet, eating eggs do not increase risk of heart attack, not even in persons genetically predisposed. Globally, many nutrition recommendations no longer set limitations to the intake of dietary cholesterol. A study shows that a high intake of dietary cholesterol, or eating one egg every day, are not associated with an elevated risk of incident coronary heart disease. In the majority of population, dietary cholesterol affects serum cholesterol levels only a little.[563]

Hidden Fat

The major sources of hidden fat are Spreads and sauces 24%, Dairy products 23%, Savoury meats 12%, Confectionery 7%

561 Institute of Medicine Committee on Qualifications of Biomarkers and Surrogate Endpoints in Chronic Disease. Evaluation of biomarkers and surrogate endpoints in chronic disease. National Academy of Sciences, 2010.

562. *Effects of dietary fatty acids and carbohydrates on the ratio of serum total to HDL cholesterol on serum lipids and apolipoproteins: a meta-analysis of 60 controlled trials. Am J Clin Nutr2003;77:1146-55.*

563 Associations of egg and cholesterol intakes with carotid intima-media thickness and risk of incident coronary artery disease according to apolipoprotein E phenotype in men: the Kuopio Ischaemic Heart Disease Risk Factor Study. *American Journal of Clinical Nutrition*, 2016; DOI: 10.3945/ajcn.115.12231

The explosive increase in Western fat intake is twice that of the rest of world:

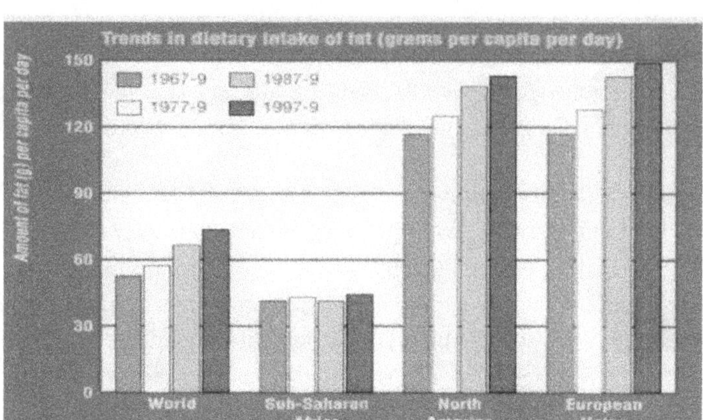

Trans Fats (TFA)

All studies agree that consumption of trans fats is associated with all-cause mortality, total CHD, and CHD mortality, according to a systematic review and meta-analysis of observational studies.[564]

Studies endorse raw, especially virgin - first pressed, vegetable oils. It is when these are hydrogenated that damaging TFA are made. Hydrogenation is an industrial process that adds hydrogen to vegetable oil, which causes the oil to become solid at room temperature. This partially hydrogenated oil is less likely to spoil, so foods made with it have a longer shelf life. Some restaurants use partially hydrogenated vegetable oil in their deep fryers, because it doesn't have to be changed as often as do other oils. A side effect of incomplete hydrogenation results in the trans isomers (TFA), which have been implicated in circulatory diseases including heart disease..

The manufactured form of TFA occurring in partially hydrogenated oil, is found in a variety of food products, including:

* *Baked goods.* Most cakes, biscuits, cookies, pie crusts and crackers contain shortening, which is usually made from partially hydrogenated vegetable oil. Ready-made frosting is another source of TFA.
* *Snacks.* Potato, corn and tortilla chips often contain trans-fat. And while popcorn can be a healthy snack, many types of packaged or microwave popcorn use trans-fat to help cook or flavor the popcorn.

[564] *BMJ.* Published online August 11, 2015

- *Fried food.* Foods that require deep frying — French fries, doughnuts and fried chicken — can contain trans-fat from the oil used in the cooking process.
- *Refrigerator dough.* Products such as canned biscuits and cinnamon rolls often contain trans-fat, as do frozen pizza crusts.
- *Creamer and margarine.* Nondairy coffee creamer and stick margarines also may contain partially hydrogenated vegetable oils.

Many countries and regions have introduced mandatory labeling of TFA on food products and appealed to the industry for voluntary reductions but in the United States if a food has less than 0.5 grams of TFA in a serving, the food label can read 0 grams trans-fat. This hidden trans-fat can add up quickly, especially when eating several servings of multiple foods containing less than 0.5 grams a serving.

Check the food label for trans-fat but also check the food's ingredient list for partially hydrogenated vegetable oil — which indicates that the food contains some TFA, even if the amount is below 0.5 grams.

Trans Fatty Acids: 'A Fat to Forget'

Trans fatty acids (TFAs) occur both naturally in foods and can be formed or added to foods during manufacture commonly used in processed foods to improve taste, texture and durability. Some TFAs are also formed during high temperature cooking. Naturally occurring TFAs are found in some animal products including butter, cheese and meat. Manufactured TFAs (also known as artificial TFAs) are formed when liquid vegetable oils are partially hydrogenated or 'hardened' during processing to create spreads such as margarine, cooking fats for deep-frying and shortening for baking. Most Western Countries have now reduced or banned trans fats completely and in June 2015 the FDA has announced food manufacturers must remove partially hydrogenated oils — the major source of artificial trans fats in processed foods — from their products within 3 years, After June 18, 2018, companies must petition the agency for approval to add partially hydrogenated oils .

TFAs have been linked to negative effects on lipid profiles, metabolic function, insulin resistance, inflammation and cardiac and general health. There is strong evidence that TFAs increase the amount of 'bad' low-density lipoprotein (LDL) cholesterol in our blood, a major risk factor for coronary heart disease. Also, TFAs may decrease the levels of 'good' high-density lipoprotein (HDL) cholesterol in blood. The World Health Organization (WHO) recommends that no more than 1% of our daily energy intake should come from TFAs whereas in the margarine and cooking-oil boom times Americans were eating 10% of their calories as trans fats from cakes, biscuits, pastries, burgers, ice-cream, chips / French fries and fried foods.[565] Depending on the country manufacturers may not be required to declare TFAs on the label. Higher consumption of dietary TFAs has been linked to worsened memory function in men 45 years old and younger.[566]

As of 2018, Australia's food labeling laws do not require trans fats to be shown separately from the total fat content. However, margarine in Australia has been mostly free of trans fat since 1996.

Limit

A trans-fat concentration of below 2% of total fat content is the limit adopted by many countries.

Australia and New Zealand have not banned Trans-Fats so here are the foods to avoid:

Food type	Total TFA (g/100g of fat)
Popcorn	18.1
Prepared Pastry	10.8
Sausage Rolls	10
Meat Pies	8.1
Custard Baked Goods	7.4
Croissant	6.7
Cream Biscuits	6.4
Desserts	6.4
Scones	5.9
Restaurant Style Takeaway Dishes	5.2
Sauces	5

565 Trans fatty acid intakes and food sources in the u.s. population:nhanes 199-2002 Kris-Etherton, P.M., *Lipids* (oct 20120; 47(10):931-40.

566 A Fat to Forget: Trans Fat Consumption and Memory. *PLOS ONE*, 2015; 10 (6): e0128129 DOI: 10.1371/journal.pone.0128129

Food type	Total TFA (g/100g of fat)
Sweet Muffins & Banana Bread	4.9
Donut	4.7
Dry Mix Pasta	4.7
Choc Chip Biscuits	4.6
Shelf Stable Cakes - No Cream	3.9
Pizza	3.8
Edible Oil Spreads*	3.4
Crumbed/Battered Fish Fillets	3.3
Dips	2.7

In summary, it would be nice to have absolute definitive evidence, but it is obvious that the very many Fats and Oils are very complex and that, all of them are not just the one fat but a mixture of many.

Furthermore, the chemical breakdown and metabolic reactions of their components are mind-blowing in their complex sequential biochemical reactions such as, just with Linoleic Acid, "the omega-6 fat linoleic acid should not be confused with conjugated linoleic acid found in pastured animal foods" and the oxidation of Linoleic Acid and its relationship to LDL involves many steps and other chemicals. Given these micro-biological metabolic reactions it will be some time before we have definitive answers and, as yet it, is not known with certainty which are absolutely beneficial, and which are absolutely bad…but evidence is accumulating.

This, however, has opened the door for the Food Industry to advertise some oils as 'Heart Healthy' just because they are vegetable oils and not even cold-pressed.

I personally stick to EVOO and fish for what I think are beneficial fats and feel the fats in grass fed beef and organic poultry are not injurious.

And my LDL is low, and my HDL is high.

RECOMMENDATIONS[567]

Limit SFA, don't use butter much, use cold pressed EVOO.

In 3.5 million person years of follow-up the risk of death was consistently lower in those who ate spicy food regularly than in those who ate such food less than once a week. But as with all food studies there is a need for caution, as it is too soon to know whether spicy food directly reduces the risk of death or is simply a marker of other dietary and lifestyle factors. Nutritional epidemiology studies are always intriguing but cannot show cause and effect.[568] They depend on self-reported recall of food intake, which is imprecise and subject to limitations of memory.

Be that as it may, high quality Observation Studies do result in recommendations that are hard to refute. For example the Nurses and Physicians Health Studies and more recently the Predimed Study: The Nurses' Health Study, established in 1976, and the *Nurses' Health Study II*, established in 1989 followed 121,700 female registered nurses since 1976 and 116,000 female nurses since 1989 to assess risk factors for cancer and cardiovascular disease.

Perhaps the biggest problem is that diet is intimately bound up with many other things that influence health, including other health behaviors as well as wealth and education and studies may reflect not causality but "a literature that is written, peer reviewed, and edited by fervent believers who will not accept any result other than what perpetuates their beliefs".[569]

"The low cholesterol, low fat diet has been the cornerstone of public health nutrition since 1980"[570] but major changes are ahead for US dietary guidelines with the type of fat rather than the quantity seeming to be most important in determining blood lipid levels. Recommendations to reduce overall fat intake have done nothing to curb the obesity epidemic and may have contributed to it. Obesity rates have risen dramatically despite reductions in fat intake, perhaps because low fat foods are not always low in calories or sugar.[571]

Attention is now focused on the benefits of the traditional Mediterranean style diet, which, as stated, has been added to and improved as the **Newtrition Micronutrient Revolution Diet.**

---

567 *BMJ* 2015;351:h4249

568 BMJ doi:10.1093/ije/dyg216.

569 http://bit.ly/1IJV4ql

570 BMJ doi:10.1136/bmj.h4034

571 BMJ doi:10.1159/000229004

COOKING WITH OILS

The idea that cooking with heat damages the oils that are highly polyunsaturated is true but not because *trans* fats are formed. What is formed under harsh circumstances such as high-temperature cooking and frying is a polymerized oil, and this is because the heat has helped to form free radicals and then various breakdown products. Polyunsaturated oils turn to trans-fat only when repeatedly reused and heated to very high temperatures.

Oils and fats liberate aldehydes when heated which are toxic.

But one experiment found that, in addition, as well as the "primary" aldehyde from heating, two new secondary aldehydes were produced when hot oil came into contact with food.

As Aldehydes are toxic the oil that produces the least should be preferred and the corollary is that those that produce the most should be avoided.

Worst to best

1. Vegetable oil (worst)
2. Sunflower oil
3. Extra Virgin Olive Oil
4. Corn oil
5. Lard
6. Goose Fat
7. Refined Olive Oil
8. Rapeseed / Canola oil
9. Butter
10. Groundnut / Peanut oil

Based on this it would seem Peanut/Groundnut oil may be the least toxic to cook with although Refined Olive Oil did, apparently, have some beneficial breakdown products.

Certain aldehydes in food are believed to be related to some neurodegenerative diseases and some types of cancer. These toxic compounds can be found in some oils, such as sunflower oil, when heated at a suitable temperature for frying and although some are volatile, others remain after frying which is why than be found in cooked food. Prolonged heating, as would occur commercially or perhaps by re-heating, was tested on three types of oil (olive, sunflower and flaxseeds). Sunflower especially and linseed oil created the most toxic aldehydes in less time.

These oils are high in polyunsaturated fats (linoleic and linolenic). Olive oil, which has a higher concentration of monounsaturated fats generated these harmful compounds in a smaller amount and later.[572] It is of interest that Peanut/Groundnut oil is used to cook with in submarines because of its high smoke point but, as avocado oil has an even higher smoke point it would seem economics played a part.

High Temperature Cooking

Foods cooked at high temperatures feature heavily in Western diets. A study that compared a diet of highly heat-treated food with one of steamed food found that after a month of the heat-treated diet, insulin sensitivity was significantly lowered, as were plasma levels of omega-3 fatty acids and vitamins C and E, while cholesterol and triglycerides increased. The results suggest that diets based on highly heat-treated food increase markers associated with enhanced risk of type 2 diabetes and heart disease in healthy people.[573]

Deleterious Effects of Reheating Cooking Oils[574]

Reheating oils and deep-frying can be fraught with problems causing damage to the cells (endothelial) that line our blood vessels, especially our coronary arteries laying the groundwork for a future heart attack. It is mandatory to use fresh oil each time and not to overheat it. Oil's smoke point is the temperature at which it will start to smoke and break down. When cooking oil starts to smoke, it can lose some of its nutritional value and can give food an unpleasant taste and worse. Oils with high smoke points, such as corn, soybean, peanut and sesame, are good for high-heat frying and stir-frying. Olive, canola and grapeseed oils have moderately high smoke points, making them good for sautéing over medium-high heat. Oils with low smoke points, such as flaxseed and walnut, are best in salad dressings and dips.

Heating oil changes its characteristics. Oils that are healthy at room temperature can become unhealthy when heated above certain temperatures, so when choosing a cooking oil, it is important to match the oil's *heat tolerance* with the cooking method.

---

[572] Aldehydes contained in edible oils of a very different nature after prolonged heating at frying temperature: Presence of toxic oxygenated α,β unsaturated aldehydes. Food Chemistry, 2012; 131 (3): 915 DOI: 10.1016/j.foodchem.2011.09.079

[573] American Journal of Clinical Nutrition 2010;91:1220-6, doi:10.3945/ajcn.2009.28737).

[574] Effects of Repeated Heating of Cooking Oils on Antioxidant Content and Endothelial Function. Austin J Pharmacol Ther. 2015; 3(2).1068.

Palm oil contains more saturated fats than canola oil, corn oil, linseed oil, soybean oil, safflower oil, and sunflower oil. Therefore palm oil can withstand the high heat of deep-frying and is resistant to oxidation compared to highly unsaturated vegetable oils. Since about 1900, palm oil has been increasingly incorporated into food by the global commercial food industry because it remains stable in deep frying, or in baking at very high temperatures and for its high levels of natural antioxidants. Palm Oil is not to be recommended.

The following oils are suitable for high-temperature frying above 230 °C or 446 °F because of their high smoke point. There are differences between the natural (cold-pressed) and refined (heat-chemical treated) smoking points of oils.

Avocado oil
Mustard oil
Refined Olive oil ("pure" or "extra light tasting)
Palm oil
Peanut oil ("groundnut oil")
Rice bran oil
Safflower oil
Semi-refined sesame oil
Semi-refined sunflower oil

Reusing cooking oil in food preparation, especially during deep-frying, is a common practice to save costs. Repeated heating of the oil accelerates oxidative degradation of lipids, forming hazardous reactive oxygen species and depleting the natural antioxidant contents of the cooking oil. Long-term ingestion of foods prepared using reheated oil could severely compromise one's antioxidant defense network, leading to pathologies such as hypertension, diabetes and vascular inflammation. The detrimental effects of reheated oil consumption extend beyond mere oxidative assault to cellular antioxidant shield. In this review, we have examined the experimental and clinical effects related to the intake of reheated oil on antioxidant contents, membrane lipid peroxidation and endothelial function. Understanding the mechanisms underlying the pathology associated with intake of repeatedly heated oil will help to set a reference for assessing the safety of cooking oil.

Repeatedly heated vegetable oil and endothelial dysfunction.

Long-term intake of diet comprising reheated vegetable oil leads to endothelial dysfunction. Repeatedly heated dietary vegetable oil promotes oxidative stress, resulting in Nitrous Oxide (NO) inactivation and reduced bioavailability. Moreover, antioxidant effect of fresh vegetable oil against free radicals may be reduced gradually as the oil is repeatedly heated. Production of free radicals and reduction of antioxidant and vitamin levels eventually lead to oxidative stress and endothelial (the cells that line our blood vessels) dysfunction play pivotal roles in the pathogenesis of cardiovascular diseases, which may be controlled by diet modification. Ingestion of repeatedly heated vegetable oil should be restricted due to the detrimental consequences on health.

Fried Food

Feeding frying oil to mice exaggerated colonic inflammation, enhanced tumor growth and worsened gut leakage, spreading bacteria or toxic bacterial products into the bloodstream. People with colonic inflammation or colon cancer should be aware of this research.[575]

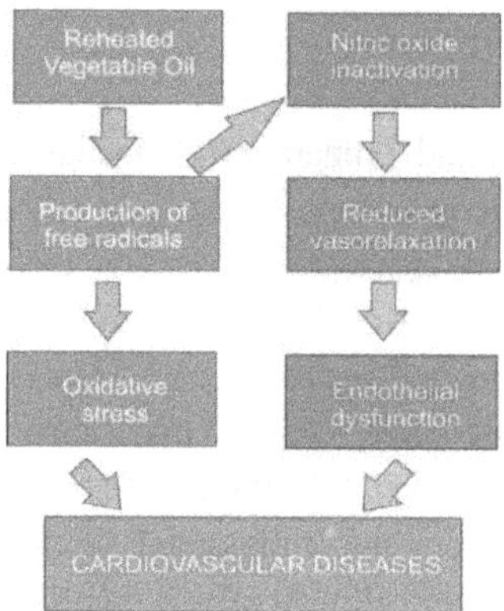

[575] Aug. 23 in ***Cancer Prevention Research***

CHAPTER 19

CHOLESTEROL, SATURATED FAT and HEART ATTACKS: Confusion and Common Sense

Jack Sprat could eat no fat,
His wife could eat no lean.
But, together both,
They licked the platter clean.
Printed in *Mother Goose's Melody* around 1765.

SUMMARY

Heart Disease and Heart Attacks – Cardio-Vascular Disease (CVD) has been our number one killer. It began as an epidemic in 1912 and some feel it is tapering off. It may well be, but the earlier diagnosis, treatments and interventions have certainly improved survival.

Since the 1950s CVD has been attributed to elevated blood cholesterol, especially the "bad" Low Density Cholesterol (LDL) which is regarded as the waste products of cholesterol metabolism, laying down debris in our coronary arteries to form plaques and then occlusions. This is the Cholesterol Hypothesis of Ancel Keys. There are a very great number of studies that show how lowering LDL results in fewer heart attacks.

Saturated Fats (SFA) were seen as culprits but recent work suggests that there is a variety of SFA and all are not bad or injurious. Ancel Keys, who proposed this cholesterol hypothesis, even noticed that *eating SFA did not elevate our blood cholesterol* but recently his hypothesis has been challenged and dietary guidelines changed. Nevertheless, replacing SFA with Unsaturated Fats has resulted, in well conducted trials of over 125,000 nurses and doctors by Harvard University over 32 years of follow-up, in reducing LDL and heart attacks.

The overwhelming evidence is that the lower our LDL the better. As we get older, many more factors determine our overall health, making the impact of high cholesterol levels less easy to detect.

The most comprehensive analysis of its kind (400,000 people from 19 countries who were followed for up to 43.5 years) suggests that there is a strong link between non-HDL cholesterol levels and long-term risk for cardiovascular disease in people aged under 45 years, not just at older ages. Looking at data for all age groups and both sexes, the authors found that the risk for a cardiovascular event decreased continuously with decreasing non-HDL levels and the risk was lowest for those individuals with the lowest non-HDL levels (classified as below 2.6 mmol non-HDL cholesterol per litre in the study).[576]

Non-HDL cholesterol includes LDL, VLDL (Very Low-Density Lipoproteins) and their remnants, intermediate-density lipoproteins and lipoprotein(a).

In other words, the Cholesterol Hypothesis is no longer a hypothesis but surely a demonstrated fact.

What Causes Heart Disease

No one knows the complete answer but the reduction in cholesterol, smoking and blood pressure has resulted in the lowering of CVD. And, it is becoming more and more evident, the ingestion of processed foods and overweight-obesity contribute.

The Cholesterol Hypothesis

The German pathologist Rudolf Virchow, around 1855, described lipid (fat molecules) accumulation in arterial walls. In 1913, a study by Nikolai Anitschkow showed that rabbits fed on cholesterol, developed lesions in their arteries similar to atherosclerosis, suggesting a role for cholesterol in atherogenesis

After the Second World War, Ancel Keys, an American physiologist, observed that, as food supplies in northern Europe became short, the death rate from coronary artery disease (CAD) dropped. This observation, coupled with reports of an epidemic of myocardial infarctions (MI) among American executives, motivated Keys to launch one of the first prospective studies in CVD epidemiology, the Minnesota Business and Professional Men's Study, which recorded the weight, blood pressure, EKG/ECG results, and cholesterol levels (mean 239 to 363 mg/dL (6.2 to 9.4 mmol/L). The only significant predictor of future heart attacks was then found to be a high total cholesterol level. Initially these observations were harshly criticized by commercial interests such as the meat and dairy industry.

---

[576] *The Lancet*, 2019; DOI: 10.1016/S0140-6736(19)32519-X

Keys then investigated the observation that rates of CAD were significantly higher in the Japanese living in Hawaii and Los Angeles than they were for native Japanese. For every native Japanese experiencing an MI, the Hawaiian Japanese had four, and those in Los Angeles had ten. This research is often unknown or forgotten but is now being duplicated as formerly primitive diets and societies are being Westernized.

Given the common genetic background of the subjects, Keys sought to examine how the "usual American mode of life" might play a role. An examination of the dietary patterns demonstrated that while native Japanese get only 13% of their calories from fats, the Hawaiian Japanese get 32% of their calories from fats, and the Los Angeles Japanese get 45% of their calories from fats. The subjects' mean total cholesterol levels corresponded to the three dietary patterns: 120 mg/dl (3.11mmol/L) for native Japanese, 181 mg/dL (4.70mmol/L) for Hawaiian Japanese, and 213mg/dL (5.50mmol/L) for Los Angeles Japanese.

In 1957 Keys began what would eventually be known as the Seven Countries Study (SCS) by surveying 12,000 men aged 40 to 59 from 18 areas of seven countries (Italy, the Greek Islands, Yugoslavia, the Netherlands, Finland, Japan, and the United States). Critics allege he was 'cherry picking' those countries which supported his hypothesis (that cholesterol was the culprit). Supporters say these critics are themselves cherry picking, and most have never read Keys' work which they admire as meticulous scientific documentation.

Keys and his colleagues were able to determine that in societies where fat was a major component of every meal (i.e., the US and Finland), both the blood cholesterol levels and the heart-attack death rates were highest. He found that saturated fat consumption was strongly associated with regional rates of heart disease, but that total fat intake was not. Indeed, total fat intake in Crete was just as high as in Finland, which had the highest rates of heart disease at that time.

Keys suggested that it was the type of fat, as well as the Mediterranean diet in general, that spelled the difference in heart disease risk.

See the next Chapter wrt Ancel Keys.

In cultures where diets were based on fresh fruit and vegetables, bread, pasta, and plenty of olive oil (i.e., the Mediterranean region) blood cholesterol was low and heart attacks were rare. The report published in 1970 had a decisive impact on CVD prevention, as it described one of the first studies to clearly show that dietary saturated fat leads to CVD, and that the relationship is mediated by serum cholesterol. In Finland "The Karelia Project" (below) significantly lowered the rate of heart attacks by lowering ingested saturated fats (plus treating blood pressure and reducing smoking).

Cholesterol is usually reported as Total, High Density (HDL- "good") and Low-Density Lipoprotein Cholesterol (LDL or LDL-C) - "bad"). Lowering cholesterol, especially LDL has resulted in the reduction of CVD world-wide. There may, of course, be other factors but the observation remains that as cholesterol fell so did heart disease. Lowering cholesterol has thus been the basis of preventive cardiovascular medicine. CVD has, and is, falling such that in some States of America it has even fallen from being the number one killer to now being second. This, as elsewhere, has been attributed to the introduction of statins - cholesterol lowering drugs. There is on-going debate as to just how low is to be recommended (see later).

Atherosclerosis:

Atherosclerosis, or hardening of the arteries, is a condition in which plaque builds up inside the arteries. Atheroma plaques are accumulations of white blood cells, especially macrophages, which have taken up oxidized LDL, fatty substances, cellular waste products, calcium and fibrin. Plaques may block the coronary artery causing a heart attack or bits flake off, travel to the brain and cause a stroke.

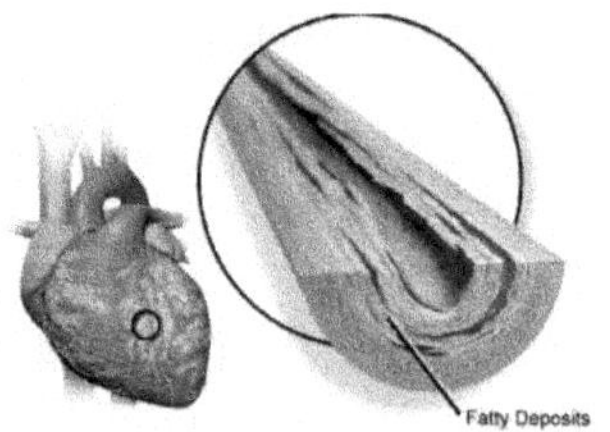

Low density cholesterol (LDL) is the major component of plaques and as such it is thought to be the major contributor to plaques and subsequent blockages and heart attacks. The result has been a great deal of research and treatments into lowering cholesterol, especially LDL.

With the Viet Nam war, autopsies were performed on 18 year old ostensibly fit soldiers whereas previously they had seldom been done on such young fit people, It was then found that many had cholesterol plaques in their coronary arteries and subsequently the coronary arteries of all young people were examined at autopsy. And now the Centre for Disease Control (CDC) reported that 21% of 6 to 19-year-olds had high cholesterol levels in the 2011-2014 National Health and Nutrition Examination Survey, and that proportion rose to 43% among the obese.

THE NORTH KARELIA PROJECT

This, to me, was and is the most impressive and influential of all studies as to the Mediterranean Diet and the effect(s) of lowering cholesterol.

In the 1960s Finnish men had the world's highest death rate from heart disease. Heart disease was a problem all over Finland, but the death rate was especially high in the province of North Karelia, an area in the eastern part of the country. The people of North Karelia had a quite high level of fitness. Smoking was not more prevalent than in other communities. However, the problem was in the diet. They liked butter and lard on their bread, whole milk, cheese, salt and sausage. Only occasionally did they eat fruit or vegetables saying they were "food for animals."

In 1972 the 'Karelia Project' introduced what was essentially a Mediterranean Diet and by the early 2000s, for men aged from 35 to 64, the number of *deaths from coronary heart disease had plunged about 75%.*

Probably the most dramatic and best population-wide improvement yet recorded.

Cholesterol lowering was attributed as the strongest contributor but other risk factors like high blood pressure and smoking were also addressed.

The diet that used to be very high in saturated fat and salt now has one of the lowest fat contents in Europe and an average salt level. As an example, in 1972, in the beginning of the project, 80% of the people used butter on bread and by the end of the study only one in ten people used butter and most people had changed to low fat spreads. Most of the population changed from drinking whole milk to the consumption of low fat or skimmed milk. The consumption of whole milk dropped from 70% to 14%. As a result of these combined efforts, cholesterol levels decreased significantly.

There was also a reduction in cancer deaths.

Dietary Changes that Lowered Cholesterol in Karalia

Dietary change	Percent
Ate more vegetables	76
Ate less fatty meats	69
Used less cooking fat	69
Changed fat spread on bread	68
Ate more fruit and berries	64
Used less spread	63
Changed cooking fat	63
Ate less full-fat cheese	61
Drank less whole milk	39
Ate less full-fat yoghurt	39
Ate more fish	32

(The 'fat spread on bread' was butter)

Benefits of Low LDL and Different Treatments

Based on results from 49 studies conducted over the past 51 years, a meta-analysis showed that:

each 1-mmol/L (38.7-mg/dL) reduction in LDL-C was associated with a 23% lower relative risk (RR) of major vascular events with statins and 25% lower risk with intensive diet, bile-acid sequestrants, ileal bypass surgery, or ezetimibe—all therapies that help clear cholesterol by upregulating the LDL receptor.[577]

This same study also found that there was a nice linear relationship (in benefit) going down to even slightly below 3.3 mom/L (60mg/dl), reinforcing the notion that lower is better.

How Low Can You Go

In fact, it was reported (December 2016) after 10 trials and 5000 patients, that LDL can trigger heart problems, but also suggests that reducing it in adults to very low levels -- to those of a new-born baby -- is both safe and beneficial.

---

[577] Association between lowering LDL-C and cardiovascular risk reduction among different therapeutic interventions: A systematic review and meta-analysis. JAMA 2016; 316:1289-1297.

Lowering levels of cholesterol reduced the risk of heart attack, stroke, angina or death from heart disease such that, for every 1-mmom/l (39mg/dL) reduction in LDL, the risk reduced by 24%.

And while most people should aim to keep their LDL cholesterol at 2.58 mmom/l (100 mg/dL) or below, this number can vary depending on a person's risk of cardiovascular disease.[578]

The IMPROVE-IT trial with ezetimibe plus statins found a continuous relationship between additional percentage reductions in LDL-C and MACE (non-fatal Major Adverse Cardiovascular Event) all the way down to a LDL-C of 0.65mmom/l (25mg/dL), which is around the level we are born with.[579]

However, rates of cataracts were significantly higher at this low level and a second meta-analysis suggested excess incidence of neurocognitive adverse events in the very low cholesterol group although the overall incidence was low (<1%). And although these results are generally reassuring, longer-term monitoring and structured assessment of neurocognitive adverse events will be needed.[580]

Measurement

It didn't really matter if LDL-C or two other lipid markers, non-HDL cholesterol or apolipoprotein B100 (apoB) were used. Once again, there was a continuous relationship between MACE and non-HDL-C and apoB levels. So there was no added benefit of either lipid marker over and above LDL-C.

---

[578] Reductions in Atherogenic Lipids and Major Cardiovascular EventsClinical Perspective. Circulation, 2016; 134 (24): 1931 DOI: 10.1161/CIRCULATIONAHA.116.024604

[579] Reductions in atherogenic lipids and major cardiovascular events: A pooled analysis of 10 ODYSSEY trials comparing alirocumab to control. Circulation 2016; DOI: 10.1161/CIRCULATIONAHA.116.024604.

[580] Safety of very low low-density lipoprotein cholesterol levels with alirocumab: Pooled data from randomized trials. J Am Coll Cardiol 2017 Feb 7; 69:471.
Increased risk of adverse neurocognitive outcomes with proprotein convertase subtilisin-kexin type 9 inhibitors. Circ Cardiovasc Qual Outcomes 2017 Jan; 10:e003153..Low-density lipoprotein cholesterol and the on-target effects of therapy: How low is too low? J Am Coll Cardiol 2017 Feb 7; 69:483.

Classification Reminder:

Saturated (SFA)	= solid at room temperature - butter, lard, palm oil
Unsaturated	
Mono-saturated (MUFA)	= Omega **9** OO, canola, avocado, peanut
Polyunsaturated (PUFA)	= Omega **6** Vegetable oils
	= Omega **3** Fish, linseed/flax, walnuts, soy

Different Fats, Different Outcomes. Some Fats are Good, Others Bad.

Effects on coronary heart disease of increasing polyunsaturated fat in place of saturated fat: a systematic review and meta-analysis of randomized controlled trials. The Nurses and Health Professionals 32 year Study

Meta-analyses found that increasing consumption of polyunsaturated fat as a replacement for saturated fat reduces the risk of coronary heart disease.

Data from the long-running Nurses' Health Study and the Health Professionals Follow-up Study data from more than 125,000 participants with a 32-year follow-up found that higher intakes of saturated fat and trans-fat were associated with increased mortality, whereas higher intakes of polyunsaturated (PUFA) and

High intake of saturated fat — when replacing carbohydrates — was associated with an 8% increase in total mortality.

High *trans* fat intake conferred a 13% mortality increase.

By contrast, high intakes of polyunsaturated fatty acids and monounsaturated fatty acids were associated with 19% and 11% reductions in mortality, respectively.

In addition, replacing 5% of calories from saturated fat with calories from polyunsaturated fatty acids and monounsaturated fatty acids was associated with mortality reductions of 27% and 13%, respectively.

Hazard ratios of total mortality:

1.13 for trans fat
1.08 for saturated fat
0.81 for polyunsaturated fatty acid
0.89 for monounsaturated fatty acid

It is estimated that replacing 5% of saturated fats with equivalent polyunsaturated or monounsaturated fats, total mortality would be reduced

Polyunsaturated fats	by	27%
Monosaturated fats	by	13%

These findings suggest that replacement of saturated fats with unsaturated fats can confer substantial health benefits and should continue to be a key message in dietary recommendations. These findings also support the elimination of partially hydrogenated vegetable oils, the primary source of trans-fatty acids.

Participants eating the most omega-6 polyunsaturated fatty acids were less likely to die than those who reported eating the least and omega-6 was associated with a lower incidence of mortality for most individual causes. Omega-3 polyunsaturated fatty acid intake was associated with a slightly lower mortality.

Linoleic acid (nuts, fatty seeds, flax seeds, hemp seeds, poppy seeds, sesame seeds, soy) intake was most robustly related with improved cardiovascular mortality. When saturated fat replaced carbohydrate intake, patients had a slightly higher cancer mortality risk, but other types of fat were not significantly associated with cancer mortality.

Conclusions for dietary recommendations:

Replace saturated fats with unsaturated fats and eliminate partially hydrogenated vegetable oils, the primary source of *trans*-fatty acids.[581,582,583] (Trans fats are banned in most countries but cooking methods can still produce them).

This approach would seem confirmed by the latest study (October 2016) of 73,147 women in the Nurses' Health Study (1984-2012) and 42 635 men in the Health Professionals Follow-up Study (1986-2010), who were free of major chronic

---

581 Evid Based Med. 2010
582 PLoS Med. 2010 Mar 23;7(3):e1000252. doi: 10.1371/journal.pmed.1000252.
583 Association of Specific Dietary Fats With Total and Cause-Specific Mortality 4*JAMA Intern Med.* Published online July 05, 2016. doi:10.1001/jamainternmed.2016.2417

diseases at baseline, which concluded that higher dietary intakes of major SFAs are associated with an increased risk of coronary heart disease. Owing to similar associations and high correlations among individual SFAs, dietary recommendations for the prevention of coronary heart disease should continue to focus on replacing total saturated fat with more healthy sources of energy (food).[584]

Lauric acid, myristic acid, palmitic acid, and stearic acid are associated with an increased risk of coronary heart disease, after multivariate adjustment of covariates. Risk of coronary heart disease is significantly lower when replacing the sum of these four major saturated fatty acids with polyunsaturated fat, whole grain carbohydrates, or plant proteins, with the lowest risk observed when palmitic acid, the most abundant saturated fatty acid, was replaced. Because intake of major saturated fatty acids are highly correlated, current dietary recommendations should focus on replacing total saturated fat with unsaturated fats or whole grain carbohydrate, as an effective approach towards preventing coronary heart disease.

Palm Oil

Palm Oil is one of, if not the most, widely used oils for commercial cooking. It is solid, delivered in large commercial paint-like drums and is pure white, which looks so clean, innocent and attractive. It is a valuable commercial crop for Asia where tropical rainforests are being destroyed to plant more and more palm trees by firstly destroying the habitat of the many native animals such as the Orangutan but downstream it may well be doing the same to humans of the affluent West as it forms the basis of most processed foods.

It is somewhat ironic to associate our own survival with that of the Orangutan but perhaps not so far-fetched as this recent study shows:

Even the one-off consumption of a greater amount of palm oil reduces the body's sensitivity to insulin and causes increased fat deposits as well as changes in the energy metabolism of the liver. The scientific investigation conducted on healthy, slim men, who were given at random a flavored palm oil drink or a glass of clear water in a control experiment. The palm oil drink contained a similar amount of saturated fat as two cheeseburgers with bacon and a large portion of French fries or two salami pizzas. The scientists showed that this single high-fat meal sufficed to cause insulin resistance and increase the fat content of the liver with metabolic

---

584 *BMJ* 2016; 355 doi: http://dx.doi.org/10.1136/bmj.i5796 (Published 23 November 2016) *BMJ* 2016;355:i5796

changes similar to changes observed in persons with type 2 diabetes or non-alcoholic fatty liver disease (NAFLD). NAFLD is the most common liver disease in the industrial nations and associated with obesity, the metabolic syndrome and an increased risk in developing type 2 diabetes. The surprise was that a single dosage of palm oil has such a rapid and direct impact on the liver of a healthy person and that the amount of fat administered already triggered insulin resistance.[585]

Saturated Fats Are Diverse

There are some 36 Fatty acids which go from a Lipid number of C3 to C38. Not all fats are equal, and it is thought the C14 Myristic and the C16 Palmitic Acids which occur in cream and its product butter may be injurious.

There are good, even essential, saturated fats. Many different saturated fats have unique properties and not all foods with saturated fat are the same. Some, such as cheese or lean meat, carry lots of nutrients, and others don't.

Fats (fatty acids) are made of varying lengths of chains of carbon (C) atoms.

1. long-chain
2. medium-chain
3. short-chain,

and many different fats in each group.

Even Extra Virgin Olive Oil, demonstrably beneficial, contains some saturated fats.

It is now apparent that not all saturated fats behave the same in the body and some fat sources are actually beneficial and unsaturated oils are still overall better than saturated fats.

Butter would seem to be 'neutral'. A study found only weak or neutral effects of butter consumption on overall mortality and cardiovascular disease (CVD) risk, suggesting that butter may not be as harmful as previously thought and may not be as harmful as the white bread and potatoes it is spread on.[586]

---

585 Acute dietary fat intake initiates alterations in energy metabolism and insulin resistance. *Journal of Clinical Investigation*, 2017; 127 (2): 695 DOI: 10.1172/JCI89444

586 June 29 in *PLoS One*

Dietary Saturated Fat

Keys himself stated, *"The evidence—both from experiments and from field surveys—indicates that the cholesterol content, per se, of all-natural diets has no significant effect on either the serum cholesterol level or the development of atherosclerosis in man"*.

The central issue or most importantly is what replaces saturated fat if someone reduces it in their diet.

If it is replaced with refined starch or sugar, which are the largest sources of calories in the U.S. diet, then the risk of heart disease remains the same.

However, if saturated fat is replaced with polyunsaturated fat or monounsaturated fat in the form of cold pressed olive oil, nuts and probably other plant oils, we have much evidence that

Saturated fat actually in the blood (and not just eating it) is a risk for heart disease. Having a lot of saturated fat in your body is not a good thing. The question is, what causes people to store more saturated fat in their blood, or membranes, or tissues? It makes more sense to focus on carbohydrate restriction than fat restriction."[587] Similarly adding eggs to the diet did not elevate serum (blood) cholesterol.[588]

When limiting overall fat intake and reducing saturated fat the consumption of carbohydrates and vegetable (polyunsaturated fats) increase[589] and substituting simple, refined carbohydrates for fat led to dyslipidemia, an increase in triglyceride levels, and a reduction in HDL cholesterol.

The danger lies in replacing saturated fat with simple-refined carbohydrates, according to findings from the Prospective Urban Rural Epidemiological (PURE) study recorded for 145,275 participants.

---

[587] Effects of Step-Wise Increases in Dietary Carbohydrate on Circulating Saturated Fatty Acids and Palmitoleic Acid in Adults with Metabolic Syndrome. *PLoS ONE*, 2014; 9 (11): e113605 DOI: 10.1371/journal.pone.0113605

[588] Medpage Today February 21, 2015

[589] *Open Heart* 2015;2: doi:10.1136/openhrt-2014-000229 Editorial

To summarize

The most adverse effect on blood lipids is from simple-refined carbohydrates; the most benefit is from consumption of monounsaturated fatty acids; and the effect of saturated and polyunsaturated fatty acids are mixed.[161]

Observational Studies

Observational studies only show associations and not the actual cause. This translates to the difference in such studies which observe there is no association between substance A and a disease, to claiming that Substance A is beneficial. In these observational studies there was no association 'observed' between saturated fat and heart disease. This cannot then be translated that saturated fat is good. It may well be but "no association" may mean that the study just didn't detect one.

The gold standard randomized controlled trial would involve thousands of people eating supervised diets of saturated, monounsaturated, or polyunsaturated fat, and a control group and then followed for decades. This is practically impossible but the PREDIMED study came close.

Doctors Can No Longer Advise

In October 2016 Doctors in all the free Government (majority) hospitals in the UK were instructed that they should no longer tell patients what treatments they need to have but must instead set out the options and let people decide for themselves. This is an attempt to avoid hospitals being sued following a ~$10 million settlement to a diabetic mother who claims she was not warned of the risks of a natural birth over a caesarian and her child was born with disabilities.[590]

What Can I Say? What Do I Advise

The cholesterol issue is complex to say the least and, given the world-wide increase in medical litigation and the above UK protocol and example, I can only present the evidence, both for and against lowering LDL and diet, and say what I, myself, do.

No one has the complete answers, but the **Newtrition** Recommendations have been updated and provide the fullest and best advice from the best studies. Beware of fad diets - they all come but they all go.

---

[590] Daily Telegraph 27 October 2016

All informed medical advice is for a Mediterranean-based diet, which should provide all essential nutrients in the correct dose and optimum delivery.

I have fixed on EVOO from a supplier I know doesn't adulterate it. We occasionally use other oils but only if cold-pressed and again from a reputable source.

I have an open mind and will watch for future studies but I still regard the Karelia Project and the dramatic effect of lowering cholesterol and the protective effect of polyunsaturates shown in the 125,000 Nurses and Health Professionals Study of 32 years, with undiminished admiration but with a low ratio Omega 3:6.

And, as I've said elsewhere, while I don't eat fat my wife does and if I thought dietary fat was bad, I would have advised her to stop. She also has low cholesterol and, as I've said, she is "a fruit-bat" and, as the latest 2,000,000 people study has found, increased consumption of fruit (and vegetables) confers greater benefits.

And the "world's Best Coronary Arteries"[591] belong to the Tsimane people of the Bolivian Amazon, who eat 72% complex carbohydrates and only 14% fat and meat. We now eat fish three times a week and lean meat at most twice a week.

In Conclusion:

There is considerable research that high cholesterol, especially LDL is associated with heart disease (atherosclerosis) and heart attacks. There is a consensus of informed medical opinion and evidence that a Mediterranean-based diet offers the best prevention and protection.

The Good News - What Works

Just as we don't know what actually causes heart attacks, we do know a hell of a lot from some 60 years of observations such as "smoking - bad', "high blood pressure - bad," and "Exercise and lowering LDL and adopting a plant-based diet - good". "More fruit and vegetables, even more good" and don't worry if you eat the fat on meat - but reduce the overall consumption of red meat and no processed meats. Increase fish to three times a week.

---

[591] Coronary atherosclerosis in indigenous South American Tsimane: a cross-sectional cohort study. *The Lancet*, 2017; DOI: 10.1016/S0140-6736(17)30752-3

We do not have to know the exact mechanisms of *how* everything works - *all we need to know is what works* and **Newtrition** is the best possible diet at our present state of knowledge and confers more health benefits than any other.

Corollary

The SAD (Sick American/Anglo/Australian Diet) and Processed Foods are bad. If you eat these, you will un-do any benefit of the good foods. To repeat the analogy, "breathing fresh air does not compensate for the damage of smoking".

A confusing anomaly: Fake News

High cholesterol was claimed in one study to be protective as we get older but it was subsequently found that this "research" was flawed:

This controversial study, led by Dr Uffe Ravnskov at the University of Lund, Sweden, argued that with a high LDL (bad) cholesterol level over the age of 60, you will live longer, there is no increased risk of cardiovascular disease and that statins will have little effect.

The researchers looked at 19 existing studies which considered the association between 'bad' LDL cholesterol levels and the overall risk of death in people aged over 60. They concluded that 92% of people with a high cholesterol level lived longer, and called for a re-evaluation of the guidelines for cardiovascular prevention, "in particular because the benefits from statin treatment have been exaggerated."

The informed opinion was that cholesterol is essential for your body to work, although too much 'bad cholesterol' (called low-density lipoprotein or LDL) can lead to fatty deposits building up in your arteries. These fatty deposits can increase your risk of developing conditions such as coronary heart disease, heart attack and stroke.

Statins lower cholesterol by reducing the production of cholesterol in the liver and therefore reduce your risk of heart disease. There is also some evidence they are anti-inflammatory and have other beneficial effects.

Only 9 of the 19 studies actually included deaths from heart and circulatory disease and two-thirds of the total number of participants in this new analysis are from one study (Bathum et al 2013). Thiis study did find that higher cholesterol (total, HDL, or LDL) in people aged 50+ was associated with a lower all-cause mortality but that taking a statin prescription provided a significant survival benefit, regardless of age, contrary to Ravnskov's team's claims because the research published in the BMJ Open journal, has been deemed unbalanced due to what John Danesh, BHF Professor of Epidemiology said was "crude study methods". This is because their analysis "relied on limited, aggregated and inconsistent information from published sources, an approach liable to bias."

Similarly, Colin Baigent, of the University of Oxford, has described the study as reaching "completely the wrong conclusion. In fact, *we know that cholesterol is just as important as a cause of heart disease in older people as it is in the young.* We know this because of the evidence from all the randomized trials of statin therapy, which have studied substantial numbers of older people."

Dr Tim Chico, a consultant cardiologist at Northern General Hospital in Sheffield, said there are several studies that has shown lowering cholesterol using a drug does reduce the risk of heart disease in the elderly. He said: "I am surprised the authors of this study do not refer to such trials, which tends to make their own paper disappointingly unbalanced."

And Professor Jeremy Pearson pointed out "The evidence from large clinical trials demonstrates very clearly that lowering LDL cholesterol reduces our risk of death overall and from heart attacks and strokes, regardless of age. There is nothing in the current paper to support the authors' suggestions that the studies they reviewed cast doubt on the idea that LDL cholesterol is a major cause of heart disease or that guidelines on LDL reduction in the elderly need re-evaluating."

The authors themselves had to admit that "We may have overlooked relevant studies as we only searched PubMed" (an online search for medical publications), and they may have excluded studies that evaluated LDL-C as a risk factor for death, if the study did not mention it in the title or abstract.

Authors note: Yeah, sure, those studies that didn't agree with our bias.

Epidemiologists and Fake News

Again, this supports my suspicions of Epidemiologists. In fact, at least five of the study authors had previously written books questioning the links between cholesterol and heart disease. The lead author Dr Uffe Ravnskov, has written a book called 'The Cholesterol Myths: Exposing the Fallacy that Saturated Fat and Cholesterol Cause Heart Disease'. Another of the authors, London cardiologist Dr Aseem Malhotra, is a prominent campaigner against statins.

Addenda:

The latest and very good research:

Statin use is associated with lower mortality risk in older adults, according to a retrospective study in JAMA.[592] Over 300,000 U.S. veterans aged 75 and older were followed for roughly 7 years. At the outset, all were free of atherosclerotic cardiovascular disease. Death rates per 1000 person-years were 79 among new statin users and 98 among non-users. After adjustment for propensity scores, the hazard ratio for statin users was 0.75 for all-cause mortality and 0.80 for cardiovascular mortality, compared with non-users.

Editorialists write that the results "provide a compelling argument for use of statins for primary prevention in older patients."

---

[592] *JAMA.* 2020;324(1):68-78. doi:10.1001/jama.2020.7848

CHAPTER 20

AMINO ACIDS

Twenty percent of the human body is made up of protein. Protein plays a crucial role in almost all biological processes and amino acids are the building blocks of it. A large proportion of our cells, muscles and tissue is made up of amino acids, meaning they carry out many important bodily functions, such as giving cells their structure. They also play a key role in the transport and the storage of nutrients. Amino acids have an influence on the function of organs, glands, tendons and arteries. They are furthermore essential for healing wounds and repairing tissue, especially in the muscles, bones, skin and hair as well as for the removal of all kinds of waste deposits produced in connection with the metabolism. In the human genome, 20 amino acids are created to build proteins and therefore termed proteinogen. Besides this, there are approximately 250 amino acids which do not form proteins. These, for example, can form sugar. When proteins are broken down, amino acids are left.

Amino Acids are classified as:

1. Essential amino acids
2. Nonessential amino acids
3. Conditional amino acids

1.Essential amino acids

Cannot be made by the body and must come from food.

The 9 essential amino acids are: histidine, isoleucine, leucine, lysine, methionine, phenylalanine, threonine, tryptophan, and valine.

2.Nonessential amino acids

Nonessential means that our bodies produce an amino acid, even if we do not get it from the food we eat. Nonessential amino acids include: alanine, arginine, asparagine, aspartic acid, cysteine, glutamic acid, glutamine, glycine, proline, serine, and tyrosine.

3.Conditional amino acids

Conditional amino acids are usually not essential, except in times of illness and stress. Conditional amino acids include: arginine, cysteine, glutamine, tyrosine, glycine, ornithine, proline, and serine.

Amino Acid Functions

Growth Amino Acids are the body's building blocks forming collagen, muscle and tissue

Nitrogen cycle:

Most proteins are a combination of increasing nitrogen complex compounds

Negative Nitrogen Balance is when the body uses this nitrogen or proteins for growth to around age 18

Then the body is in dynamic balance – unless we overeat (and get fat)

Breakdown Food (enzymes)
Build Protein

- Amino acids build proteins.
- Nitrogen forms amino acids then polypeptides then proteins
- When cells need protein, they follow instructions from DNA that define the specific amino acids and the order in which they must connect to build the protein. DNA depends on another macromolecule -- RNA -- to make the protein. RNA takes a copy of the code from the DNA, leaves the cell, finds the amino acids and brings them back to the cell, where they bind into a chain. Each amino acid must be available at the time it's needed, or the protein won't be synthesized. When the chain is complete, it twists and folds into a specialized shape. The chemical structure of each amino acid controls the final shape, and the shape determines the function of the protein.

Produce antibodies, hormones

- Hormones = Growth Hormone, testosterone, insulin, others,
- *Enzymes,*
- *Collagen*
- *Antibodies*

Repair damaged tissues

Synthesize Neurotransmitters

- Several amino acids produce neurotransmitters e.g: *tryptophan* and *tyrosine.* Tryptophan produces serotonin, which regulates mood and makes the hormone melatonin. Tyrosine is used to synthesize norepinephrine and adrenalin. Tryptophan and tyrosine compete with each other for access to the brain. When you eat a lot of carbs, more tryptophan gets into your brain and makes you sleepy. A meal high in protein increases the amount of tyrosine in your brain, which gives you more energy.

Protect Cardiovascular Health

- The body uses the amino acid arginine to make nitric oxide which helps lower blood pressure by relaxing muscles in blood vessels. It's produced in heart muscles, where it regulates contractions. It may also prevent atherosclerosis by inhibiting the development of plaque. Nitric oxide is the active ingredient in nitroglycerin, a medication used to relieve angina, or chest pain caused by coronary heart disease.

Metabolism and Other Roles

Energy: Carbs and fats are preferentially metabolized for energy, but when necessary, amino acids can also be recruited.
Glutamic acid, cysteine and glycine -- combine to form glutathione, which is an antioxidant.
Histidine makes enzymes used to produce red blood cells and maintain healthy nerves.
Tyrosine is needed to synthesize thyroid hormones, while
Methionine makes SAMe, or S-adenosylmethionine. SAMe is essential for the metabolism of DNA and neurotransmitters.

Recommendations and Sources

Humans can make 11 of the amino acids needed. The other nine must come from ingested food.

Complete Proteins:

Foods that contain a specific amount of all nine amino acids are called complete proteins

Complete proteins are found in animal products, soybeans and quinoa.

Most plant-based foods lack a sufficient amount of one or more of the nine amino acids. What one food lacks, will be obtained from another by eating a variety of foods and consume the recommended dietary allowance of protein: 46 grams daily for women and 56 grams for men.

CHAPTER 21

VITAMINS

The 13 vitamins and their year of discovery.

There are four fat-soluble vitamins: A, D, E, K

and nine water-soluble C and eight B group

1. A (1939)

B Group

2. B1 thiamin (1926)
3. B2 riboflavin (1933)
4. B3 Niacin (1937)
5. B5 Pantothenic acid (1931)
6. B6 Pyridoxine (1936)
7. B7 Biotin (1939)
8. B9 Folic Acid (1939)
9. B12 Cyanocobalamin (1948)
10. C (1926)
11. D (1931)
12. E (1936)
13. K (1939)

Humans cannot synthesize A, B1, B2, B5, B6, B7, B9, B12, C, E and K

VITAMINS

Vitamins are organic (carbon atom containing) compounds (more than one chemical) which occur naturally in food and are produced by living things. There is no real definition as they are different from each other and not one class or the same group of chemicals even though the originator of the word, Polish biochemist Casimir Funk, thought they were amines and in 1912 coined the word "vital amine". As is too often tragically the case in medicine, jealousy reared its head and his colleagues, and the journals eschewed the name but finally one London biochemist suggested the "e" be dropped and the word "vitamin" has become one of the most successful and evocative in all medicine.

Most vitamins have to be obtained from the diet, either because humans do not have the enzymes necessary to make them or because we cannot produce them in sufficient quantities. They act as catalysts necessary to make metabolic and other reactions in the body go better or faster. They don't provide energy themselves but rather control chemical processes in the body that convert food to energy and help the body use that energy.

There are 13 vitamins but humans cannot synthesize 11 of these which then have to be obtained from food and are then known as "essential" but we are able to synthesize some vitamin B3 (niacin) and D. The human recommended daily intake for vitamin C (60 mg) is the highest among all vitamins.

The significance of these previously unknown ingredients was suggested when a Dutch doctor in Java, between 1886 and 1895, had to treat many cases of beriberi which caused a swollen heart and heart failure and peripheral neuropathy - nerve damage especially to the legs. Some soldiers came down with the illness while others mysteriously did not. Then some Military martinet (no surprises there but actually it was the replacement cook) found that the kitchen was serving the left over white rice, meant for the soldiers (I think it was “Officers only”), to the chooks. And the chooks were also suffering from beriberi and peripheral neuropathy. The new cook immediately put a stop to it and the chooks had to go back and eat the natural unprocessed brown rice, and they subsequentially recovered - which the Dutch doctor noted.

White rice was "polished" and the husk removed to make it more attractive - "pure white". This may be regarded as one of the first examples of processing food to make it unnatural as the husk contained the essential vitamin, and lack of this led to a swollen heart (beriberi) and nerve damage (peripheral neuropathy). This was later analysed and this essential, vital ingredient identified as thiamin - vitamin B1.

Until then most Dietary Deficiency Diseases were thought to be caused by germs. The germ theory of disease had become popular in not only the medical field but also the public's consciousness. As a result, the germ theory was often generalized to far more ailments than it actually caused.

In 1914, Dr Joseph Goldberger was asked by US Surgeon General to investigate pellagra, then an endemic disease in the Southern US. Previously it had been rather rare in the United States, but an epidemic broke out in 1906, primarily in the South, and continued until the 1940s. By 1912, South Carolina alone had 30,000 cases, and with a death rate of 40% pellagra had devastating effects on the region

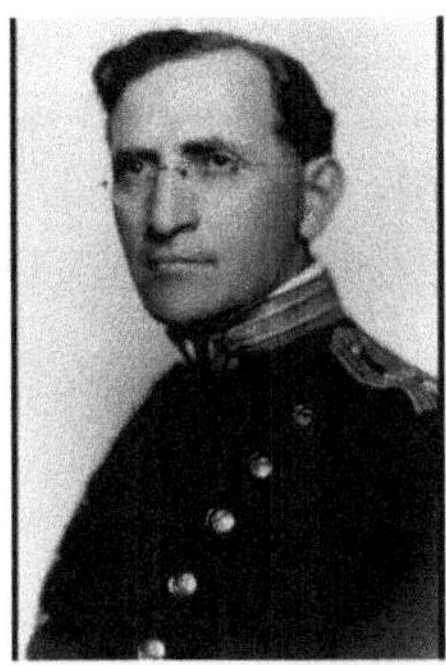

Goldberger concluded the cause was a deficiency in the Southern Diet. But the proud (but ignorant) Good Ol' Boy Southerners ran him out of town for criticising their food.

Goldberger persisted performing increasingly disgusting experiments on himself, his wife and some volunteers, to eventually prove his proposition. He didn't actually identify the deficient chemicals, vitamin B3 (Niacin) and tryptophan, but by administering small amounts of yeast people were cured and thousands, if not millions, of lives saved.

Today, poor quality, processed foods or restricted choices can lead to vitamin deficiencies. The impoverished are obviously at risk as are the elderly living alone or in poor quality nursing homes; but not so obvious may be those on a restricted diet such as vegans or the well-to-do who frequently eat fast or processed foods. In fact, as will be seen later, it has been suggested that 100% of Americans need supplements, as their diets are so poor. Here, of course, vitamin supplementation has its place.

It was interesting to my wife and I that, with the Covid-19 pandemic and the world-wide ransacking of super-markets, that it was all the junk food (and toilet paper?) that was taken. Because we were working in my surgery we were completely out flanked by these marauders and thought when we finally could get to the shop there would be nothing left. How wrong we were: All the junk food was gone, and we were left with high quality fruit, veg and meats.

Covid-19 confirmed that the publics knowledge of hygiene and nutrition is not very good.

There are then problems with manufacture with many fast foods not containing what their label alleges. The best vitamin supplements are made from hydroponic natural sources with guaranteed content.

In her charming and informative book "Vitamania" (Penguin Press) Catherine Price points out, "Today, we're still vitamaniacs, such believers in vitamins' inherent goodness...We don't notice the ways that food marketers and dietary supplement makers use synthetic vitamins to add a veneer of health to otherwise unhealthy products; nor do we acknowledge the extent to which we use vitamins and these other vitamin-inspired nutrients to give ourselves a free pass to overeat foods of all kinds. And we certainly don't recognize the irony of our vitamin obsession that by encouraging the idea that isolated dietary chemicals hold the keys to good health, our vitamania is making us less healthy".

Or, to put it another way: If you put Rolls Royce wheels on a jalopy it's still a jalopy: If you add vitamins to junk food, it's still junk.

Vitamins are Necessary

Vitamins are essential for good health. When people are deficient in them, they cause profound illnesses and then their addition or administration works like a dramatic miracle.

This, unfortunately, has led to them being regarded as miracles for conditions other than their deficiency, when they are not.

Using them to promote our health, as an prophylactic against illnesses, or "just in case" or in the hope they will extend our life is completely wrong but ruthlessly exploited by the vitamin industry who infer all the above and so disturb and distress the gullible into taking them. If you have access to fresh foods, especially fruit and vegetables, you get, not only all the vitamins you need, but also the minerals and especially the incredible array of micronutrients which also benefit us.

That said, as detailed elsewhere, because, even in first world rich nations, we eat so much processed foods, we may not be eating enough fresh foods nor a great variety. So it's time to change and stop eating processed/fast foods.

In the BMJ of 16-17 March 2017 the following case with photos was documented:

"A 79 year old man was referred to the medical assessment unit by his general practitioner. Over the previous four weeks he had experienced progressive discoloration of both lower legs. His GP had given two courses of antibiotics for possible cellulitis but there was no clinical improvement. He was systemically well and had no history of fever. He denied any trauma to the legs and had no dermatological history. He was taking no regular medication. The man lived alone and was fully independent. His diet lacked fruit and vegetables".[593]

In fact, he had scurvy, and this was 2017 in a first world nation. Even as a medical student in one of the world's richest nations (Australia) with easy, and affordable access to a cornucopia of fresh fruit and vegetables, I remember cases at the Royal Children's Hospital of both scurvy and rickets! (I can still see the classic x-ray changes in the child's legs).

Not only do we have to eat fruit and vegetables every day, but the latest evidence is that we have to eat a lot more than the "five serves" most countries recommend. The old, the poor and the institutionalized are obviously at risk and they may need supplements.

The Green Drought

Without any nutritional science, advertising agencies, vitamin manufacturers and pills, our ancestors worked out that apples, oranges, berries, nuts, meat and such were beneficial.

It was only when humans were deprived, such as sailors being taken to sea and not able access fresh fruit or, as in Java, when the husks were taken off rice, to 'make it look better', that scurvy and beriberi developed. It was only when the industrial revolution took children from the country, out of the sun (vitamin D) and without a variety of food especially milk (calcium) that rickets developed.

Now, in a bizarre twist, we are subjected to similar unnatural deprivations but now disguised as excess with junk food high in calories but low in essential nutrients,

---

[593] *BMJ* 2017; 356 doi: https://doi.org/10.1136/bmj.j1013 (Published 16 March 2017) Cite this as: *BMJ* 2017;356:j1013

much like 'a green drought' for livestock where the fodder looks great but has no nourishment and the animals effectively starve.

Today, as in a green drought, there appears to be enough food, but it is an oversupply of similar low nourishment processed junk food.

To add insult to injury, vitamins and supplements are then added (back) to this junk along with emulsifiers, preservatives, coloring agents, flavorings, taste enhancers, sodium (salt), sugar and goodness knows what else, so that it continues to be popular and continues to cause the present epidemic of the Diseases of Affluence.

The Vitamin Scam

The vitamin, mineral and supplement "Industry" is, however, a massive confidence scam. There are some 100,000 supplements on sale in the USA. What for? A good balanced diet as per **Newtrition Foods** gives all the necessary vitamins, minerals and supplements we need. But, better still, in the correct doses and with the best bioavailability facilitated by micronutrients.

Eating a variety of fresh foods donates not only all the vitamins, minerals and micronutrients we need (except B12, carnosine and zinc) but, in the long term, it is also cost effective as it minimizes illnesses and compresses morbidity allowing us to live longer and healthier. Fresh produce supplies not only the protein, carbohydrates and fats but also the vitamins in the correct dose and provides the best bio-available formula along with many co-factors to enhance their efficacy. These are the flavonoids, trace minerals, phytochemicals, carotenoids, odorants and perhaps other micro ingredients yet to be discovered which no manufactured tablet can provide.

There are some 70 known and an estimated 400 ingredients in an orange including Vitamin C. It would seem obvious that some, if not all, of the 69 or 399 other ingredients must help the orange's Vitamin C be better absorbed, metabolized and utilised by the human body and that common sense would suggest that fresh foods are the best source of vitamins and essential nutrients...after all we have had two million years of practical experience and experimentation.

Americans spend, or rather waste, $30Billion a year on vitamins and supplements. The "umbrella review," in the Annals of Internal Medicine in 2019,[594] is a

[594] Effects of nutritional supplements and dietary interventions on cardiovascular outcomes. Ann Intern Med. 2019;171:190-198.

comprehensive reporting of randomized trials of vitamins and supplements that examined their effects on cardiovascular disease and overall mortality and included studies of 24 different interventions comprising 277 randomized trials and nearly a million patients which has provided the best data on vitamins and supplements to date.

Sadly, for those with expensive urine there was no high-quality evidence that any vitamin or supplement has a beneficial effect on overall mortality.

It did find some low-quality evidence that omega-3 fatty acids might protect against myocardial infarction and heart disease, and that folic acid might protect against stroke, and moderate-quality evidence that a combination of calcium and our vitamin D increased the risk for stroke.

With vitamins there is both the placebo effect and "healthy user bias" in that, people who take vitamins invariably engage in a healthy lifestyle.

Ripest Best

Vitamins and other nutrients are maximal when the fruit or vegetable is ripest.

But Fresh Not Always Best[595]

It has been found that levels of the cancer-fighting phytonutrient in Rocket (sulforaphane) plummet after picking only to recover and peak between five to seven days, peaking at seven, after being left in the fridge. Thereafter it declines. Sulforaphane is found in other green leafy vegetable and its high-level intensity gives rocket its peppery flavor

Supplementation

The only people who need vitamin supplements are people without access to an adequate supply of fresh food - either from ignorance, laziness or circumstances such as people who can afford fresh food but prefer fast-food junk, fad dieters such as vegans who may need supplemental iron and B12, the starving in famine areas or refugees, the elderly in poor quality nursing homes serving the inmates splodge or, as above, the isolated lone old person eating a diet lacking fruit and vegetables.

595 University of Reading

IF you eat enough variety of foods you should get all the vitamins you need. There are claims that our fruit and vegetables, because of intensive farming practices, exhausted soils and storage, don't contain the amounts of vitamins or nutrients they used to. So OK, have two. But natural foods have many more ingredients than just the vitamins and these micronutrients must surely be beneficial too. Food processing, especially heat-treating, destroys many nutrients that would normally be consumed if the food were eaten in its natural state.

There are six claimed common nutritional deficiencies in our modern commercial foods: Calcium, copper, folic acid, magnesium, pantothenic acid (vitamin B5) and selenium.

Why We May Need Vitamin Pills

As pointed out "IF you eat enough variety of foods you should get all the vitamins you need". Unfortunately it would seem a mighty big "IF": USA research in 2011 stated "large percentages of vitamins A, most Bs, C and D and iron were from fortification" with synthetic vitamins and that "100% of Americans would fail to meet the Estimated Average Requirement (EAR) for vitamin A, C, D, E thiamine, B6 and folate"[596]

Refining of Grains: The Loss of Nutrients

Refining consists of when the bran and germ are stripped off all that is left is nutrient poor starch in the form of white flour (or white rice). Grains were originally refined to extend its shelf life. However, grains consist of fiber-rich bran and nutrient-rich germ, which is lost in the refining.

Wheat is the most eaten grain in Western diets and 98% of this wheat is eaten in the form of nutrient deficient white flour.

---

596 Foods, Fortificants and Supplements: Where Do Americans Get Their Nutrients" Journal of Nutrition, 141, no 10 ((2011):1847.

% of Nutrients Lost by Refining

- Protein 25%
- Fiber 95%
- Calcium 56%
- Copper 62%
- Iron 84%
- Manganese 82%
- Phosphorous 69%
- Potassium 74%
- Selenium 52%
- Zinc 76%
- Vitamin B1 73%
- Vitamin B2 81%
- Vitamin B3 80%
- Vitamin B5 56%
- Vitamin B6 87%
- Folate 59%
- Vitamin E 95%

Enriching / Fortification: Only chemically adds 5 of the lost 25 nutrients back (only 17 listed above)

No Need

My point, however, remains: Natural vitamins from fresh produce work better because of the micronutrients and, in a first world country, we should make more of an effort to access these fresh quality products. This relative vitamin deficiency can again be shafted back to the first world eating so much processed foods.

As Catherine Price points out enriching or fortifying processed foods *"is a damning indictment our diets, especially when you consider that most of us are consuming more calories than we require"*. Rather than quantity, think quality and variety.

We must really make an effort to seek fresh (the riper the better) foods and great variety of such as it would seem in many cases and, in the vast majority of cases in the USA, vitamin supplements are needed - but not necessary. The greatest impediment to fresh food is cost as fast foods and drinks are invariably cheaper...but only in the short term.

I would emphasize again that these recommendations are for countries where a variety of fresh food is available and where people can afford it. There are, however, many impoverished countries where synthetic supplements are still needed. But a December 2016 Global study found most supplements necessary in poor countries for the healthy growth of infants from 6 to 24 months of age, did not contain enough essential ingredients nor what was stated on the labels. Only 15% met benchmarks for fat content, and less than 25% met standards for iron and zinc -- two essential nutrients not present in sufficient levels in breast milk for healthy infant growth after six months of age, the critical time point for introducing solid foods.[597]

The Paradox: The 'Health Halo'

As processed food became "the flavor of the month" - then the decade, and now the millennium, synthetic vitamins had to be added to fortify this deficient processed food. This gave processed food a veneer of respectability and claims as to being healthy, which enabled them to prosper and be profitable. But these now acceptable and preferred foods with added vitamins are still injurious and cause health issues such as Diseases of Affluence and as Catherine Price observes, *"synthetic vitamins enable the very products and dietary habits that are making us sick".*

Short Term: Long Term

Processed fast junk food and drinks are invariably cheaper but the short-term financial savings of a diet of cheaper processed foods don't compensate for the long-term disabilities or premature death from the Diseases of Affluence. Spend more on your health: Eat the best.

Synthetic Vitamins Manufacture

Synthetic vitamins, in most cases, have the exact chemical compositions as natural ones. They are, however, due to the cost of extracting them from natural food, mostly made from some amazing sources:

Vitamin C is mostly made from sorbitol fermented with bacteria.
Vitamin A from nylon 6.6 used in carpets, zip ties, conveyor belts and, I think, my surgical sutures.
Vitamin B1 from coal tar chemicals
Vitamin D from lanolin

---

[597] Nutrient composition of premixed and packaged complementary foods for sale in low- and middle-income countries: Lack of standards threatens infant growth. *Maternal & Child Nutrition*, 2016; e12421 DOI: 10.1111/mcn.12421

Big Pharma Profits and Price Gouging

The big Vitamin Companies went for profits such that,

* In 1999, Hoffman-La Roche were fined $500 million in the USA for their part in a global cartel for price fixing vitamins.
* BASF had to pay $223 million,
* Takeda paid $72 million.
* In Europe eight companies were fined a total of $1 billion in criminal fines and more than $1 billion in civil judgments for similar price fixing.
* a group of Chinese companies were fined $162.3 million in 2013 for price fixing.

Vitamins, as above, are not expensive to make - just to buy. Now most of the world's vitamins come from China.

Every day I am surprised by the new patients I see who, in their Registration Form list the many vitamins and supplements they take, and research shows most don't admit to taking them, so I suspect there are even more. They cost a considerable amount of money (many are young women on low salaries) and when I ask why they are taking them or what for, most have no answer. But when I point out how fresh foods supply all needs, I detect that they don't quite believe me... *"Scams sell and science sucks"*.

Only one, a physiotherapist (physical therapist), thanked me, he had stopped them and *"saved a fortune"*. And I have to admit, on his subsequent visits he was not suffering from beriberi, peripheral neuropathy, scurvy, rickets, problems with his vision, pellagra or any other vitamin deficiency syndromes and he appeared fit and well nourished.

Amazing! (Sarcasm intended).

Ignorance

In the small country towns around where I live, and even to a lesser degree in the capital city, the young checkout attendants at the super-market frequently can't recognize much of the fruit or vegetables and have to ask, "What's this"?

Laziness

Perhaps it is not laziness in many instances where people are working longer and harder. With former generations women stayed at home and cooked and men had vegetable gardens and chooks. Now the women often don't get home until seven at night after leaving before 8 in the morning. Not only is there little time to shop but who then wants to turn around and cook?

On the other hand, studies have shown that the lower socio-economic groups prefer fast or prepared meals even if they are not working.

Altered Tastes

The addition of artificial flavorings has so altered natural foods that many younger generations have never tasted natural poultry or meats such that when presented with range fed organic produce, they prefer the Fried Chicken or the meat smeared with BBQ sauce.

My wife gave some of our eggs to a friend who recoiled in horror that "there was something wrong with them as they were so yellow"! An even crazier extreme, reminiscent of the "pure white rice" mistaken belief, is where people prefer white fat on beef. Natural fat is yellow, especially on animals that absorb the carotenoids from eating grass. I have also never operated on a patient with white fat.

So insidious and pervasive are these intrusions that it even took me some years to regain my taste for natural, grass-fed beef. I thought it was most odd and surprising when my wife said she couldn't finish her steak at the award-winning restaurant but I knew she was no prima donna, never made a fuss and didn't ever send a meal back (she just explained to the waiter that it was delicious but she had had a big lunch).

What had happened, however, was that by breeding Royal Show winning beef carcasses, she had refined, rather than developed, an exquisite palate as to how the best grass-fed beef should taste and I then realized (with something of a jolt to my ego) that it was I who had had my taste buds corrupted like the kids who prefer chicken-chain fried chicken to organic ones, I didn't know what "real" steak should taste like. But, trust me, by diligent effort I soon regained my taste for the best foods, which, I insist, are not expensive in the long run and none of this is meant to imply any undue affluence or affectation as, after all, the Blue Zones, where people live longest, are peasant communities where such natural foods are the norm and what we should emulate. (But, like them, don't eat too much meat).

While the wonderful advance of freezing and air-transport have made all produce available all year it nevertheless deprives us of the lusciousness that tree or vine ripened fruit have over their frozen, nitrogen ripening-room cousins.

Vitamins and Minerals are essential

It was their lack in poor or altered foods or even the absence of the correct foods that caused vitamin deficiencies. Giving these essential nutrients back to these patients worked like a miracle and the vitamin craze was born. There are, however, only 13 vitamins but most 'health' shops sell close to 2,000 items with 8,000 supplements also available.

An excess of vitamins can be harmful as was the case in Mawson's 1912 Antarctic Expedition when Sir Douglas Mawson and his companion Mertz had to eat a dog's liver to survive. Canine livers, however, accumulate toxic (to human) levels of vitamin A. Mertz then suffered dizziness, nausea, abdominal pain, mucosal fissuring, skin, hair, and nail loss, yellowing of eyes and skin, irrationality, went mad and died.

But overdoses are usually from synthetic supplements (pills). It is also thought that supplements may block the absorption of naturally occurring vitamins or that they may have a negative effect such as reported from vitamin-E or they may reduce HDL (the good cholesterol).

The body has an elegant "Feedback Mechanism" such that, if one essential hormone or whatever is low, it signals the brain, or rather the brain detects this low level in the circulating blood, and the brain then signals the appropriate organ to restore it to normal levels. If, however, our circulation is flooded with artificial supplements the brain detection system is overwhelmed and closes down. It then may have trouble re-booting.

It is just common sense that humans evolved to find what foods firstly didn't poison us, then which ones sustained us and finally which made us prosper. We then worked out which we could utilise and metabolize most efficiently. This took tens of thousands of years if not longer.

A large cohort study (8,640 women and 4,983 men) with long follow-up (1981–2013), found there was no consistent substantial relationship between antioxidant vitamin intake (supplemental, dietary, or total) and mortality. The conclusion was that there is no justification for the general and widespread intake of supplemental vitamins A, C, and E to increase longevity among persons with a nutritionally adequate diet.[598] However, 1000 IU of Vitamin D supplement a day is associated with a reduced All-Cause-Mortality.[599]

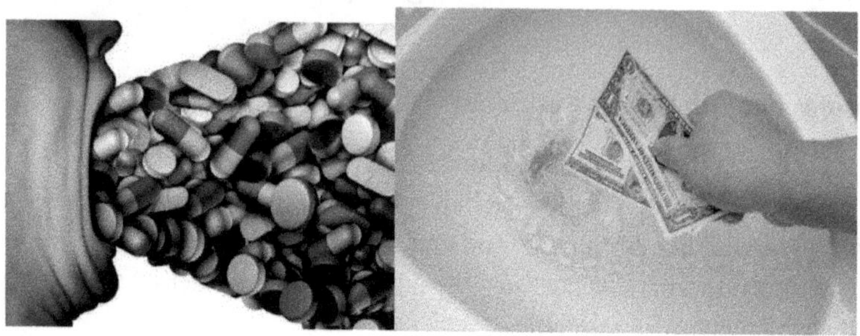

Vitamins: The most expensive urine money can buy.

[598] Am J Epidemiol. 2015;181(2):120-126. © 2015 Oxford University Press
[599] Arch Int Med 2007:167:1730-37

VITAMIN PILLS AND SUPPLEMENTS ARE A SCAM

(Unless you have a *proven* deficiency or a very poor diet)

Do not trust the "Health" shop. Do not listen to any advice other than a qualified medical practitioner and even then, I'd be cautious if he, or she, was "alternate"

EAT THE NEWTRITION MICRONUTRIENT REVOLUTION DIET FOODS

They provide ALL nutritional needs AND donate health benefits

There are only 13 vitamins but today there are over 100,000 "supplements" on the market. Most have not been tested and most have dubious, if any, benefit. Whereas a variety of fresh food provides all, in the right dose and more efficiently absorbed and metabolized.

WE CANNOT PROCESS PROCESSED FOODS

LYDIA E. PINKHAM'S

VEGETABLE COMPOUND.

Is a Positive Cure

for all those Painful Complaints and Weaknesses so common to our best female population.

It will cure entirely the worst form of Female Complaints, all ovarian troubles, Inflammation and Ulceration, Falling and Displacements, and the consequent Spinal Weakness, and is particularly adapted to the Change of Life.

It will dissolve and expel tumors from the uterus in an early stage of development. The tendency to cancerous humors there is checked very speedily by its use.

It removes faintness, flatulency, destroys all craving for stimulants, and relieves weakness of the stomach. It cures Bloating, Headaches, Nervous Prostration, General Debility, Sleeplessness, Depression and Indigestion.

That feeling of bearing down, causing pain, weight and backache, is always permanently cured by its use.

It will at all times and under all circumstances act in harmony with the laws that govern the female system.

For the cure of Kidney Complaints of either sex this Compound is unsurpassed.

LYDIA E. PINKHAM'S VEGETABLE COMPOUND is prepared at 233 and 235 Western Avenue, Lynn, Mass. Price $1. Six bottles for $5. Sent by mail in the form of pills, also in the form of lozenges, on receipt of price, $1 per box for either. Mrs. Pinkham freely answers all letters of inquiry. Send for pamphlet. Address as above. *Mention this Paper.*

No family should be without LYDIA E. PINKHAM'S LIVER PILLS. They cure constipation, biliousness,

a's pills and lozenges asily recognized, by the most gullible of us, ;cam.

t is more difficult is to ze the fantastic ntation, advertising)seudo-health claims of 's vitamin pills and lements are the direct ndants of Lydia.

are all scams despite pseudo-medical 'health .

ll your vitamins, rals, amino acids and onutrients from fresh – mostly fruit and ables.

CHAPTER 22

MINERALS

Major minerals

1. calcium
2. phosphorus
3. potassium
4. sodium
5. magnesium

Trace Minerals

1. Boron
2. Cobalt
3. Chromium
4. Copper
5. Fluoride
6. Iodine
7. Iron
8. Manganese
9. Molybdenum
10. Selenium
11. **Zinc**

Ultra Trace Elements

1. Silicon
2. Bromine
3. Arsenic
4. Chromium

Silicon and boron are known to have a role but the exact biochemical nature is unknown. Arsenic and chromium are suspected to have a role in health, but with weaker evidence. Bromine has recently been found to have a biochemical role in the body in the synthesis of collagen, but these findings have not yet been confirmed.

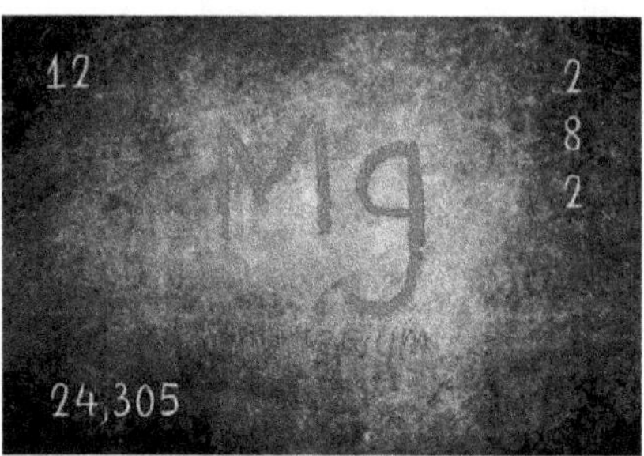

The Placebo Effect

In an article on magnesium by an American Specialist Physician, he explained how we don't know too much about magnesium's metabolic pathway and how he was taking one tablet a day and "felt better" for it. Thus encouraged I then took one a day - and felt no different - but I felt great to begin with. In subsequent studies magnesium does seem to donate some benefits (see "Notes").

Be that as it may the Placebo Effect can donate a 60% improvement. I am sure that if my American colleague was given an identical pill with no active constituents but told it was magnesium, he would feel the same "improvement".

If you buy a vitamin let alone a multivitamin you are going to feel better even though your body vitamin stores were already saturated. If you now look on fresh fruit and vegetables and other produce with the same reverence and expectations you will achieve the same feeling better - but this time I contend your metabolic pathways will be more exquisitely supplied with the correct dose of vitamins, minerals but importantly the micronutrients too.

Herewith an interesting extract from a chapter on Depression in one of my books: "A systematic review of 252 trials of drugs for depression published between 1978 and 2016 has found (only) one drug that consistently works for 35-40% of participants It is called placebo. Contrary to expectation, the effect size did not vary over more than 25 years".[600]

---

600 *Lancet Psychiatry* doi:10.1016/S2215-0366(16)30307-8.

CHAPTER 24

DAIRY

DAIRY, DAIRY ME

The following was written by a Dietician / Nutritionist employed by the Dairy Industry which documents the case for dairy products. It is obviously a complex and incomplete problem but, for the moment, I still recommend no (or little) butter and no cream but fermented products, such as yoghurt and cheese, no matter their fat content, are fine and even beneficial. Once again it is eating the whole food and not just one ingredient. I have retained this article referenced separately below:

Article

Full fat dairy products are higher in saturated fat, which was thought to increase cholesterol and hence heart disease risk. However, the latest research indicates a change in thinking when it comes to dairy foods.

There is evidence that higher levels of saturated fat increase levels of LDL cholesterol[1] and cholesterol-lowering medications that lower LDL can lower cardiovascular disease (CVD) risk,[2] but the evidence for saturated fat reducing CVD risk is less clear.[3—8] This is particularly so for studies that use dairy products as sources of saturated fat.

Whole dairy foods such as milk, cheese and yoghurt are a complex food matrix of nutrients. Saturated fats, protein, calcium, vitamin D, potassium, magnesium, and so on, together do not have the same impact on CVD[8] as saturated fat alone.

Meta-analyses indicate dairy consumption is either linked to a lower risk of CVD, CHD and/or stroke or there is no association.[9-13] No significant link has been found between high and low fat dairy for CHD,[10] although low fat dairy has specifically been linked with a reduced stroke risk.[9,11]

There is also no difference between high and low-fat dairy and biomarkers of CVD.[14,15]

A meta-analysis of three studies assessing butter consumption and CVD found no statistical difference,[12] similar to more recent studies.[11,16]

Cheese consumption is also inversely associated with CHD[9] and stroke.[11,17] Fermented dairy foods which may include cheese, yoghurt and milks/buttermilk, also showed no change or improved biomarkers of CVD.[11,14,18,19]

While butter is rich in saturated fat and can increase total cholesterol it also increases HDL cholesterol and hence reduces the total cholesterol/HDL cholesterol ratio. A lower ratio means a lower risk for heart disease.[1,13]

Regardless of fat content, milk, cheese and yoghurt also reduce total and/or LDL cholesterol.[20—23] Dairy calcium appears to affect fat absorption and increase fat fecal excretion, which may explain these cholesterol effects.[24—26]

References:

1. Effects of dietary fatty acids and carbohydrates on the ratio of serum total to HDL cholesterol and on serum lipids and apolipoproteins: a meta-analysis of 60 controlled trials. Am J Clin Nutr. 2003;77:1146–55.
2. Quantifying effect of statins on low density lipoprotein cholesterol, ischaemic heart disease, and stroke: systematic review and meta-analysis. BMJ. 2003;326:1423.
3. Meta-analysis of prospective cohort studies evaluating the association of saturated fat with cardiovascular disease. Am J Clin Nutr. 2010;91:535–46.
4. A systematic review of the evidence supporting a causal link between dietary factors and coronary heart disease. Arch Intern Med. 2009;169:659–69.
5. Dietary fat and coronary heart disease: summary of evidence from prospective cohort and randomised controlled trials. Ann Nutr Metab. 2009;55:173–201.
6. Effects on coronary heart disease of increasing polyunsaturated fat in place of saturated fat: a systematic review and meta-analysis of randomized controlled trials. PLoS Med. 2010;7:e1000252.
7. Reduced or modified dietary fat for preventing cardiovascular disease. Cochrane Database Syst Rev. 2011;CD002137.
8. An update on the cardiovascular pleiotropic effects of milk and milk products. J Clin Hypertens (Greenwich). 2013 Jul;15(7):503-10.
9. Dairy consumption and risk of cardiovascular disease: an updated meta-analysis of prospective cohort studies. Asia Pac J Clin Nutr. 2015;24(1):90-100.
10. Milk and dairy consumption and incidence of cardiovascular diseases and all-cause mortality: dose-response meta-analysis of prospective cohort studies. Am J Clin Nutr. 2011;93:158–71.
11. Dairy foods and risk of stroke: a meta-analysis of prospective cohort studies. Nutr Metab Cardiovasc Dis. 2014 May;24(5):460-9.
12. The consumption of milk and dairy foods and the incidence of vascular disease and diabetes: an overview of the evidence. Lipids. 2010;45:925–39.
13.Influence of dairy product and milk fat consumption on cardiovascular disease risk: a review of the evidence. Adv Nutr. 2012 May 1;3(3):266-85.
14. Effects of low-fat or full-fat fermented and non-fermented dairy foods on selected cardiovascular biomarkers in overweight adults. Br J Nutr. 2013 Dec;110(12):2242-9
15.Effects of high and low fat dairy food on cardio-metabolic risk factors: a meta-analysis of randomized studies. PLoS One. 2013 Oct 11;8(10):e76480
16. Consumption of dairy products and associations with incident diabetes, CHD and mortality in the Whitehall II study. Br J Nutr. 2013 Feb 28;109(4):718-26.
17. Association between dairy food consumption and risk of myocardial infarction in women differs by type of dairy food. J Nutr. 2013 Jan;143(1):74-9.
18. Impact of buttermilk consumption on plasma lipids and surrogate markers of cholesterol homeostasis in men and women. Nutr Metab Cardiovasc Dis. 2013 Dec;23(12):1255-62.
19. Effect on blood lipids of two daily servings of Camembert cheese. An intervention trial in mildly hypercholesterolemic subjects. Int J Food Sci Nutr. 2014 Dec;65(8):1013-8
20. Effect of cheese consumption on blood lipids: a aystematic review and meta analysis of randomised controlled trials. Nutr Rev 2015 advance access pg 1-17
21. Cheese consumption in relation to cardiovascular risk factors among Iranian adults- IHHP Study. Nutr Res Pract.

2014 Jun;8(3):336-41.
22. The effect of a probiotic milk product on plasma cholesterol: a meta-analysis of short-term intervention studies. Eur J Clin Nutr. 2000 Nov;54(11):856-60.
23. Dairy products and metabolic effects in overweight men and women: results from a 6-mo intervention study. Am J Clin Nutr. 2009 Oct;90(4):960-8.
24. Effect of dairy calcium from cheese and milk on fecal fat excretion, blood lipids, and appetite in young men. Am J Clin Nutr. 2014 May;99(5):984-91.
25. Effect of dairy calcium on fecal fat excretion: a randomized crossover trial. Int J Obes (Lond). 2008 Dec;32(12):1816-
26. Milk minerals modify the effect of fat intake on serum lipid profile: results from an animal and a human short-term study. Br J Nutr. 2014 Apr 28;111(8):1412-20.

Butter

We all love butter and for those of us who cook there is often nothing better. However, the consensus of informed opinion is that "long term health will be better with olive and other (than butter) oils" and "foods that we know improve health and butter is not one of them".

Another study found that patients who consumed the most butter after a heart attack had x 3 times the risk of dying within 42 months compared to those eating the Mediterranean Diet.[601]

Yet another claimed that butter would seem to be 'neutral'. A study found only weak or neutral effects of butter consumption on overall mortality and cardiovascular disease (CVD) risk, suggesting that butter may not be as harmful as previously thought and may not be as harmful as the white bread and potatoes it is spread on.[602]

Butter contains most of the damaging SFAs

Palmitic acid: 31%
Myristic acid: 12%
Stearic acid: 11%

Common name	Carbon chain length	Typical food sources
Lauric acid	12	Coconut oil
Myristic acid	14	Coconut oil, dairy fat
Palmitic acid	16	Palm oil, meat and dairy fats
Stearic acid	18	Meat fat, cocoa butter

[601] JAMA 2000;284 Dec 13
[602] June 29 in PLoS One

I use Extra Virgin Olive Oil but whatever you use make sure it is cold-pressed, as all others are heat or chemically processed. In addition, Italian Olive Oil has been found to be the most adulterated in the world. Make sure you know your brand.

There are exceptions when nothing tastes better than butter and a little, now and then is not going to hurt us. It is the daily use, as with lard in North Karalia, that would seem to be a problem.

When cheese was added to a low-fat diet the cholesterol and lipid levels didn't alter but added butter did elevate them.[603]

The French paradox:

Countries where people eat more cheese have less heart disease than in the U.S. The French eat 24 kg of cheese a year and have a third the heart attack rate of the British and Americans who eat 13kg annually. Most cheese contains 30 to 40% fat of which most is saturated. Only 1% is cholesterol. Cheese has now been shown to have a protective effect on heart disease and mortality.[604] Just 12g (0.42oz) a day (the butter on two slices of toast) doubled the risk of developing diabetes 2.[605]

Nutrition Experts Opinions Summary[606]

Do you agree that it's still a good idea to avoid butter and other animal fats?

"The occasional piece of buttered toast isn't going to kill anyone but opting for poly- and mono-unsaturated fats like olive oil is likely the healthier choice".

Walter C. Willett, MD, DrPH, Harvard T.H. Chan School of Public Health

"I agree it is a good idea to avoid excessive amounts of butter and animal fats, just as it is in general a good idea to avoid excess of just about anything in our daily diet."

Christopher D. Gardner, PhD, Stanford University

---

[603] Cheese intake in large amounts lowers LDL-cholesterol concentrations compared with butter intake of equal fat content. Am J Clin Nut;94:1479-84, 2011.

[604] Dairy and Cardiovascular Disease. A Review of Recent Observational Research. Curr Nutr Reo;3:130-38 (15 Mar 2014).

[605] American Journal of Clinical Nutrition Marta Guasch-Ferre, Harvard T.H. Chan School of Public Health in the US Feb 17, 2017.

[606] MedPage Today February 17, 2017

"The goal for limiting animal fats is more of a moderation rather than a 'must avoid.' Just as important is boosting carbohydrates in place of fats but choosing polyunsaturated fats instead of animal fats will help lower LDL-C".

Connie Diekman, MEd, RD, LD, FADA, Washington University in St. Louis

"The important factor is the relative amount of unsaturated to saturated fat, in favor of the former and limited in the latter. What should be avoided is the replacement of animal and dairy fat with refined carbohydrate".

Alice H. Lichtenstein, DSc, Tufts University

"I do think it's wise to avoid butter and animal fats. TIME magazine reported that "butter is not linked to a higher rate of heart disease" but neglected to mention that it IS directly linked with all-cause mortality, which is even more important".

Dean Ornish, MD, Preventive Medicine Research Institute

I would add here that most of the above are pro-vegan anti-dairy.

Addendum: Dairy, Butter and Cream

The landmark Mediterranean Diet of 1994 that has saved so many lives prohibited butter and cream, which are high in saturated fats. It also promoted olive oil, a monosaturate. While olive oil would seem beneficial and high saturated fats in our bloodstream bad, the recent findings that ingesting saturated fats and high cholesterol foods did not elevate blood levels would seem a second look at this advice is warranted.

This has warranted the separated chapter on cholesterol.

Butter, for those who have cooked with it and eaten it, as I have (and do), is immeasurably superior to any margarine – which is, of course, a processed food. If you have a high LDL, I would not recommend butter and I avoid it by using EVOO (extra virgin olive oil – totally unprocessed) or no spread at all, like the Italians use garlic or tomato as a spread on bruschetta.

We don't have all the answers (yet) and butter and cream may not be the villain in all cases, but the epidemic of heart disease is reducing by using the Mediterranean Diet which does not use butter or cream or by the use of EVOO.

Nutrition science research continues, and all is not clear especially with these new recommendations as to eating saturated fats. In fact, SFA consumption, especially from animals, has subsequently increased due to this data suggesting less correlation with heart disease than previously suspected. But SFA are not all created equal in terms of their effects on lipids, likely due to differing chain lengths, other aspects of their composition or other components of the (whole) foods they are contained in – we seldom just eat the fat.

A review from Cochrane[607] looked to assess the mortality and cardiovascular morbidity effect of reducing saturated fat intake via replacement with carbohydrates, unsaturated fats, or protein in randomized controlled trials (RCT) that had a variety of interventions. It found that reducing saturated fat does reduce serum cholesterol. The trials long-term data showed that cardiovascular events were reduced by 17% mostly due to replacing SFAs with polyunsaturated fats (PUFA) though effects on overall mortality were less evident. It goes on to recommend '*Lifestyle advice to all those at risk of cardiovascular disease and to lower risk population groups should continue to include permanent reduction of dietary saturated fat and partial replacement by unsaturated fats. The ideal type of unsaturated fat is unclear'*.

While this Cochrane report couldn't recommend the type of unsaturated oil to use, the DIVAS study[608] did show a MUFA-rich diet (olive oil) or n-6 PUFA-rich diet (safflower oil) compared with SFA-rich diet (butter) resulted in much lower LDL/non-HDL values in the MUFA/PUFA groups than the SFA group.

Another study[609] showed favorable effects of olive oil versus butter on LDL-C and non-HDL-C in a randomized crossover design. It concluded: 'Moderate intake of butter resulted in increases in total cholesterol and LDL cholesterol compared with the effects of olive oil intake and a habitual diet (run-in period). Furthermore, moderate butter intake was also followed by an increase in HDL cholesterol compared with the habitual diet. We conclude that hypercholesterolemic people should keep their consumption of butter to a

---

607 Reduction in saturated fat intake for cardiovascular disease Lee Hooper1,*, Nicole Martin2, Asmaa Abdelhamid1, George Davey Smith3
Editorial Group: Cochrane Heart Group Published Online: 10 JUN 2015 Assessed as up-to-date: 5 MAR 2014 DOI: 10.1002/14651858.CD011737

608 Replacement of saturated with unsaturated fats had no impact on vascular function but beneficial effects on lipid biomarkers, E-selectin, and blood pressure: results from the randomized, controlled Dietary Intervention and VAScular function (DIVAS) study1,2 * First published May 27, 2015, doi: 10.3945/ ajcn.114.097089 Am J Clin Nutr ajcn097089

609 Butter increased total and LDL cholesterol compared with olive oil however resulted in higher HDL cholesterol than habitual diet1 Sara Engel* and Tine TholstrupFirst published July 1, 2015, doi: 10.3945/ ajcn.115.112227 Am J Clin Nutr ajcn112227

minimum, whereas moderate butter intake may be considered part of the diet in the normo-cholesterolemic population'.

Dairy may cut the risk of suffering a stroke by up to ten per cent

A major study by Oxford University found eating cheese, yoghurt and milk may reduce the likelihood of suffering a stroke in later life. They studied 400,000 people to come to the conclusion that for every extra glass of milk each drank a day, the risk of an ischaemic stroke caused by a blood clot fell by 5 per cent, and it dropped by 9 per cent for every small pot of yogurt.

The results, however, cast doubt on 'going to work on an egg', as those who ate more eggs were more likely to have a rarer haemorrhagic stroke. The most significant results showed that those who ate lots of fiber, along with fruit and vegetables, were significantly less likely to have a stroke.

But the study also suggests dairy foods may be important, although opinion is divided on this since their high saturated fat content has been said to make the food group bad for the heart. There was no difference in cancer risk between full fat versus reduced or non-fat milks, all three spiked the disease's prevalence.

The research found no association between dairy-free milk alternatives such as almond, oat or soy milk and cancer.

CHAPTER 25

SUGAR

SUGAR vs Fat

Evidence for Saturated Fat and Sugar Related to Coronary Heart Disease.[610]

In 1980, the United States issued its first dietary guidelines for the nation, recommending that Americans avoid too much fat, saturated fat and cholesterol for better heart health. The guidelines also mentioned to avoid consuming too much sugar -- but not for the heart, rather because "the major health hazard from eating too much sugar is tooth decay"

As at 2016 Dietary Guidelines continued to recommend restricting intake of saturated fats. This recommendation follows largely from the observation that saturated fats can raise levels of total serum cholesterol (TC), thereby putatively increasing the risk of atherosclerotic coronary heart disease (CHD).

However, TC is only modestly associated with CHD, and more important than the total level of cholesterol in the blood may be the number and size of low-density lipoprotein (LDL) particles that contain it.

As for saturated fats, these fats are a diverse class of compounds; different fats may have different effects on LDL and on broader CHD risk based on the specific saturated fatty acids (SFAs) they contain.

Importantly, though, people eat foods, not isolated fatty acids. Some food sources of SFAs may pose no risk for CHD or possibly even be protective. Advice to reduce saturated fat in the diet without regard to nuances about LDL, SFAs, or dietary sources could actually increase people's risk of CHD.

When saturated fats are replaced with refined carbohydrates, and specifically with added sugars (like sucrose or high fructose corn syrup), the end result is not favorable for heart health. Such replacement leads to changes in LDL, high-density lipoprotein (HDL), and triglycerides that may increase the risk of CHD.

---

610 Prog Cardiovasc Dis. 2016 Mar-Apr;58(5):464-72. doi: 10.1016/j.pcad.2015.11.006. Epub 2015 Nov 14.

Additionally, diets high in sugar may induce many other abnormalities associated with elevated CHD risk, including elevated levels of glucose, insulin, and uric acid, impaired glucose tolerance, insulin and leptin resistance, non-alcoholic fatty liver disease, and altered platelet function.

A diet high in added sugars has been found to cause a 3-fold increased risk of death due to cardiovascular disease, but sugars, like saturated fats, are a diverse class of compounds. The monosaccharide, fructose, and fructose-containing sweeteners (e.g. sucrose) produce greater degrees of metabolic abnormalities than does glucose (either isolated as a monomer, or in chains as starch) and may present greater risk of CHD.

Dietary guidelines should shift focus away from reducing saturated fat, and from replacing saturated fat with carbohydrates, specifically when these carbohydrates are refined.

To reduce the burden of CHD, guidelines should focus particularly on reducing intake of concentrated sugars, specifically the fructose-containing sugars like sucrose and high-fructose corn syrup in the form of ultra-processed foods and beverages.

Experts are still debating what the role of sugar and heart disease is, even though there was evidence going back to the '50s and '60s that a segment of the population with high triglyceride levels should potentially be concerned about their sugar consumption and people who had this triglyceride level would have been counseled much earlier.

Now, as above, it turns out that *added sugars* might be more of a risk factor for coronary heart disease than saturated fats and a diet high in added sugars can cause a three-fold increase in the risk of death due to heart disease.

In the latest dietary guidelines issued by the Office of Disease Prevention and Health Promotion, the government put a limit on sugar for the first time, recommending that added sugar make up only 10% of your daily calories.

What Are the Added Sugars

On the Food Label, Nutrition Facts added sugars include any ingredient with the words

- *"sugar,"* such as white granulated sugar, coconut sugar, brown sugar, beet sugar, raw sugar, or sugar cane juice
- *"nectar,"* such as agave nectar, peach nectar, or fruit nectar
- *"syrup,"* such as corn syrup, high fructose corn syrup, carob syrup, maple syrup, brown rice syrup, or malt syrup
- An ingredient ending in *"-ose,"* including sucrose, dextrose, glucose, fructose, maltose, lactose, galactose, saccharose, and mannose
- *cane juice*/evaporated cane juice/cane juice crystals
- *caramel*
- *corn sweetener*/evaporated corn sweetener
- *fruit juice*/fruit juice concentrate (but whole fresh fruit OK)
- *honey*
- *molasses*
- *muscovado*
- *panela (raspadora)*
- *sweet sorghum*
- *treacle*
- *golden syrup*

New recommendations from the American Heart Association say children 2 to 18 should consume no more than about 6 teaspoons of added sugars in their daily diets.

- Sugar per se, *in small amounts*, is OK. Per se it is not injurious and does not cause diabetes or heart disease
- It is the incredible adding of excess sugars to processed foods resulting in a (very) high daily intake - often unknown and unrealized.
- As to obesity a meta-analysis of randomized controlled and prospective cohort studies found absolutely no effect on body weight when sugar is replaced with the same calories from other carbohydrates.[611] The inference is that fatter people tend to eat more of everything, including sugar and sugar-sweetened beverages (SSBs)

---

611 Dietary sugars and body weight: systematic review and meta-analyses of randomised controlled trials and cohort studies. BMJ. 2012;346:e7492. doi: 10.1136/bmj.e7492.

- Both SSBs and artificially sweetened "diet" versions cause tolerance to unnatural sweetness, which promotes weight gain, mainly by promoting consumption of very sweet, energy-dense foods. Obese people prefer sweeter tastes and sweet, high-fat foods and children who eat more fast foods prefer sweeter tastes.
- However, there has been an incredible explosion in total consumption which exceed guidelines and contributes to obesity
- The problem is that today we are swamped with high sugar processed foods and sugared drinks and are consuming too much
- Sugar is in virtually every processed food: White bread, ketchup, barbeque sauces, salad dressings, canned soups, peanut butter and even canned tomatoes (where elsewhere I recommend them - just don't get ones with any added sugar)
- Sugar – Sucrose - is 50% Glucose (good) and 50% Fructose (bad). Since the 70s cheaper high-fructose corn sweeteners have progressively been used. Fructose does not stimulate the same hormone response and thus is more likely to be converted into fat.
- The bottom line is an overall rise in total consumption of soft drink. Kids are now consuming >30% of their daily calories mostly as soft drinks
- Even Toddlers in Edinburgh were getting 30% of their total calories and up to half their food from sugar
- Up to 22% of British children are currently consuming less than the minimum safe amounts of vitamins and 50% of girls are consuming less than the minimum safe amount of minerals (iron & magnesium)
- Increasing evidence that sugary drinks and inactivity contribute to epidemic of obesity
- Target = < 10 % dietary Calories
- Although glucose is an essential nutrient necessary for the function of every cell in our bodies, it is technically not essential in our diets, being readily generated from other foods. There are health benefits from sugar-containing fruits and vegetables, but sugar added during manufacturing confers no physical benefits

A Fermenting Problem

If we consider harms from addictions and lifestyles in contemporary societies, sugar is high on the list of offenders. Ecological analyses show that humans have evolved to be active and functional in seeking out sugar from food sources primarily fruits and honey.

No wonder then that when sugar is so easily available in such refined and potent form we take so much of it—a global average of 50 g per person a day; no wonder that the heavy sustained use of sugar is similar in some respects to that of alcohol and other drugs. And, no wonder because our bodies are not used to taking so much of it, sugar causes so many health problems— increasing dental caries, cardio-metabolic risk, overweight and obesity (and subsequent effects on cancers), diabetes, and liver dysfunction.

To reduce the harm done by sugar, the World Health Organization launched a consultation on revised sugar guidelines, noting that consumption below 5% of total daily energy intake (around 25 g for an adult of normal body mass index) would bring health gain.

There are calls for effective sugar regulation, similar to those for alcohol, but initiatives such as taxes on sugar sweetened drinks or regulation of serving sizes are often vetoed because of lobbying by the sugar industry. This has led some to call for food producers to voluntary reduce sugar content, similar to salt reduction initiatives.[612]

U.S. adult consumption of added sugars increased by more than 30% over three decades.[613]

The wrong white crystals: not salt but sugar as etiological in hypertension and cardio metabolic disease[614]

Cardiovascular disease is the leading cause of premature mortality in the developed world, and hypertension is its most important risk factor. Controlling hypertension is a major focus of public health initiatives, and dietary approaches

---

[612] BMJ 2015; 350 doi: http://dx.doi.org/10.1136/bmj.h780 (Published 11 February 2015) Cite this as: BMJ 2015;350:h780

[613] Obesity Society. "U.S. adult consumption of added sugars increased by more than 30% over three decades." ScienceDaily. ScienceDaily, 4 November 2014. <www.sciencedaily.com/releases/2014/11/141104141731.htm>.

[614] Open Heart 2014;1: doi:10.1136/openhrt-2014-000167

have historically focused on sodium (salt). There is little debate that the predominant sources of sodium in the diet are industrially processed foods.

Processed foods also happen to be generally high in added sugars, the consumption of which might be more strongly and directly associated with hypertension and cardio metabolic risk.

Added sugars, particularly fructose, may increase blood pressure, increase heart rate and myocardial (heart) oxygen demand, and contribute to inflammation, insulin resistance and broader metabolic dysfunction.

The benefits of reducing consumption of processed foods are highly appropriate and advisable but might have less to do with sodium—minimally related to blood pressure and perhaps even inversely related to cardiovascular risk—and more to do with highly-refined carbohydrates.

It is time for us to shift focus focus greater attention to the likely consequential food additive: sugar.

A reduction in the intake of added sugars, particularly fructose, and specifically in the quantities and context of industrially-manufactured consumables, would help not only curb hypertension rates, but might also help address broader problems related to cardio metabolic disease.

- Sugar may be more related to blood pressure than sodium (salt).
- Higher sugar intake significantly increases both systolic and diastolic blood pressure.
- Ingesting one 24 ounce soft drink has been shown to cause an average maximum increase in blood pressure of 15/9 mm Hg and heart rate of 9 bpm (beats per minute).
- Those who consume 25% or more calories from added sugar have an almost threefold increased risk of death due to cardiovascular disease.
- Fructose has been shown to stimulate sympathetic tone directly, and indirectly by inciting insulin resistance and hyperinsulinemia.
- A high-fructose diet for just 2 weeks not only significantly increased 24 h ambulatory blood pressure and increased pulse rate by 8%, but also increased triglycerides and fasting insulin.
- Excess fructose intake has also been shown to double the prevalence of the metabolic syndrome.
- Current US per capita intake of added sugars is approximately 2–8 times higher than current recommendations by the American Heart Association

(AHA) and WHO. Considering adolescents specifically, current consumption might be as much as 6–16 times higher.

- Ingestion of sugars, including fructose, in their naturally occurring biological contexts (eg, as whole fruits) is not harmful and is likely beneficial.

Dietary sugars and cardio-metabolic risk:

Dietary sugars influence blood pressure and serum lipids independent of effects of sugars on body weight.[615]

Global Deaths

In the first detailed global report on the impact of sugar-sweetened beverages they are linked to an estimated 184,000 adult deaths each year worldwide. In 2010, the researchers estimate that sugar-sweetened beverages consumption may have been responsible for approximately:

- 133,000 deaths from diabetes
- 45,000 deaths from cardiovascular disease
- 6,450 deaths from cancer

The impact of sugar-sweetened beverages varied greatly between populations. At the extremes, the estimated percentage of deaths was less than 1% in Japanese over 65 years old, but 30% in Mexican adults younger than 45. Of the 20 most populous countries, Mexico had the highest death rate attributable to sugar-sweetened beverages with an estimated 405 deaths per million adults (24,000 total deaths) and the U.S. ranked second with an estimated 125 deaths per million adults (25,000 total deaths.[616]

The West Indian Sugar Ships to Glasgow: Worse Teeth Than Cambodia.

I thought it was a joke against Glasgow, given the rivalry between it and Edinburgh, where I specialized, but I had heard it before and that was *"In Glasgow, for a 14th birthday the child had either its upper or lower teeth completely removed and for its 18th birthday those remaining were extracted. And*

[615] Am J Clin Nutr July 2014 vol. 100 no. 1 65

[616] Estimated Global, Regional, and National Disease Burdens Related to Sugar-Sweetened Beverage Consumption in 2010. Circulation, June 2015 DOI: 10.1161/CIRCULATIONAHA.114.010636

there could be no finer Glaswegian 21st birthday or a bride's wedding present, than a full set of "choppers" (dentures)."

But it was true! As reported in the Guardian:[617] A girl would often have all her teeth pulled when she was 18, and get a nice set of dentures, so as not to be a trouble to her husband when she married.

This may sound like legend, but it's a fact that in 1972, when I was in Edinburgh, an amazing 44% of Scots over 16 had no teeth at all. Even today the Scots are fairly toothless - one in six women and one in seven men have lost all their teeth by their mid-50s.

It developed because the West Indian sugar ships mostly sailed up the Clyde to dock in Glasgow. The Clyde was the center of the trade in the nineteenth century and, after sugar-import taxes were halved in 1874, the business got even bigger.

By 1878, 16 of Scotland's 17 sugar refineries were around Glasgow: the Clyde town of Greenock was known as 'Sugaropolis' and it was there that Abram Lyle, later of Tate and Lyle, invented Golden Syrup, as a way of using up surplus sugar at a time of glut.

This surplus of sugar witnessed the eruption of "Sweetie Shops" practically on every corner and the Scots, but especially the Glaswegians, addiction to sugar such that, some years ago, Glasgow had the worst dental hygiene in Europe and the "cure" was the complete extraction of their rotten teeth.

For 200 years there was a lot of cheap sugar around the Clyde. Glasgow, followed by the west of Scotland and then the whole country, put it to use, developing the astonishing range jams, puddings, cakes and sweets whose remnants we see today.

Sugar, the cheap, easily-digested energy source, fueled Scotland. By the beginning of the 20th century, jam - which is up to 65% sugar - had become a staple in the diet: the 'Jilly piece', a jam sandwich, the basis of a working man's lunch.

Glasgow, I thought, had cleaned up its act but in 2006 it was reported that, "Scottish children have the worst teeth in Britain. Over the last 20 years, their sugar intake has doubled. And the statistics are shaming. Scottish children consume more fizzy drinks than anyone else in Europe and they have the worst teeth in Britain - with an average 'd3mft' count (that's the average number of

---

617 The Guardian, The Rot Starts Here", Sunday 28 May 2006.

decayed, missing or filled teeth) of 2.36 at five years old, rising to over three in Glasgow. (In England generally the d3mft figure is 1.47, and less than one in places like Surrey and Sussex). Almost half of all Scottish five-year-olds suffer from tooth decay and a Glaswegian 12-year-old has teeth similar - according to the World Health Organization - to those of a 12-year-old in Kazakhastan or Cambodia. Glaswegians aren't ignorant of the problem - they've long called lemonade and chips 'the Glesca diet'.

The sugar content in soft drinks is one of the junk food industry's great dirty statistics - even 'healthy' apple or blackcurrant juices can contain as much as 14mg of sugar per 100ml. The blackcurrant Ribena that we all happily glugged on as children - 'because it's good for you' - has more sugar in it (34.56g, or seven teaspoons, in the modern 288ml carton) than does Coca-Cola. The fact that Ribena's parent, Glaxo Smith Kline, also sells 600 million tubes of toothpaste a year, is one of mega-industry's charming ironies.

But it's not all due to sugar. Americans eat a lot more sugar than the British - 40kg per annum to 34kg in the UK. Having disease-free teeth is about a lot of factors - hygiene, dental care, orthodontics, genetics, fluoridation and sugar.

Scotland and the North of England still have more dental caries and rotten teeth than most places. The Sugar Ships have been replaced by the Sugar Supermarkets with rows and rows of sugary sweets and mothers who buy them for their kids to shut them up or as a dreadfully wrong "reward".

If it doesn't make you fat, give you diabetes 2 and the metabolic syndrome, sugar will, at least, rot your teeth.

Sugar, Fructose and High Fructose Corn Syrup

We are actually eating less than before but gaining weight such that there is now an obesity epidemic.

Enter Fructose: Fructose is a sugar found naturally in fruit.

As it was not regulated by insulin, it was thought to be the ideal sweetener for diabetics. In 1966 the Japanese invented High Fructose Corn Syrup (HFCS) and by 1980 USA soft drink companies were using it in their products. Our human consumption in 1970 was less than 250 grams a year. However, it has now zoomed up to 25 kg a year i.e. *100 times more!*

The childhood obesity epidemic began in 1980 and shadows this introduction of fructose into our diet, especially in soft drink, fruit drinks and as a sweetener in almost everything in a packet. The problem with fructose is that only our livers can take it up, whereas Glucose, the essential body energizer, is used by every organ in our body. In fact, glucose is the only food our brain can use.

The increase in obesity, however, is attributed to sugar from any source as, at this time, there's insufficient evidence to say that high-fructose corn syrup is any less healthy than other types of sweeteners. What is known, however, is that too much added sugar — not just high-fructose corn syrup — can contribute unwanted calories that are linked to health problems, such as weight gain, type 2 diabetes, metabolic syndrome and high triglyceride levels. All of these boost your risk of heart disease.

The American Heart Association recommends that women get no more than 100 calories a day from added sugar from any source, and that most men get no more than 150 calories a day from added sugar. That's about 6 teaspoons of added sugar for women and 9 teaspoons for men.

Fructose occurring naturally in fruit or food is fine because of the fiber. An orange is 20 calories, 10 of which are fructose, but it also has high fiber. Whereas a glass of orange juice takes six oranges, contains 120 calories or 60 calories of fructose and has no fiber.

The American diet: 44% of the added sugar is sucrose, 42% is high-fructose corn syrup and the remaining 14% includes honey, molasses, juice concentrates and agave -- all of which also combine fructose and glucose (which also is known as dextrose). Yet worldwide, high-fructose corn syrup represents only about 8% of added sugar consumption.

In just 10 days, restricting the amount of fructose children consumed through sugary drinks and juices resulted in "dramatic" reductions in liver fat. When fructose is ingested in large quantities, such as in fruit juices or in sodas (soft drink), it causes almost a tsunami in the liver, forcing it to produce more fat according to this study.[618]

Matched calorie for calorie with the simple sugar glucose, fructose causes significant weight gain, physical inactivity, and body fat deposition in mice. Because of the addition of high-fructose corn syrup to many soft drinks and

---

[618] "Isocaloric fructose restriction for 10 days reduces hepatic de novo lipogenesis and liver fat in obese Latino and African American children" ENDO 2015.

processed baked goods, fructose currently accounts for 10% of caloric intake for U.S. citizens.[619]

BEVERAGE	**QUANTITY**	**SUGAR Grams**
MILK		
Skim	8oz glass	11
Silk Vanilla Soymilk	glass	8
Silk Almond Milk Original	glass	7
Ditto unsweetened		0
JUICES		
Smoothie Bolthouse Farms Berry Boost	15.2oz bottle	24
Minute Maid 100% Apple	15.2oz bottle	49
Sunny D Original	16oz bottle	28
SPORTS DRINKS		
Gatorade Thirst Quencher Cool Blue	32oz bottle	56
Powerade Mountain Berry Blast		56
ENERGY DRINK		
Red Bull	16oz can	52
Monster Energy	16oz can	54
SODA / SOFT DRINKS		
Coca-Cola	20oz bottle	65
Pepsi	20oz	69
COFFEE		
Starbucks Iced Flavored Latte		28
Dunkin Donuts Iced Caramel Latte	16oz	37

619 Fructose decreases physical activity and increases body fat without affecting hippocampal neurogenesis and learning relative to an isocaloric glucose diet. *Scientific Reports*, 2015; 5: 9589 DOI: 10.1038/srep09589

Sugar Content of Top USA Selling Beverages[620]

According to a 2018 analysis published in the journal *Nutrients*, soft drinks were the main sugar-sweetened beverages (SSB) for adolescents, teens, and adults, but sweetened fruit drinks were the key contributor for children. Sports and energy drinks were increasingly prevalent in the nine and up age groups, but especially for nine- to 18-year-olds.

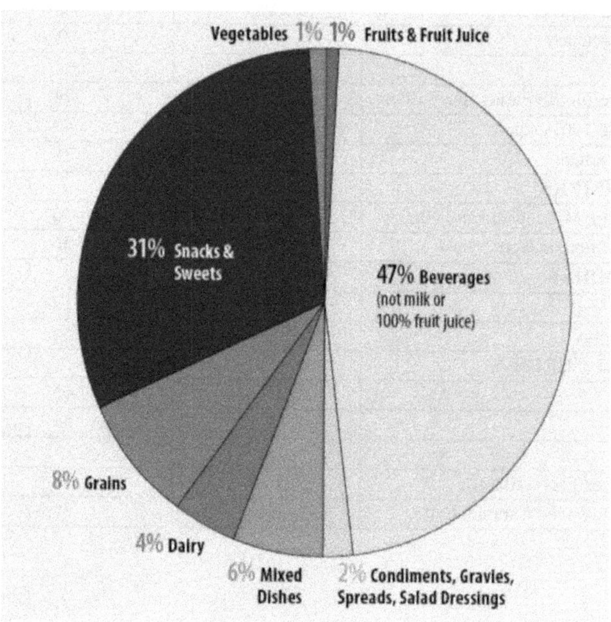

Recommendations

No sweetened Fruit Juice, no soft drink / sodas and avoid all sugar including HFCS. No added sugar.

NOTE: Corn syrup found on supermarket shelves is only a distant cousin to the high-fructose corn syrup used commercially. The HFCS process is much more complex and results in a different chemical structure.

[620] Source: Beverage Industry magazine's 2013 State of the Industry Report
One teaspoon of sugar weighs slightly less than 4 grams.

CHAPTER 26

SALT

Reducing salt is the most cost-effective measure to lower blood pressure and reduce the number of people suffering from strokes and heart disease, the commonest causes of death in first world countries.

Linear Relationship Between Sodium Consumption and Mortality

Trials of Hypertension Follow-up (TOPH) phase 2 is the largest clinical trial to date to evaluate a sodium reduction intervention. Consistent evidence shows a direct relationship between dietary sodium intake and blood pressure.

It found that for every added 1000 mg/day of sodium (the equivalent of about half a teaspoon per day), the risk for premature death went up by 12%. People with the lowest intake of sodium have the lowest rates of total mortality, according to a study spanning more than 20 years published in the October issue of the *Journal of the American College of Cardiology*. There is greater detail in Part C Notes Dietary guidelines are for levels below 2300 mg a day.

Industry Regulation of Salt and Sugar: or Who's Guarding the Guards? The "Fox to Guard the Hen House."

Industry-funded research has been found five times likelier to observe no relation between sugar-sweetened beverages and obesity or weight gain than industry-independent work. Worried about government regulation, global food-and-drink companies are increasingly funding research, especially on sugar, according to a four-part feature in the *BMJ*. One government-funded organization looking to address obesity in the U.K. — the Scientific Advisory Committee on Nutrition — has had 40 scientists as members over a 12-year span. Only 13 of the 40 have not had to declare potential conflicts of interest over industry ties. Both Coca-Cola and PepsiCo have declared, in filings with the U.S. Securities & Exchange Commission, that research on the adverse health effects of their products is worrisome. Such fears, according to a Union of Concerned Scientists report, have led to a funding strategy that "could produce systematic biases in nutrition research."

Voluntary agreements between industry and government (including the UK public health responsibility deal) have been shown repeatedly to be ineffective.

The best hope of achieving ongoing reductions in the salt and sugar content of processed foods lies in mandatory regulation and taxation in specific areas. Data from Mexico showing that a 10% tax on sugar sweetened beverages (equivalent to 1 peso (4p) per litre of sugary drink) was associated with a decline in purchases averaging 7.6% over two years, with the biggest effect on the poorest households.

Industry arguments often fall back on ideas of personal freedom. Strategies include reframing soft drinks or fat taxes as issues of consumer rights and examples of the alleged excesses of the "nanny state" and then promoting public-private partnerships and corporate social responsibility deals that allow the "fox to guard the hen house."

A report from Consensus Action on Salt and Health (CASH) shows that only one out of the 28 food categories surveyed are on track to meet Public Health England's (PHE) 2017 salt reduction targets. The food industry will also fail to hit a PHE target to achieve a 20% reduction in sugar content across nine food categories — including breakfast cereals, cakes, and yogurts — by 2020, confirming the long held view of some experts that voluntary agreements aren't working and we should now move from soft to hard regulation.[621]

Many foods we take for granted or even consider 'healthy' are, in fact, "salt mines": Bread and breakfast cereals are big offenders, but even crumpets, widely considered to be a healthy breakfast or teatime treat, contain high amounts of salt. The average salt level per crumpet was 0.62g, nearly the same amount of salt as one-and-a-half packets of ready-salted crisps. Salt levels in branded crumpets were much higher on average (1.31g per 100g) compared with supermarket own-label crumpets which contained 1.10g of salt per 100g. Gluten-free crumpets were, on average, 15% saltier than normal crumpets.

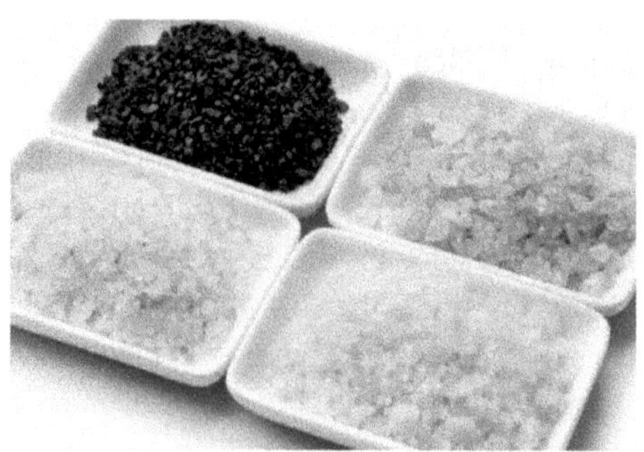

Commercial hummus and dips are also "salt mines".

[621] BMJ 2017;357:j1709

CHAPTER 27

MEAT

In the Medically Beneficial Diets, I detail how a Vegetarian Diet is "one of the healthiest". Be that as it may, very, very few early populations have ever willingly adopted it because most could have died out as humans need essential supplements, such as vitamin B12, choline and zinc not readily available from plants. Nevertheless, some societies and individuals did without any seeming effects.

Vitamin B12 is produced by bacteria, not animals or plants. As such, animals, including humans, must obtain it directly or indirectly from bacteria-laden manure and unsanitized water. Today, however, with modern hygienic practices more effectively cleaning and sanitizing produce, along with soil being exposed to more antibiotics and pesticides, most plant foods are no longer reliable sources of this bacterial product nor, as a result, are the grazing animals. Further, in many countries, factory-farmed animals are kept indoors and never even see soil during their lifetimes. These animals then need supplementation. In fact, it is claimed that some 95% of all B12 supplements manufactured are now actually given to farmed animals.

Today, people, regardless of whether they ate meat, are at risk for B12 deficiency.

Even if Hindus never ate dead animals, their drinking water and soil particles (and bugs) on their produce had plenty of it. Not all Hindus abstain from meat, but the ones who do were actually vegetarians who also ate animal products like milk, ghee and curds. The Jains were closer to vegans. They claim there never was a deficiency of B12 until modern ultra-sanitation, which protects us from things like cholera and dysentery, but destroys B12. And that today even meat eaters can easily be deficient in B12 because of both the chemical abuse and sterilization of our soils, and the fact that in factory farms, the animals are fed prepared grains instead of their natural diet of grass from pastures. One step forward, three back!

The earliest records of vegetarianism as a concept and practice are from ancient India, especially the Jains and ancient groups in southern Italy and Greece. All were concerned with animal welfare. But not everyone who refused to participate in any killing or injuring of animals also abstained from the consumption of meat and there are two schools of thought as to Buddhist vegetarianism. One says that the Buddha and his followers ate meat offered to them by hosts or alms-givers if they had no reason to suspect that the animal had been slaughtered specifically for their sake. The other one says that the Buddha and his community of monks were strict vegetarians and the habit of accepting alms of meat was only tolerated later on.

Today Indian vegetarians, primarily lacto-vegetarians, are estimated to make up more than 70 percent of the world's vegetarians. They make up 20–42 percent of the population in India, while less than 30 percent are regular meat-eaters.

Surveys in the U.S. have found that roughly 4% of adults eat no meat, poultry, or fish.

It can be seen how omnivores are a combination of grinding herbivore teeth (molars) and meat tearing carnivore (canine) teeth. In humans our canine teeth differ as to their prominence and sharpness, but nevertheless provide the evolutionary evidence that humans were (and are) meat eaters.

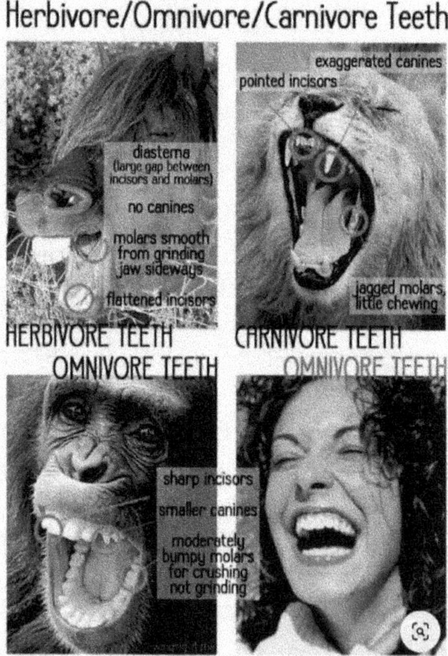

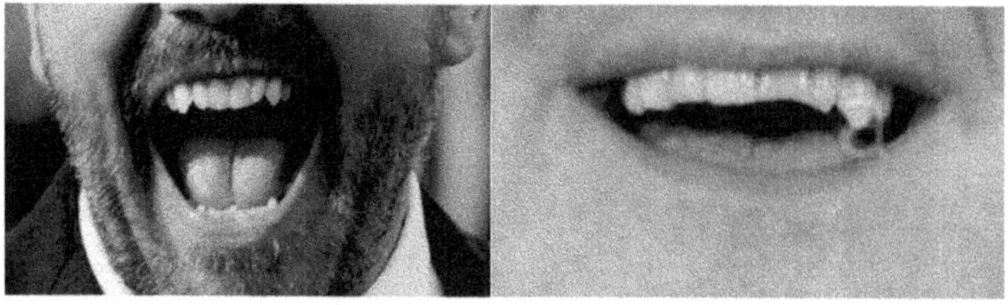

Humans have flat teeth (molars) that evolved to crush rather than grind; but we also have pointed incisor and tearing "canine" teeth, which identify us as meat-eating animals.

One of the world's biggest studies the EPIC (European Prospective Investigation into Cancer and Nutrition) of 448,568 participants from 10 different European countries followed for 12.7 years found that *"red meat posed no detectable risk as judged by all-cause mortality*". It did, however, find an association with processed meat.[622]

And, most recently, the world's best coronary arteries yet studied were in the Tsimane people of the Bolivian Amazon have the lowest reported levels of vascular aging and the lowest prevalence of coronary atherosclerosis of any population yet studied and they eat meat[623].

Some 14% of their diet is meat but you can bet it's lean, with no growth promoters or antibiotics and mostly grass or plant fed.

Meat has gained a bad reputation, but I think this is mainly because what the animal is fed, how it is prepared and cooked how and that we eat too much. Searing and char is carcinogenic (cancer causing), much is fed an abnormal feed-lot diet which, in some countries also includes "growth promoters" aka steroids, and antibiotics and, on top of this we eat too much.

If you think about it our ancestors didn't get much meat. They had to chase a beast for days or weeks, so they were fit and lean but so was their kill! So, they only ate lean meat occasionally...and it was grass fed or had eaten other meat eaters. Meat shortened the human gut, so we didn't have to eat all day like Herbivores and cooking it provided protein for our brains to grow bigger than any other animal. Meat was fundamental to human nutrition and survival. It isn't today if you take the various supplements especially B12. But, if you eat meat, make sure it's grass fed, lean and a small, not overcooked, steak only a couple of times a week.

Processed meat such as bacon, ham and sausages are definitely bad for us and associated with cancer of the colon. I don't know if it were always thus and suspect the modern preservatives such as the nitrates may be carcinogenic. Poultry seems OK and so does pork.

---

[622] Meat consumption and mortality - results from the European Prospective Investigation into Cancer and Nutrition *BMC Medicine*2013**11**:63**DOI:** 10.1186/1741-7015-11-63

[623] Coronary atherosclerosis in indigenous South American Tsimane: a cross-sectional cohort study. *The Lancet*, 2017; DOI: 10.1016/S0140-6736(17)30752-3

However, it is to be emphasized that there's growing evidence that *high-protein food choices* do play a role in health—and that eating healthy protein sources like fish, chicken, beans, or nuts *in place of red meat* (especially processed red meat) can lower the risk of several diseases and premature death. A high ingestion of red meat increases the risks for cardiovascular disease, diabetes, cancer and osteoporosis.

How Much Red Meat is OK?

No one knows but a hell of a lot less than most people, eating the present Western Diet, consume. At the most I would suggest a steak no bigger than one's hand, twice a week and grass fed with no char on cooking.

Animal sources of protein tend to deliver all the amino acids we need.

Other protein sources, such as fruits, vegetables, grains, nuts and seeds lack one or more essential amino acids.

Vegetarians need to be aware of this. People who don't eat meat, fish, poultry, eggs, or dairy products need to eat a variety of protein-containing foods each day in order to get all the amino acids needed to make new protein.

The Vegetarian Six - Hour Gut

To survive Humans obviously worked out which foods nourished them from what was available. If our ancestors were originally vegetarians this would have necessitated having a long, large intestinal tract as, for herbivores (plant eaters), it requires a six-hour-a-day, chewing marathon to obtain enough nutrition to survive.

Cooking, Meat, Bigger Brains and Shorter Guts

Cooking and meat altered the need for this prolonged digestion. Cooking food breaks down its cells, meaning that our stomachs need to do less work to liberate the nutrients. Without cooking, an average person would have to eat around five kilos of raw food to get enough calories to survive. It is accepted that the introduction of meat into our ancestors' diet caused their brains to grow and their intelligence to increase. Meat - a more concentrated form of energy - not only meant bigger brains for our ancestors, but also an end to the need to devote nearly all their time to foraging and eating to maintain energy levels. The increase in brain-size mirrors the reduction in the size of the gut. The reduction in the size of our digestive system was found, as previously noted, to be exactly the same amount by which our brains grew - by some 20%.

The modern human brain is two to three times larger than that of our closest relatives, chimpanzees. Humans also have the largest cerebral cortex of all mammals, relative to the size of their brains. This area houses the cerebral hemispheres, which are responsible for higher functions like memory, communication and thinking. Our brain accounts for ~2% of our body weight but it consumes ~20% of glucose-derived energy making it the main consumer of glucose at ~5.6 mg glucose per 100 g human brain tissue per minute and to supply energy to such metabolically demanding tissue, a distinct trade-off in energy allocation had to evolve. In 1992, researchers proposed that this gradual expansion of the ancestral brain was made possible by switching from a vegetative diet to a meat-rich, fat-rich diet. As meat became a dietary staple, the gut shortened, and the brain no longer needed to rely on fuel from muscle and fat stores in the body. A shorter gut requires a great deal less energy than the lengthy gut of herbivores. Drawing on the extra energy resources from a fatty diet, and a shorter gut, the brain could afford to grow.

Bigger Brains and Saliva

The second great boost to the human brain is thought to be the development or increase in salivary amylase. This enzyme breaks down grains allowing their nutrients, often a source of glucose and essential vitamins like thiamine, to be released and digested by humans. The human brain uses 25% of the body's total energy needs and 60% of total blood glucose requirements to function effectively. The glucose needs of the brain cannot be met on a low-carb diet. It is not likely that the human brain could have evolved without our ancestors consuming a lot of carbs (but I hasten to add these were unrefined natural fruits and vegetables).

There was a spurt in the development of the brain from around 800,000 years ago. Our ancestors started eating cooked food from just before this period. Cooked starch products are more easily digested than their raw forms. So it is likely that humans were eating cooked starch during the centuries before their brain started to develop in rapid bursts. However, genetic and archaeological studies revealed a critical finding: Salivary amylase genes started multiplying in humans from about a million years ago. Salivary amylase is instrumental in breaking down starch rapidly and making it available to the body for absorption and humans have more salivary amylase gene copies (approximately six, but the number varies across individuals) than any other primate (only two).

As well as better nutrition it is proposed that competition with others, cooperation and reward for complex tasks may have been instrumental in driving brain evolution to refine and develop it further[624] which would seem self-evident to me.

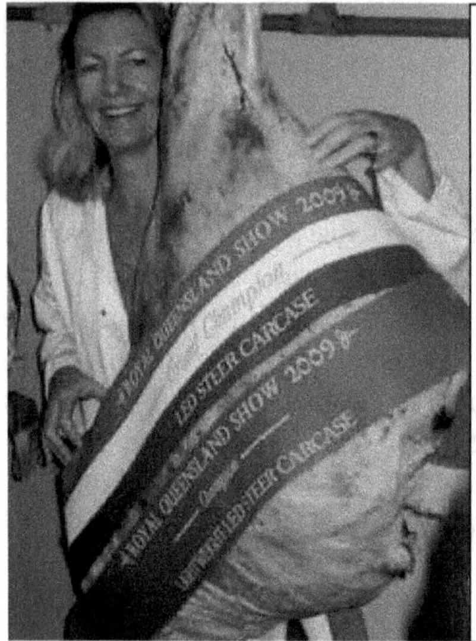

Today we are probably eating too much but, after humans eating it for 2.8 million years, a little grass-fed meat would seem beneficial. It contains the essential vitamin B12 and other beneficial micronutrients.

It is thought that meat and cooking promoted the human brain to be the biggest.

The healthiest coronary arteries, yet found in the world, are in meat eaters.

Preserved meats, however, are not recommended

The woman in this photo bred this prize winning carcase. She eats meat. She is slim. Her LDL is low and she loves animals.

Growth Promoters and Antibiotics

In 1964, as a medical student at an august seminar with all the senior professors and doctors I brought up the problem of antibiotic resistance (yes it's that old) and pointed out that farm animals and poultry were being fed 'preventive' antibiotics over which there was no control and no information as to any remaining in the produce we ate, let alone the obvious dangers of resistance. It was met with silence which I attributed to skepticism or ignorance or both.

HGP (Hormone Growth Promoters) are not illegal in most countries but many Supermarkets now refuse to stock such HGP meat. Prophylactic animal antibiotics are being legislated out in many countries.

Some years ago, in the UK, farmers were feeding their cattle on other dead cattle with the potential for a long-incubating virus which attacks the brain being passed to humans. The UK egg market was also nearly ruined in 1988-89 by an outbreak

[624] A Dominant Social Comparison Heuristic Unites Alternative Mechanisms for the Evolution of Indirect Reciprocity. Scientific Reports, 2016; 6: 31459 DOI: 10.1038/srep31459

of Salmonella. A good resume of the use of antibiotics in poultry can be found at Is Your Meat Safe? - Antibiotic Debate Overview | Modern Meat - PBS

www.pbs.org/wgbh/pages/frontline/shows/meat/safe/overview.html

Fish farms are the way of the future and it would seem the fish now also receive prophylactic antibiotics.

Not only that, their valued Omega 3 oil content has halved.

We can only depend on the diligence and standards of our National Health services, which are obviously of a high standard. But keep alert! While the Government Agencies are good, they often have to wait, gathering information and then investigating. In the meantime, hundreds of thousands are getting food poisoning, with thousands dying, each year. So, if you read of any "outbreak", be it animal or vegetable, cease that food or source immediately until the problem has been fixed. A sad case in point for me was in the 90s when people fell ill from contaminated oysters. I had just bought 12 dozen for the family Christmas and even though they were ostensibly from another area they had the common factor that they were river oysters, and so I felt I had to throw them all out (as I thought upstream contamination and slow tides would provide good conditions for bacterial or viral inoculation). I was right: People who ate these oysters also became very ill.

CHAPTER 28

MAN THE MEAT EATER

OK, Women too – it's just a catchier heading.

But humans have always eaten meat otherwise the human race would have died out from lack of essential nutrients especially vitamin B12 which was then only available in nutritional amounts in meat.

However, humans have adapted, perhaps more than any other species, to thrive on a number of diets from the vegetarian diet of India's Jains, the meat diet of Inuit, the fish-heavy diet of Malaysia's Bajau, the insect diet of the Nochmani off the coast of India,

But nutritional scientists and anthropologists think meat and the cooking of it is also how humans developed a shorter gut and a bigger brain.

And, even today, with the Vegetarians and Vegans, zealously proclaiming their benefits, the healthiest coronary arteries in the world – and coronary artery disease is what kills most of us – are to be found in meat eaters.

We are, nevertheless, eating too much meat.

And, it is my contention, we are not only eating too much, but abnormally, artificially fed meat on grains not grass, and artificially fattened, some laced with antibiotics or growth promoting steroids and then we cook it at high temperatures which cause cancer causing heterocyclic amines, all of which help give meat a bad profile. And processed "deli" meats are thought to be carcinogenic probably due to preservatives.

The vegetarian-vegan diets are healthy but require supplements. There are, however, religious zealots trying to turn us all into being vegetarians and they publish studies to promote their bias some of which I find cruel, offensive and totally lacking in any medical basis such as one alleging the part meat and milk play in causing diabetes.

A little lean, grass-fed meat, as the Tsimane Indians of Bolivia, who have the world's best coronary arteries, may be good for us and certainly not as injurious as the veggies would have us believe.

Meat and cooking are thought by some anthropologists and nutritional scientists to have been crucial to the evolution of our ancestors' smaller gut and larger brains.

Meat and marrow are nutrient and calorie-dense compared with the low-quality plant diet of apes, humans' closest relatives and direct ancestor. Beginning some 2 million years ago this higher quality diet and less bulky plant fiber would have allowed these humans to have much smaller guts and the increased energy such a meat diet liberated allowed for our bigger brain which requires 20%of a human's energy when resting when an ape's brain requires only 8%. We also have relatively smaller guts some 60% of the size that you would expect for a primate of our body size.

But further, it is thought that the biggest revolution in the human diet came not when we started to eat meat but when we learned to cook, sometime between 1.8 million and 400,000 years ago.

Cooking was preceded by pounding and then the cooking "predigests" it, so our guts spend less energy breaking it down, absorb more than if the food were raw, and thus extract more fuel for our brains. Today humans can't survive on raw, unprocessed food alone. We have evolved to depend upon cooked food.

Around 10,000 years ago agriculture developed with the domestication of grains which made for the first time a relatively reliable food supply. Even given the contingencies of floods, famines and pestilence this new plentiful food supply saw increased reproduction with farmers' wives having babies every 2.5 years compared with every 3.5 years for hunter-gatherers.

Very, very few tribes, communities or societies eat, or can eat, meat exclusively. Firstly, with just spears and bow and arrows they were never guaranteed 'supply' and secondly few developed the genes. The exception are the Inuit of the Artic who get as much as 99% of their calories from seals, narwhals, and fish. While the progress of agriculture has seen the Hunters relegated to a few marginal areas such as the Amazon and Africa.

And while grains were domesticated only some 10,000 years ago humans, from anthropological studies, may have been eating grains, as well as tubers, for at least 100,000 years—long enough to have evolved the ability to tolerate them such as the development of salivary amylase – the enzyme necessary to digest grain. Populations that traditionally ate more starchy foods have more copies of the gene than the Yakut meat-eaters of Siberia, and their saliva helps break down starches before the food reaches their stomachs.

But we can't digest raw grains. However, when starch has been cooked, the granule swells and it takes up water in a process called gelatinization and then the amylases can easily break down the di- and tri-saccharides and start to create sugar, which is why cooked vegetables taste sweeter than raw.

Humans also then developed a mutation in the myosin component of the jaw muscle that effectively limits bite force such that our chewing and chewing power became reduced compared to chimpanzees. As humans relied more and more on softer plant foods our teeth, jaws, and faces have become smaller, and our DNA has changed since the invention of agriculture.

But research into this reduction in chewing muscles concluded that "by simply slicing meat and pounding, hominins would have improved their ability to chew meat into smaller particles by 41%, reduced the number of chews per year by another 5%, and decreased masticatory force requirements by an additional 12%. Although cooking has important benefits, it appears that selection for smaller masticatory features in *Homo* would have been initially made possible by the combination of using stone tools and eating meat".[625]

Lactose tolerance is an exquisite study in this evolutionary process: All humans digest mother's milk as infants, but weaned children no longer needed to digest milk. As a result, they stopped making the enzyme lactase, which breaks down the lactose into simple sugars. But after humans began herding cattle, it became tremendously advantageous to digest milk, and lactose tolerance, or lactase persistence, evolved independently among cattle herders in Europe, the Middle East, and Africa. Groups not dependent on cattle, such as the Chinese and Thai, the Pima Indians of the American Southwest, and the Bantu of West Africa, remain lactose intolerant. But further, migration to the colder climes saw humans skin go paler so as to absorb more vitamin D to promote calcium absorption and the need for calcium from dairy products resulted in lactase persistence. In fact, lactase persistence is 100% in the Finns and Irish.

The Diseases of Affluence, Obesity and its downstream effects of CVD, High lipids, Blood Pressure, Diabetes and such are mostly absent in primitive diets such as the Caveman and this has seen the promotion of the Paleolithic diet that focus on meat.

The fact is that there was never "one" caveman/paleo diet. Again, humans adapted to eat whatever was available and what they could get and such diets don't replicate the diversity of foods that our ancestors ate—or take into account the

[625] Nature volume 531, pages500–503(2016)

active lifestyles that protected them from heart disease and diabetes and it is argued that the real hallmark of being human isn't our taste for meat but our ability to adapt to many habitats—and to be able to combine many different foods to create many healthy diets.

In other words, there is no one ideal human diet but to propose vegetarian or vegan diets as preferred substitutes for our former active hunter lifestyles and to hypocritically promote their processed, sugar laden breakfast cereals is more based on religious zealotry than actual facts.

As evidenced by the splendid coronary arteries of the Tsmaine and the lack of CVD and diabetes in meat eating primitive tribes, a little, lean meat is not the problem.

Our modern Western Diet obtaining some 60% from processed foods is the problem, and this includes 'processed', artificially fed and processed meats. Processed foods are so ubiquitous that for the first time in human evolution, humans are getting more calories and of poor quality, than they can burn off.

But to promote a diet based on an 1863 "vision" of the Lord, by an uneducated "prophetess" with absolutely no medical or scientific training, that excludes meat and wine, when our Lord drank wine, milk and ate meat and fish, is frankly Looney Land.

Counterfactual Crusade

Many may argue that this was a "miracle" but, to me, the real miracle is how intelligent medical graduates of today can be so seduced by this hog-wash and promote it. As an article in the Washington Post pointed out (there is the) "ideological veganism, the kind that goes beyond diet and lifestyle wisdom to a sort of counterfactual crusade. For this crowd, it has become an article of faith that not only is meat-eating bad for humans, but that it's *always* been bad for humans—that we were never meant to eat animal products at all, and that our teeth, facial structure and digestive systems are proof of that".[626]

The vegetarian-vegan diets are, due to modern day supplements, now healthy – but they are not the only ones – just ask the Tsmaine.

---

[626] "Sorry Vegans: Here's How Meat-Eating Made Us Human", The Washington Post, 2016.

CHAPTER 29

THE NUTRITION PIONEERS: THE BIG DEBATE

The evil that men do lives after them,
The good is oft interred with their bones.

Shakespeare: Julius Caesar

Ancel Keys vs John Yudkin: Fat vs Sugar

Ancel Keys was a Minnesota physiologist who fostered and promoted the Mediterranean Diet as he thought dietary saturated fats caused CVD.

John Yudkin was a Doctor and Professor of Nutrition in London who didn't think it was these fats but sugar.

This chapter outlines their research and the dramas that attended much of it, as it leads to, in my opinion, a more balanced conclusion as emotions among these gurus ran high, especially for Keys who took no prisoners.

This has taken me only some 50 years to write having been appointed to the World's First Coronary Care Unit, becoming intensely interested in blood lipids, before the Seven Nations Study was published, and studying and following the Framingham Studies (you'll have to look that up) and witnessing the vociferous argy-bargy and debates.

I would add, at the outset, that my Father cut off all the fat on his steaks and practised medicine until he was 84 years old, whereas his brother, a Banker, who had a heart attack aged 54, "had a bowl of cream and sugar on his porridge every day for breakfast," my Father told me while he mused as to the cause of his brothers early death and his longevity.

I was only a schoolboy but I connected the dots: It was *both* the cream and the sugar that my Father implicated.

I too don't eat much fat – and my cholesterol and my triglycerides have been normal-low for over 50 years. My wife, however, who is slim, eats all the fat off the steak and off mine as well, has low cholesterol and low triglycerides too. And, between us 'we lick the platter clean'.

I also had a friend who was an International sportsman who "had a turn" when in his 30s' He lived on shell fish, steak and eggs and at that stage these were "high cholesterol foods" (and still are) such that an angiogram (to look inside his coronary arteries) was done and they were "as clean as a whistle"

So it was that, before all this hub-bub, I had decided that eating the fat on steaks, or eating shellfish, did not affect one's cholesterol or triglyceride levels and I did not advise my wife to change these aspects of her diet (just others) and both of us don't add sugar to anything.

The champion of the Mediterranean Diet was this Minnesota Physiologist, **Ancel Keys**, who had done nutrition research, into starvation, in WW2 and developed a more portable and non-perishable ration that would provide enough calories to sustain soldiers in the field for up to two week and was instrumental in the development of the famous (or infamous) K-Ration ("K" for Keys or more likely "Kommando").

He became interested in cardiovascular disease (CVD) prompted, in part, by observing that American business executives, in Minnesota, presumably among the best-fed people in the world, had high rates of heart disease; while in post-war Europe, CVD rates had decreased sharply in the wake of reduced food supplies. He then postulated a correlation between cholesterol levels and CVD and initiated a study of Minnesota businessmen which was a pioneering first prospective study of CVD.

He observed that southern Italy had the highest concentration of centenarians in the world and hypothesized that a Mediterranean-style diet low in animal fat protected against heart disease and that a diet high in animal fats led to heart disease.

The results of what later became known as the Seven Countries Study (SCS) appeared to show that serum cholesterol was strongly related to CVD mortality both at the population and at the individual levels.

The Seven Countries Study (SCS for short) was the first major study to investigate diet and lifestyle along with other risk factors for cardiovascular disease, across contrasting countries and cultures and over an extended period of time. There have been many criticisms of it subsequently, most of which are ill-informed or by someone trying to attract publicity, but the pioneering concept and achievements of this SCS set the example for most, if not all, subsequent studies. It is easy to improve on something but it is difficult to initiate the prototype.

The Seven Countries Study (SCS) was begun in 1956 and first published in 1978 and then followed up on its subjects every five years thereafter. As the world's first multi-country epidemiological longitudinal study, it systematically examined the relationships between lifestyle, diet, coronary heart disease and stroke in different populations from different regions of the world. It directed attention to the causes of coronary heart disease and stroke, but also showed that an individual's risk can be changed.

Keys encountered considerable criticism mainly because it was claimed that he cherry-picked only seven of an actual 22 countries originally studied whose results supported his hypothesis. Keys responded that due to WW2 the countries deleted had incomplete or unreliable records and France withdrew.

There were many other methodological errors and his study would not stand up to today's standards but that can be said of any pioneering novel study. It was the first in the world and a massive undertaking without any precedents or computers to do the number crunching or statisticians running around checking numbers.

Keys himself didn't think eating high cholesterol foods raised our blood cholesterol finding that, no matter how much dietary cholesterol he fed volunteers, the level in their blood was unchanged. *"The evidence – both from experiments and from field surveys – indicates that cholesterol content, per se, of all-natural diets has no significant effect on either the cholesterol level or the development of atherosclerosis in man."*

Nevertheless, by eating less saturated fat, but probably more importantly to my reasoning, changing to the Mediterranean Diet, CVD fell.

So Ancel Keys is regarded highly by many and a meta-analysis by the Cochrane Collaboration found that reducing saturated fat intake did reduce the risk of cardiovascular disease and recommended "population groups should continue to include permanent reduction of dietary saturated fat and partial replacement by unsaturated fats." [1] And based on the total body of scientific literature, American College of Cardiology/American Heart Association Guidelines of 2019 recommend that dietary saturated fat intake be replaced by monounsaturated and polyunsaturated fat for prevention of heart disease.[64]

There is no doubt that high blood lipids deposit plaque in our coronary arteries which leads to a coronary occlusion or heart attack. And if you have high lipids you should reduce them – especially LDL cholesterol.

Finally, Keys' work and the SCS were analyzed in detail in 2017 by a panel of august academics and, for those interested, this should be read. Keys comes out of this investigation extremely well:

Ancel Keys and the Seven Countries Study: *An Evidence-based Response to Revisionist Histories.* With emphasis on primary source material, historical records, and review/critique by *Seven Countries Study* investigators

http://www.truehealthinitiative.org/ *August 1, 2017*

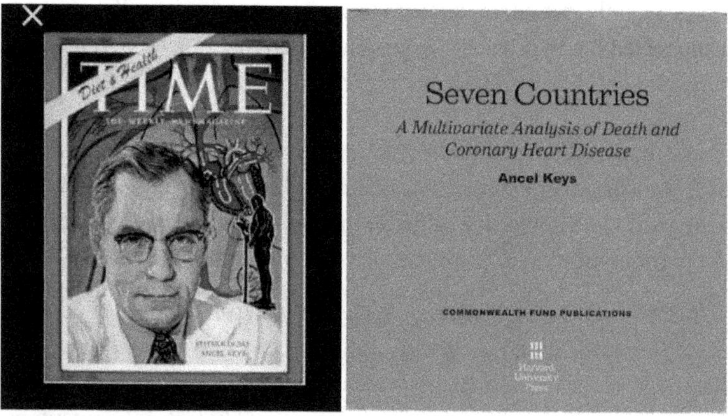

But if dietary fat doesn't elevate our lipids what does?

As flagged, not all fats are created equal and saturated fats would seem to contain both good and bad and these latter do contribute to heart disease. And, as we don't yet know which is which, all saturated fats should be avoided if you have high lipids. I am also a fan of monosaturates and EVOO.

So, we don't know the complete reasons - but that doesn't matter as we do have the cure: The Mediterranean Diet plus no processed foods, added sugar and salt.

Pure, White and Deadly

The other big alleged culprit causing CVD, and the cause of a very bitter fight, was sugar.

Keys was, by all reports, belligerent, aggressive and "direct to the point of bluntness", politically skilled and had gathered around him an army of supporters (as well as opponents).

This was in stark contrast to **John Yudkin.**

Yudkin had studied biochemistry, physiology then medicine at Cambridge and after serving in WW2 was appointed Professor at Queen Elizabeth College, London, where he established the department of nutrition science. Yudkin thought it was sugar, not saturated fat, that was causing this epidemic of CVD and, oh dear, Keys didn't like this.

Yudkin knew sugar was metabolized in the liver to fat and thence into the blood stream as lipids. He also knew humans were carnivorous and had only increased their consumption of carbohydrates since the dawn of agriculture 10,000 years ago, compared with the 2miilion hunter years before. But what was more, refined carbohydrates, especially sugar, had only been available for 300 years.

Saturated fats are an essential content of breast milk and in human diet for 2.8 million years of evolution. Yudkin thought that it was this new refined sugar causing this new epidemic of heart disease and not the diet that humans had existed on, relatively CVD free, for 2.8 million years.

But Keys attacked Yudkin unmercifully accusing him of promoting the interests of meat and dairy that his theory was "a mountain of nonsense" and "propaganda". That's OK, he attacked anyone else who had the temerity to question his dogma.

Yudkin was apparently a gentler personality and didn't respond in kind.

An historical search[689] has unearthed letters and documents that suggest that the Sugar lobby moved any suggestion that sugar was implicated in heart disease on to fat as being the culprit. This, it would seem, helped Ancel Keys (cholesterol) win the argument against John Yudkin (sugar).

While this maybe the dirty politics of the sugar lobby there is no doubt that the cholesterol theory still applies. The higher the LDL the more heart attacks; the lower the LDL (natural genetics, diet, weight or statins) the less heart attacks.

But sugar, or to be more accurate, too much sugar also elevates triglycerides which cause heart attacks. So too much sugar is bad too.

The unnoticed, insensible addition of sugar, salt and fats to our everyday processed foods, even to what seems benign and healthy such as our bread and breakfast cereals, is a deadly combination leading to high blood pressure, high cholesterol and triglycerides and the other Diseases of Affluence (obesity, diabetes 2, cardiovascular disease being the most obvious with depression, arthritis and possibly Alzheimer's being further downstream results).

Research published in 2016 analyzed the letters and other heart disease research-related public documents -- from symposium proceedings to annual reports -- from the 1950s and 60s.

The researchers discovered that executives in the sugar industry funded research in the 1960s and '70s that, upon the executives' request, cast doubt on the health risks of sugar while promoting the risks of fat. As fat was slowly reduced in the American diet, sugar was used more often to keep foods tasty.

Whatever happened to Yudkin's theory? Researchers suggest that when the sugar industry "manipulated" the scientific debate on heart disease, his theory -- along with other sugar consumption research -- was swept under the rug. After all the Yudkin hypothesis was not supported by animal experiments and was not found to be an independently associated factor in population-level studies. There were no consistent case-control study results to support the idea. There was no autopsy evidence in its favor. No intervention studies had demonstrated any effect of the removal of sugar from the diet. Whereas Keys would say *"I've got 5,000 patients. How many have you got?"*.

Keys may have won the battle, but the war goes on and now the Sugar Hypothesis holds sway at least as to replacing salt as the new villain.

To make the long story short, Keys effectively destroyed Yudkin, despite the latter's book *'Pure, White and Deadly',* and he retired in 1971 considered an eccentric and ignored by the nutritional scientists. Only today are his views being embraced.

Yudkin died aged 85; Keys lived to be 100.

Who was right?

That's easy: Both.

There has been enormous controversy and many articles attempting to debase Key's Seven Countries Study, but it was the first major multi-country epidemiological sturdy in the world before computers could crunch the numbers and statisticians scurrying around with their 'lies and damn lies'.

Keys, to my research, found that people with high cholesterol had more heart attacks – correct. He did not claim eating saturated fat caused this.

But, what he also did was draw the world's attention to the Mediterranean Diet which 70 years later has become recognised as the best. I wonder if any of his carping critics, or inflammatory journos living off his work, can ever claim such a contribution to world health.

The Mediterranean Diet Keys proposed is associated with less CVD and refined carbohydrates are, indeed, 'pure, white and deadly'.

Yudkin was also on the ball and made a great contribution – sadly only recognised recently and posthumously.

Are they (cholesterol and sugar) both the cause of CVD? Yes, but not the only cause.

OTHER GURUS

Nathan Pritikin was not a medical practitioner but when diagnosed with heart disease in 1957, he began searching for a treatment. Based on studies indicating that people in primitive cultures with primarily vegetarian lifestyles had little history of heart disease, he introduced his low-fat diet that was high in unrefined carbohydrates like vegetables, fruits, beans, and whole grains, along with a moderate aerobic exercise regime and established the Pritikin Longevity Center & Spa in 1976 providing controlled diet, counseling in lifestyle change, and exercise in a resort/spa-type setting. In the early 1980s, he began to suffer severe pain and complications related to leukemia and committed suicide on February 21, 1985 aged 69 years. However, his autopsy revealed his arteries were "like those of a child and a heart like that of a young man".

Roy Walford, was a medical graduate but spent his life in research mostly underfeeding mice who dramatically prospered and lived longer compared to his mice on a normal diet and he pioneered the hypo-caloric diet. He then disciplined himself to live on just a Spartan 1600 calories a day year after year after year. I saw how he seemed to take forever to slowly cut up a lettuce. His research convinced him he could live to 120 years (the title of his book) but he never made it. He died aged 79, a good age, but he suffered for many of these final years with amyotrophic lateral sclerosis commonly known in the USA as Lou Gehrig's or motor neuron disease-MND, severely incapacitating his former vigorous life.

While both of these diets have merit, to me and most of my patients, they impose a Spartan or somewhat Zealot lifestyle which is hard to stick to but, even if you can and do, like Pritikin and Walford, you may not live as long as todays statistical average age of death. Long living people would, in the vast majority, have not followed any diet but did eat well and probably little, by default or environment.

Dr Aitkin recommended a low-carb, high-fat diet (*Dr. Atkins' Diet Revolution)* in 1972. When he slipped on black ice, hit his head and died aged 72 years, weighed 117 Kg or 258 pounds but had suffered a cardiac arrest in April 2002 and had a viral cardiomyopathy (infection of the heart).

Conclusions

Many of these gurus recommended restricted diets or emphasized one food group over another. I feel these diet pioneers were admirable zealots who lived a lifestyle far and beyond the normal discipline that I and what I've observed most of my patients are able to stick to.

Whereas, the latest research reveals there is a more gentle, acceptable diet and lifestyle which provides more benefits because it accesses the new evidence that has now become available as well as culling the best evidence from the past.

For example

A survey of 1810 people followed for 18 years found 'Even among the oldest (85 years or older) and people with chronic conditions, the median age at death was four years higher for those with a low risk profile compared with those with a high risk profile'. Identifying these high risks and changing them to low risks, no matter how old (or young), increases the lifespan. And the clincher is that none of these changes are punitive, Spartan or difficult to change to.

But whatever: As I said, we may not know the reasons, but we do have the answers and they are:

1. Newtrition Micronutrient Revolution Diet
2. No Processed Foods
3. No added sugar
4. No added Salt
   And
5. No smoking
6. Low LDL
7. Optimum weight
8. Exercise
9. Blood Pressure control
10. My books, **"What's Going to Kill You This Year"** and **"Successful Aging"** also to be published in this Live Longest Series, completes the medical and Lifestyle picture (even a dog, gardening and retail therapy help!).
11. The Golden Rules early in this book also give the more complete preventive diet spectrum.

CHAPTER 30

LABELS

Color coding has been tested and found to be the best way to label foods but the FFI have so nobbled Governments that this is not done much, if at all. So they are written in impossibly small font, smeared with obliterating colors or glued down to make it as difficult as possible to read, it is important you now learn some basics. Always be suspicious if the labels are difficult to read – what are they trying to hide? The easiest way is to look at the 100g column. The other column is usually a "per serving" but serving sizes differ whereas 100g is a known constant. Then it is handy to remember the following:

The 3 main ingredients to know are Saturated fats, sodium and sugar.

RECOMMENDED LEVELS: LESS THAN per 100g	
Total Fat:	10g per 100g
Milk, yoghurt, ice-cream	2g
Cheese	15g
Saturated fat	3g
Trans Fats	0
Sodium	400 mg < 120 mg best
Sugar	4 g
Fiber should be *more* than	3 g / 100g
Serving size	143 Cals (600 Kj)

Other Names Used as Disguises

To try and fool you even further the food processors use 'friendly' names that sound innocent or even beneficial such as 'vegetable oil' which is invariably potentially harmful Palm Oil and so on, disguised as follows:

Saturated fats

Animal fat/oil, beef fat, butter, chocolate, milk solids, coconut, coconut oil/milk/cream, copha, cream, Ghee, dripping, lard, suet, palm oil, sour cream, vegetable shortening

Sugars

Dextrose, fructose, glucose, golden syrup, honey, maple syrup, sucrose, malt, maltose, lactose, brown sugar, caster sugar, palm sugar, raw sugar

High Salt Ingredients

Baking powder, celery salt, garlic salt, meat/yeast extracts, monosodium glutamate (MSG), onion salt, rock salt, sea salt, sodium, sodium ascorbate, sodium bicarbonate, sodium nitrate/nitrite, stock cubes, vegetable salt

Serving Sizes:

1 serve =

Fruit	=	1 medium apple, citrus, banana = 150g
Vegetables	=	1 medium potato = 75g
	=	1/2 cup cooked or 1 cup if leafy
Bread	=	1 slice
Meat	=	80g
Fish	=	150g
Cereal	=	1 cup
Nuts	=	1/3 cup
Rice/Pasta	=	1/2 cup

Note: Different countries recommend different amount of daily servings of fruit and vegetables usually based on what it is thought that society will tolerate e.g.: France = 10; Japan = 9; Denmark = 6; Canada 5 to 10; UK = 5, but whatever they all recommend eating more than that countries usual 'default' mark.

Remember: The skin of fruits such as apples and pears contain more than 90% of the good nutrients.

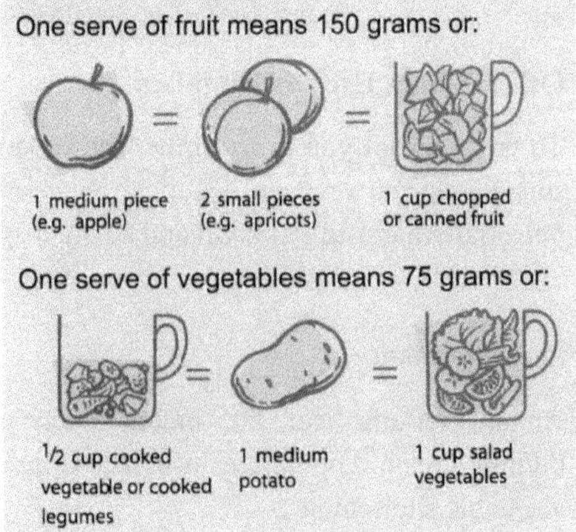

CHAPTER 31

COOKING and HYGIENE

Brief basic and essential bits of advice:

Some foods are less nutritious raw because they contain substances that destroy or disarm other nutrients and heating disarms the enzyme inhibitor. Meat, poultry, and eggs are potentially dangerous when consumed raw (or undercooked).

Some nutrients are lost when foods are cooked. Simple strategies such as steaming food rather than boiling, or broiling rather than frying, can significantly reduce the loss of nutrients when you're cooking food.

Cooking can break down cells and make nutrients more available. It also can kill unwanted germs. We don't hear too much about the disasters from such events, but they are horrific and often fatal.

Food poisoning is more common than we realize but most of these events are from eating out or not cooking poultry adequately. Here we are concerned with cooking at home and maximizing nutrients

- Wash your hands
- Use paper towels
- Tea towels and cloths are fomites - reservoirs for germs
- Unless you are absolutely sure as to the food chain for your meat and poultry it should be well cooked. Medium at least. Semi-raw hamburger meat in the USA has resulted in deaths
- Brazil has been exporting rotten meat and poultry with corrupt bribed food clearance certification[627]
- No high temperature cooking unless it is brief and use fresh oil each time. Peanut oil best if high temperature needed.
- Don't char meat
- Marinate meat for a BBQ or wipe with beer, wine or vinegar
- Hot food hot > 60 ^{0}C; cold foods cold < 5^{0}C
- Wash each lettuce leaf and stalks and leafy vegetables individually
- Use separate knives and chopping boards for meats and vegetables

627 BBC News 17 March 2017

- Look at the expiry dates
- No single cooking or preparation method is best but overall microwaving vegetables is best.
- Microwaving or steaming preserves vitamins and micronutrients best. Microwaved and pressure-cooked vegetables retained 90% of their vitamin C. Boiling destroys vitamins
- Certain foods actually benefit from cooking. With carrots, spinach, and tomatoes heat facilitates the release of antioxidants by breaking down cell walls, providing an easier passage of these nutrients from food to body.
- Fat soluble vitamins: When the salsa or salad was served with fat-rich avocados or full-fat salad dressing, the diners absorbed as much as 4 times more lycopene, 7 times more lutein and 18 times the beta carotene than those who had their vegetables plain or with low-fat dressing.
- Raw and plain vegetables are not always best. A raw diet resulted in normal levels of vitamin A and relatively high levels of beta carotene but fell short when it came to lycopene.

Plastic containers:

- Plastic can leach endocrine disrupters with hormonal interference in humans. The two main ones are bisphenol-A (BPA) which makes plastic hard and phthalates which makes it soft.
- These can migrate into foods stored or cooked with them
- The Government Agencies are aware of this and conduct regular tests
- The "Microwave Safe" Label is pretty accurate (most don't have these additives)
- Don't use plastic-wrap to microwave
- Take-Away food, margarine or such containers are not microwave safe
- As are plastic storage bags
- Throw away old containers that have been microwaved a number of times
- Always never cover completely - allow venting of steam
- This is covered in detail in Successful Aging Book 3.
- Styrofoam cups and containers are safe (and microwavable)
- Glass and ceramics are best

Smoking of Foods

There is concern that eating smoked foods can increase cancer risk. There is some weak evidence that high intakes of smoked meats and fish increase the risk of stomach cancer. Smoked fish contains nitrates and nitrites, byproducts of the smoking process. Some brine solutions can also contain sodium nitrite. The concern is that nitrites and nitrates can be converted in the body to N-nitroso-compounds, which have been shown to cause stomach cancer in lab animals.

However, humans have been eating smoked meats and fish for the last 400,000 years or longer with anthropological discovery of hearths. Obviously, an open fire produces much less exposure to smoke than deliberately smoking food, but people have most likely smoked foods for quite a while and no explicit connections of cause and effect has yet been made. In other words, any risk involved eating smoked meat or fish is probably quite small and would seem applicable only to regular and high consumption.

Here I confess to an unresolved gap in my knowledge as I can't find any definitive research:

1. Does just the pure and only salting of meats, such as Prosciutto, as distinct from the Preserved Meats, which contain nitrates and other chemicals, such as sausages and which are implicated in increased cancer of the colon, incur the same risk(s)?

and

2. Does the smoking of meats and fish pose any evidenced risks?

I confess that I love prosciutto wrapped around a fresh fig or a juicy piece of rock melon (cantaloupe) and I do eat a lot of smoked salmon, so I await the trials, if any, with interest. My rationalization, however, is the sheer centuries old duration of salting and smoking as pre-refrigeration preservatives with no seeming mass outbreaks of cancers or heart disease.

What Takes Nutrients Out of Food

Nutrient	Heat	Air	Water	Fat
Vitamin A	X			X
Vitamin D				X
Vitamin E	X	X		X
Vitamin C	X	X	X	
Thiamin	X		X	
Riboflavin			X	
Vitamin B6	X	X	X	
Folate	X	X		
Vitamin B12	X		X	
Biotin			X	
Pantothenic acid	X			
Potassium			X	

Virtually all minerals are unaffected by heat. But potassium escapes.

CHAPTER 32

THE COMPLEAT HISTORY OF DIETS

The 4,600 YEARS OF SCAMS and FADS

These are mostly weight loss diets which is ***not*** the purpose of Newtrition.

Newtrition is for optimizing for your long-term good health and minimising illnesses, however, it does stabilise your weight and is phenomenally simple – just five different food groups a day fruit, vegetables, nut, grains and protein. All obtainable from foods you like either meat eaters or vegans.

I have, however, written a weight-loss book "Slim 4 Life" which I may put on Kindle and Amazon. I point out in it, however, that it is only for those who were once slim but have insidiously put on weight and is not for the morbidly obese.

This History of Diets is staggering with 4,600 years of desperate scam after desperate scam. And they are all so complicated! This, of course, is how they work: They make the poor dupe, who tries them, so busy weighing or working out the percentages or proportions or silly restrictions that they don't work out they are just reducing their calories.

Why I have researched and written this chapter is because it is such a wretchedly boring scandal like watching some cheap side-show or incompetent magician, stuffing it up.

I don't think anyone could read it in one go and if it, itself, were a single book, I would have chucked it out the window. There is just so much one can tolerate of cheap confidence tricks,

But scanning this History will, hopefully, make you more aware, more discerning to choose wisely and be more determined to eat properly.

One sad note for me were the number of charlatan Doctors who tried to exploit this gravy (or is it now the plant) train. It was, however, intriguing how most were not trained in nutrition, some were obstetricians, some were not even medical doctors.

The vast majority of diet authors were Loonies, Zanies, Crazies or very shrewd scammers who exploited the gullible.

By contrast, **Newtrition** is based on the world's best medical and university studies, trials and evidence.

The few diets that stand out in this tsunami of historical rubbish are the Mediterranean Diet, Yudkin who identified refined sugar and processed foods as a problem, the Doctor who first advocated counting calories, Lulu Hunt Peters, in 1917, high fiber as advocated by Dr Denis Burkitt, Intermittent Fasting as popularised in his 5:2 by Dr Michael Mosley and the nutritionally correct meal suppliers.

While I acknowledge the achievements of Weight Watchers for losing weight, I cannot comment on the nutrition they recommend.

And this is the point of **Newtrition**: It is not just weight control but recommending the foods that optimise our health and optimising our weight is just part of this.

THE 4,600 YEARS OF SCAMS and FADS

Most of these diets below are for losing weight. What then has this History of Diets got to do with you living longest, healthiest?

Well, the point is, to warn you off all these Fads and Scams and make you more aware and alert to the next one coming to you this week on the Internet via some Celebrity or Influencer. And if you don't know how to identify and recognise what are scams you may be tempted to try and try and try them: There have been, arguably, more scams and books on diets than on any other health subject.

So, may I suggest you just run your eye over these and come back to them if you are ever tempted to try the latest Fad.

Here are 4,620 years of diets which keep being repeated and resurrected.

Why?

Because they didn't work to begin with.

Self-control, however, is not the only answer: Knowing the best foods is also necessary and **Newtrition** is not only concerned with weight control but on optimising our health and preventing illnesses.

The problem with common sense is that it is not very common as Churchill observed, but use your common sense to glance through this history to see how history repeats itself and how these diets have been being peddled and re-presented to new gullible generations after generations (the Cabbage Soup diet has grabbed every generation since 175BC!).

Fasting Diets, which unlike most, are to be commended because of their health benefits, are as old as God's dog. The Daniel Fast is drawn from the Book of Daniel, which appears in the Old Testament. Daniel decides to avoid the rich, indulgent foods that surround him and have nothing but vegetables to eat and water to drink for 10 days. A later reference says, Daniel, mourned for three weeks. I ate no choice food; no meat or wine touched my lips; and I used no lotions at all until the three weeks were over. At the end of the fast, he was healthy. According to scholars the Book of Daniel gives clear internal dates such as the third year of the reign of king Jehoiakim, î (1:1), which is 606 BC.

Research by the University of Memphis found that the Daniel Diet, after just three weeks, can begin to lower risk factors for metabolic and cardiovascular disease, such as high blood pressure and cholesterol, and reduce oxidative stress. Maybe he was also healthy before his fast, but he sure was thinner by an estimated 6 pounds or 2.7 kg from duplicate studies.

It is interesting how Daniel renounced "choice food" as this theme keeps re-occurring with some foods linked by the sexually disturbed religious zealots as causing lascivious urges. Dr Kellogg, a Seventh Day Adventist, even thought his Corn Flake would cure the curse of masturbation and Ellen White one of the founders of the Seventh Day Adventists (SDA), was obsessed how meat would inflame the "base desires". I am not sure if they all agreed as to which were the foods that so inflamed the desires, but, of course, it was not only the religious zealots interested in naughty desires but every schoolboy reading as much as he can about aphrodisiacs. And, while I don't know of any, I do seem to remember a marvellous scene in the movie Tom Jones where such a feast between Tom (Albert Finny) and Molly Seagrim (Diane Cilento) was a simply erotic romp where the suggestive meal was better than witnessing the actual inevitable event.

The Keto Diet: Using starvation to treat seizures can be found in the Bible and in references as far back to 500 B.C. In 1911, two physicians in Paris tried starving 20 persons and found that seizures improved. In 1921, the Ketogenic diet was evolved as a long-term treatment for epilepsy without actual starvation. With the development of modern epilepsy drugs, the Keto Diet lapsed, only to now be revived.

Fad diets, the current short-term craze, are usually with little or pseudo-scientific basis, but advertising extravagant claims. They are generally restrictive, obsessive and unsustainable.

In the 6th century BC Olympic athletes followed specific fads such as favouring cheese, figs and grains but avoiding pork, fish and beans. It is claimed that the famous Olympic wrestler Milo of Kroton of this era would consume up to 40lb (18kg) of meat and bread in one sitting. He was obviously not dieting in the modern usage of the word.

The Father of Medicine, the Greek physician Hippocrates in the 3rd century BC, recommended a diet of light and emollient foods, slow running, hard work, wrestling, sea-water enemas, walking about naked and vomiting after lunch.

The Greeks believed that being fat was morally and physically detrimental, the result of luxury and corruption, so food and living should be plain with nothing to unduly stir the passions or arouse the appetites. This was the first documented diet or diatia.

The following, I assure you, are just the highlights of a very big, obese iceberg of silly diets. Today, as you read this, there will be over 100 such Fad diets inviting you to fail with new ones on the way.

2800 BC: Archaeological evidence suggests that humans hunted the bison that roamed North America's Great Plains and blended their meat, fat, and marrow into energy-dense patties with a serious shelf-life. A single pound of pemmican lasted for years and might've packed as many as 3,500 calories. It later became the favourite and essential for Arctic explorers.

2,600BC The Daniel Diet – see above

500BC The Keto Diet - see above

500BC: Olympic Athlete Fad Diets

175BC: The Cabbage and Urine Diet

Cato the Elder was a Roman statesman, writer and public speaker who was a massive fan of cabbage; he not only promoted eating plenty of cabbage but also drinking the urine of people who had a diet high in cabbage. It is reported that Cato continued to believe in the power of cabbage even after this diet failed to save the lives of his wife and son. It had a big resurgence in the 1950s and even today some advocates still urge cabbage soup diets.

300AD Fasting:

John Chrysostom claimed fasting promotes health.

The Friday Fast is a Christian practice of abstaining from animal meat, other than fish, on Fridays, or holding a fast on Fridays, that is found mostly in the Eastern Orthodox, Catholic, Anglican and Methodist traditions. According to Pope Peter of Alexandria, the Friday fast is done in commemoration of the crucifixion of Jesus Christ on Good Friday. Abstinence is colloquially referred to as "fasting" although it does not necessarily involve a reduction in the quantity of food. (?!).

And I thought it was just a clever way to get some protein, via fish, into the poor!

Tribal Survival

Some religions and sects such as the Jews, Muslims Seventh-day Adventists along with the Eritrean Orthodox Church, the Ethiopian Orthodox Church and many Yazidis in Kurdistan consider pork taboo.

This was pure tribal survival, made universal by the threat of excommunication, hell or whatever, in that pigs were then riddled with the pig worm, Ascaris lumbricoides, which could be fatal. Bottom feeding fish had the same disease implications making them taboo too.

In the same way most tribes found what foods made them thrive, which were poisonous and even how to de-toxify some of them.

Nutrition science has been notoriously slow. The Scottish surgeon in the Royal Navy, James Lind, is generally credited with proving that scurvy can be successfully treated with citrus fruit in 1753. Nonetheless, it would be 1795 before the British Royal Navy to routinely give lemon juice to its sailors and the magic ingredient, vitamin C, was not discovered until 1926.

1087 Liquid (Alcohol) Diet:

Dieting does not seem to have been recorded between and 1087 when it was mentioned how William the Conqueror had become too heavy to ride his horse, so he decided that he would stop eating solid foods and only partake in a liquid diet that consisted only of alcohol in an attempt to lose weight. It must have worked as he later died from a fall off his horse but was still too big for the casket. This may be the first recorded instance in which an individual changed his or her food intake habits to lose weight.

1558: The First Diet Book – still in print

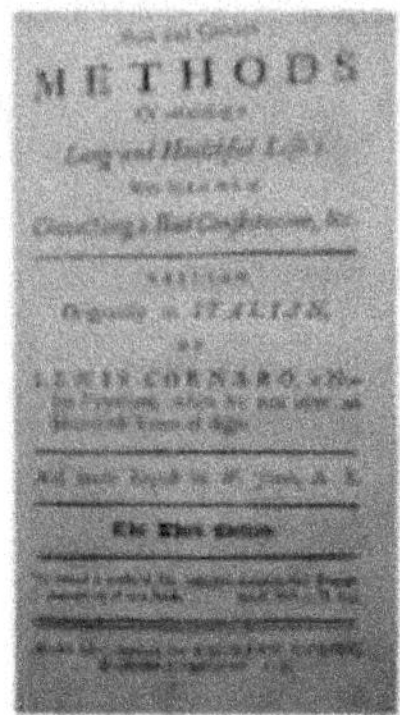

METHODS

17th Century Chocolate, Coffee, Tea and the Vatican

The introduction of chocolate to Europe created such a craze among the upper classes that the Catholic Church was forced to declare the drinking of liquids like chocolate, coffee, and tea acceptable to the fast. Monasteries were among the major consumers of chocolate, buying the drink in large quantities. The Cistercian monastery of Piedra, in Aragon, is said to be the first place in Spain where chocolate was prepared and became a firm favourite among the monks there but not all religious orders approved. The Jesuits believed that it went against the precepts of mortification of the flesh and poverty.

The question as to whether such a rich beverage should be drunk during periods of fasting sparked a theological debate between defenders and detractors of the chocolate habit. The 17th-century theologian Cardinal Francesco Maria Brancaccio gave a definitive answer to the vexed question in his now famous decree: “Liquidum non frangit jejunum” - Liquid does not break the fast.

1724 - Veganism

Yes, sorry! It was not invented just now but in 1724, when very overweight Doctor George Cheyne decided to eat nothing but milk and vegetables. He then wrote arguably the world's first diet book (but the first Fad diet is accredited to 1820). Cheyne recommended avoiding "luxury foods" such as meat and bread, and to take long walks in the countryside for good health.

Lord Byron (the poet) used the Vinegar Diet (yes it’s back today too) of potatoes flattened and drenched in apple vinegar or drinking water mixed with apple cider vinegar. It also caused vomiting and diarrhea. But he also purged himself and wore heavy clothing all day to cause sweating.

1825 Lo-Carbs: Physiologie du gout (The Physiology of Taste):

French lawyer and physician Jean-Anthelme Brillat-Savarinís pioneered the low-carb diet observing Tell me what you eat, and I will tell you what you are.

Late 1820s: The First Fad Diet.

Sylvester Graham was a Presbyterian Minister who combined his strict religious beliefs and temperance proposing a plain vegetarian diet to prevent the over-stimulation of other foods which caused immoral behaviour, gluttony and promiscuity. He invented the cracker and had a huge following including John Harvey Kellogg (see later). He claimed his diet would prolong life to 100 years but died aged 57. Thereafter Sanitorium health spas of the Seventh Day Adventists took over from the Presbyterians such as that of Dr Kellogg of Corn Flake and anti-masturbation fame.

But before then there were odd diets which, had there been the mass media, would have been fads then as some have been re-discovered to be come modern day fads. For example, as above, low carb diets date back at least to 1825.

1830: Tapeworms

Victorians and later1920s Hollywood (see) swallowed tapeworms which not only competed for the ingested food but could cause serious, even fatal, results.

1863: Lo-Carb Diet.

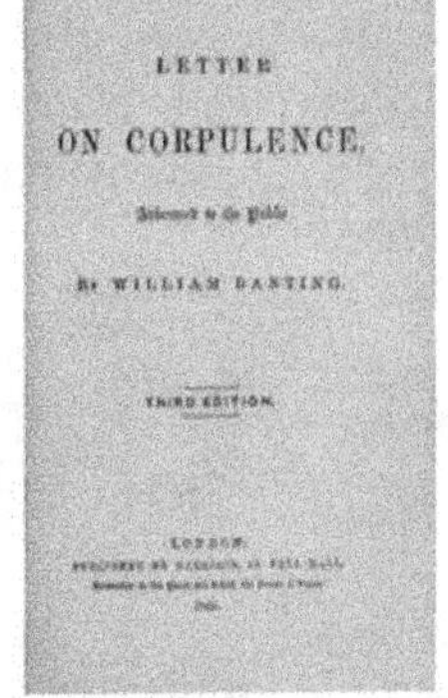
LETTER

ON CORPULENCE,

BY WILLIAM BANTING.

THIRD EDITION.

LONDON.

William Banting was a notable English undertaker. Formerly obese, he was advised to lose weight by his doctor and to begin journaling about his diet i.e. keep a diet diary. His diet was worked out by Dr William Harvey but Banting, while acknowledging this, privately published his diet and became the first to popularise a weight loss diet based on limiting the intake of carbohydrates, especially those of a starchy or sugary nature. Just as did Brillat-Savarin, and now popular again today. He recommended four meals a day consisting of simple food like meat, vegetables, fruits and wine. You were also asked to avoid all sugar and bread altogether...which sounds very close to the modern way of thinking.

1863 Seventh Day Adventist Vegetarianism

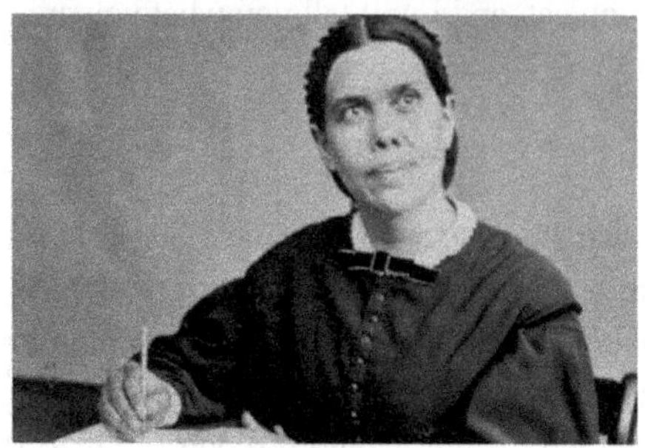

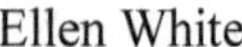

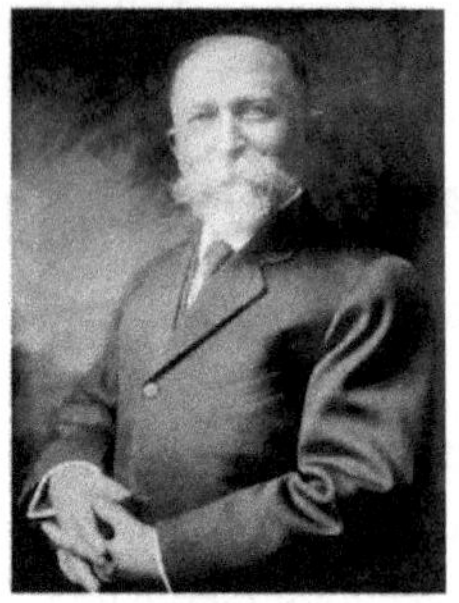

Ellen White John Kellogg

But while the SDA revere Ellen they do not ordain women (?!). They also ban dancing, jazz, rock, alcohol, caffeine and so on. They also didn't recognise mental illness, which is why they reassured one of my patients, a Psychiatrist, that his patient was healthy, well and with no problems – that is until he shot his wife, four kids and himself.

They also don't seem to know Jesus drank wine and ate meat.

They don't believe in evolution.
I also wonder how they reconcile the edict:

"Every moving thing that liveth shall be meat for you."- Genesis 9:3

The SDA church is now reputedly the fifth biggest Christian denomination with unequalled missionary evangelism such that their programs aired on 853 radio stations and 441 television stations in 80 different countries wherein the 'health message,' diet continues to be a most important aspect of the church's evangelistic efforts

Vegetarians and the SDA of Loma Linda in California do live longer than average. But so do the Mormons and so does anyone who eats well, including meat, fish and dairy, don't smoke and so on, as the Live Longest Series recommends.

1917: Breakfast becomes the Most Important Meal of The Day

Dr John Harvey Kellogg, who co-invented corn flakes in the hope it would cure the curse of masturbation was another Adventists advocating vegetarianism and, guess what, being more an astute businessman than a medical brain, he saw a way to sell his Corn Flakes so, in the issue of Good Health magazine of 1917, edited by Kellogg himself, he states "In many ways, the breakfast is the most important meal of the day, because it is the meal that gets the day started".

1880 High fat, low carb diet

Germany. Popularized again by Dr Atkins in 1972

1885 No breakfast and Raw Food

Raw food faddists make a comeback. The cooking of food makes available many nutrients that raw food cannot and is credited as allowing the evolution of the human gut to be shorter and our brains bigger than or ape ancestors.

Late 1800s: Arsenic Diet Pills

These Victorian diet pills were advertised as miracle cures which could speed up the metabolism. Although the amount of arsenic within the pills was small, these were still very dangerous and posed the risk of arsenic poisoning; especially when the pills were taken in high doses. It also didn't help matters that the labels of these pills didn't always declare that they contained arsenic5!

Early 1900s: The Tapeworm Diet

This was first recorded (as above) in 1830, reputedly reached maximum vogue in the Hollywood of the 1920s and last recorded when the opera singer Maria Callas, the paramour of Aristotle Onassis, see below. People would voluntarily ingest tapeworms in order to decrease nutrient absorption and promote vomiting and diarrhea to achieve weight loss. This has multiple risks associated with it such as: organ swelling, anaphylaxis, infections of the digestive system, appendicitis, damaged vision, meningitis, epilepsy, dementia or even death in severe cases. It doesn't seem quite worth the risk to drop a few pounds.

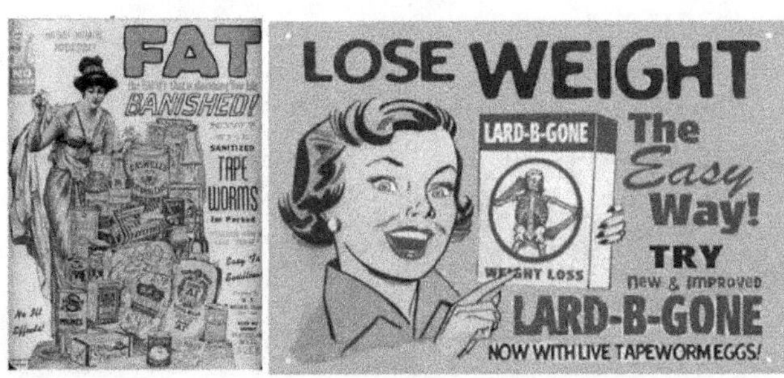

1895-1919: Fletcherism Diet 'Chew and spit'.

Fletcher, The Great Masticator, was an ex-whaler, pirate, sharp-shooter, opera manager, businessman (art dealer) and self-taught nutritionist who became the 20th century's first diet guru with John D. Rockefeller, Franz Kafka and Henry James as adherents. Chewing food thoroughly until liquid (32 to 100 to 700 times) and then spitting it out was the idea behind the Fletcherism Diet. Fletcherites were also urged to eat only when they were really, really hungry and to never eat when their emotions were running high.

Authors note: Not bad advice really and a small 2011 study showed that higher chewing counts reduced food intake.

1903: President William Howard Taft

Pledges to slim down after getting stuck in the White House bathtub.

He apparently then kept a daily log and adopted a low-calorie, low-fat diet.

Some feel that this was the start of today's obsession with dieting and looking slim.

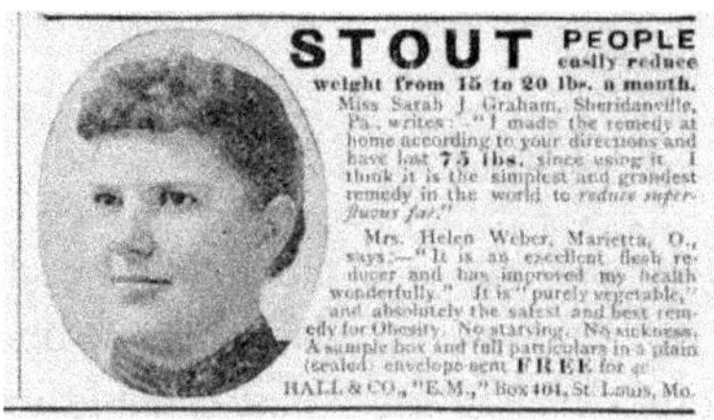

1911: Hereward Carrington The Fasting Cure

Carrington embraced different food fads and experimented with fasting, fruitarianism and raw food diets. His book Vitality, Fasting and Nutrition is over six hundred pages and was negatively reviewed in the British Medical Journal. He died aged 78.

1911 The Ketogenic diet:

Two physicians in Paris tried starving 20 persons and found that seizures improved. In 1921, the Ketogenic diet was evolved as a long-term treatment for epilepsy without actual starvation

1914 - The Sun-Kissed diet

An Australian diet advocating only eating food and meat that was "kissed by the sun every day" with nothing out of the ground like potatoes and carrots and only eating eggs and above-ground plants and fruits. The idea was that it would bring sunshine into participants "interior" and give them wonderful health.

1916: Amelia Summerville, author of the book called "Why be Fat?"

Wrote "I would die sooner than be fat."

1917 Dr Lulu Hunt Peters published Diet and Health

She introduced the concept of counting calories and so new was the concept she even included how to pronounce it. It sold more than two million copies and became the first best-selling American diet book. Dr Peters urged readers to view the calorie as a measurement and rather than judge meals by portion size. It was recommended that the amount of calories in any given food were counted and totalled each day. She concluded that to lose weight it was important to stay under 1,200 calories a day.

Authors Note: She was correct! But portions have now increased 10fold. It has been observed that counting calories has worked in the past. But modern-day-calories have changed because the nutrition contained in a calorie has diminished.

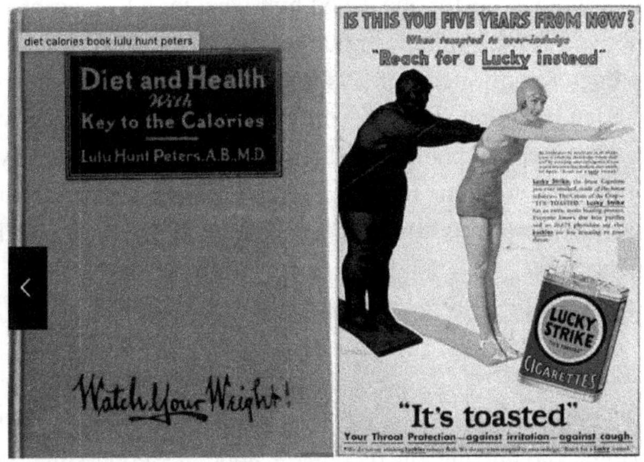

The calories that most of us consume are just not the same from a nutritional standpoint as those calories from decades and centuries before. Though it can be argued that a high-calorie diet will cause weight gain and a low-calorie diet will lead to weight-loss, the body's health does not solely rely on this aspect of nutrition. If the body is constantly supplied with calories that have no nutritional value, the body will want to eat more, causing weight gain, obesity and disease.

1920 The Hay Diet also known as The Food Combining Diet

A nutrition method developed by the New York physician William Howard Hay in the 1920s and became one of the most famous early fad diets. It claims to work by separating food into three groups: alkaline, acidic, and neutral. Acid foods are not combined with the alkaline ones. Acidic foods are protein rich, such as meat, fish, dairy, etc. Alkaline foods are carbohydrate rich, such as rice, grains and potatoes. It has been copied a number of times. Among Dr. Hay's thousands of followers were car manufacturer Henry Ford and artist Man Ray. There is nothing scientific about his claims, although they endure today.

1920s: Cereal, Bacon and Eggs for Breakfast

Well, before the 1920s, most people, at least in North America, ate oatmeal and porridge for breakfast.

In the 1920s, Bernays was approached by the Beech-Nut Packing Company ñ producers of everything from pork products to the nostalgic Beech-Nut bubble gum. Beech-Nut wanted to increase consumer demand for bacon. Bernays turned to his agency's internal doctor and asked him whether a heavier breakfast might be more beneficial for the American public. Knowing which way his bread was buttered, the doctor confirmed Bernays suspicion and wrote to five thousand of his doctors' friends asking them to confirm it as well. This study of doctors encouraging the American public to eat a heavier breakfast ñ namely Bacon and Eggs was published in major newspapers and magazines of the time to great success. Beech-Nut's profits rose sharply thanks to Bernays and his team of medical professionals.

1925-9 The Cigarette Diet

The Lucky Strike cigarette brand launches the Reach for a Lucky instead of a sweet campaign, capitalizing on nicotine's appetite-suppressing superpowers. This advertising campaign advised customers to Reach for a Lucky Instead of a Sweet and Light a Lucky and You'll Never Miss Sweets that Make You Fat was a very successful campaign at the time reputedly boosting sales by 200%.

1926 Dr. Leonard Williams

His diet book said being fat was about "self-indulgence, greed and gormandising" and accused American women of overfeeding their husbands to make them docile.

At the 1926 American Medical Association's Convention, doctors spoke out against silly but dangerous diet cures and insane female regimes designed to diet away natural body curves, a fad they said could jeopardize a woman's ability to conceive a child. As one doctor put it, "It's prepostorous. Is there no humbug too raw? Women should not follow beauty ideals to endanger motherhood."

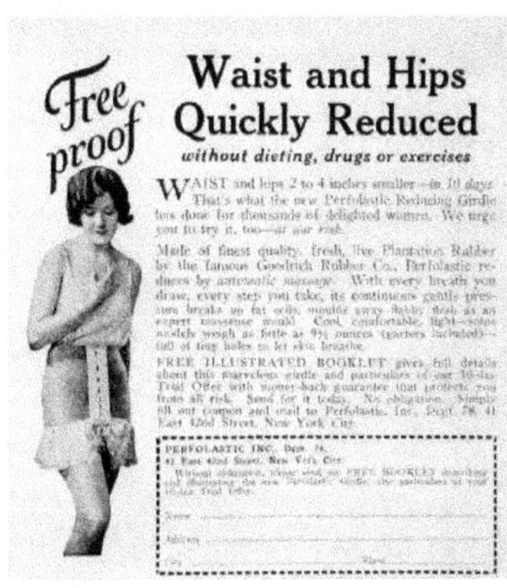

“Dietotherapy" by William Fitch, wrote that fat people turn their stomachs into "an overfed boiler that burns out."

The "Inuit Diet”

Introduced by a Swede who lived in the Arctic, Vihjalmur Stefansson, who preached that Eskimos ate high calorie diets of whale blubber, caribou, and raw fish along with very little fruit or vegetables, and yet they remained healthy and slim.

This was emulated in 1979 (see) by Dr Hugh Macdonald Sinclair.

1929: Dr. Morris Fishbein

"Malnourished women are deeply unattractive," he wrote, "and they threaten male and female norms, encouraging the rise of lesbianism. Female fat is necessary for societal survival. This nonsense is the result of feminism."

Dr. Harlow Brooks: "A woman who is naturally sweet-tempered, good-natured and competent," he wrote, "transforms into a different person (on a diet). She becomes petulant, unreasonable and hard to get along with, and might even end up as a lesbian."

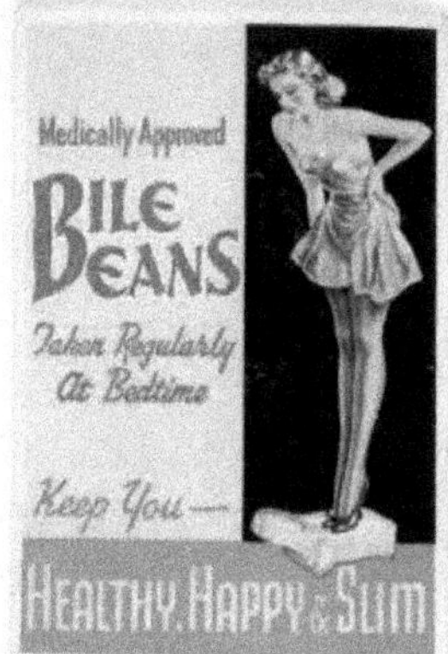

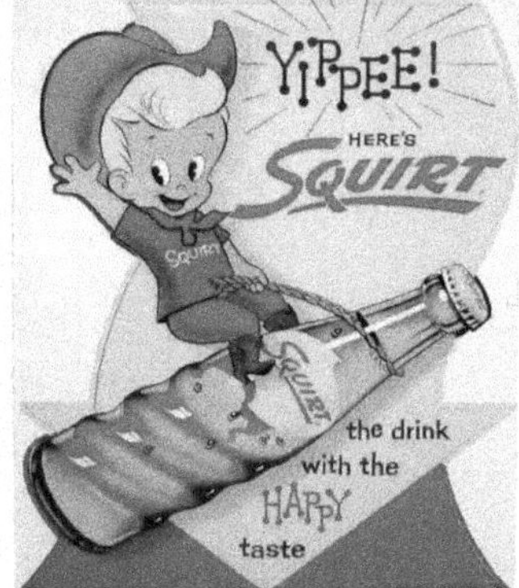

1929: The Great Depression

Suddenly people were going hungry. Overindulgence in food was seen as immoral and insensitive while others were starving. This paradoxically saw how the demand for diets, cigarettes, and weight loss cures did not go away, and may have even increased.

All kinds of products were for sale, such as La-Mar Reducing Soap, Slends Fat Reducing Chewing Gum, Slenmar reducing brush, and Lesser Slim Figure Bath Oil. Over $50 million was spent every year on laxatives, which were used as an ingredient in "reducing breads." The first diet drink, named Squirt, also went on the market.

1930s: Grapefruit Diet

The Grapefruit Diet a.k.a. the Hollywood Diet, a forerunner of the Scarsdale and similar ones in the 1970s, equals a half grapefruit, egg, and one Melba toast for breakfast, six slices of cucumber for lunch, and a half grapefruit, two eggs, lettuce and one tomato slice for dinner and only 800 calories a day.

Of course, it is trotted out every decade or so.

Bananas and Skim Milk
Another fad diet also dates from the 30s.

1930: Dr Stoll's Diet Aid and liquid Diets
Sold in beauty salons from 1930 it was the first explicitly designed liquid meal replacement (as distinct from the good old cabbage soup diet) and composed of a teaspoon of chocolate, starch, whole wheat and bran blended in a cup of water for breakfast and lunch. It pioneered the immensely profitable liquid diet industry, but many people gave up because they were both drinking the shakes and eating normally at the same time, causing an ironic increase in weight.

1936: "You Are What You Eat."
Author Victor Hugo Lindlahr has 26,000 join his radio "reducing party".

1936 Men- Body Building Craze Starts
Angelo Siciliano, an Italian immigrant, was at the beach at Coney Island when a bully kicked sand in his face. The "97-pound weakling," as Siciliano described himself, had no defence against the bully. Siciliano got into weight-lifting, and by the 1930s he was winning body building competitions and posing for artists. He changed his name to "Charles Atlas," and took out ads in men's magazines and newspapers to promote his body building secrets. All the ads had a similar theme: after a bully insults a weakling, his girlfriend laughs and leaves him. They had titles like: "The Insult That Turned a 'Chump' Into a Champ" and "How Jack the Weakling Slaughtered the Dance-Floor Hog." Over six million kits were sold. Mahatma Gandhi supposedly ordered a Charles Atlas kit, but unfortunately the company couldn't ship to India.

In 1936 Jack LaLanne started the first health club in Oakland, California, and designed the first leg extension machines and other fitness equipment. He immediately faced opposition from the medical establishment, and later told an interviewer, "The doctors were against me—they said that working out with weights would give people heart attacks and they would lose their sex drive." Nevertheless, his health clubs were successful and eventually licensed as Bally Total Fitness.

By the mid-1950s, ads for diet cures began to air on television. Daytime shows by Jack LaLanne and other fitness experts featured exercises you could do along with them.

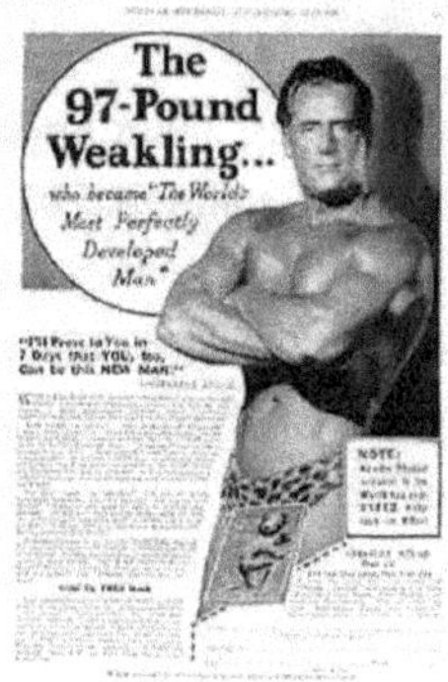

1930s: Dr. Eustace Chesser's book, "Slimming for the Million"
Advised overweight people to avoid "fat-forming foods" and eat eggs and bacon for breakfast, meat, vegetables and fruit for lunch and dinner.
Meanwhile scientists and other experts continued to write mean things about overweight people.

1935: Professor Charles Lambie
Believed obesity is most common in people with "sluggish habits."
Dr. Ernest Blaxton remarked that "noble savages" are never fat so it is unnatural. "Why do we laugh at the fat man?" he asked. "Because they look funny and have an intrinsic lack of dignity."

1937: Amphetamines
Used as diet drugs until the 70s

1939: Gaylord Hauser's Eat and Grow Beautiful
He arrived in Hollywood with a fake doctorate degree, but with his good looks and charismatic personality, he was able to convince movie stars like Marlene Dietrich, Paulette Goddard, and Gloria Swanson to follow his advice. He later worked with Ingrid Bergman, the Duchess of Windsor and Grace Kelly. His most famous client was Greta Garbo, who was also his lover.

Hauser wrote that "there is a real tragedy in fat" because fat women never reach their potential and "sleep is their only pleasure." He was the first to use juice diets to "cleanse" the body. His diet was extreme: a small fruit for breakfast, salad for lunch, and one meat with chilled vegetables and small fruit for dinner. He dropped his claim to holding a medical degree after he was investigated and was prosecuted by FDA for fraudulent claims but lived a wealthy man in Hollywood to age 89.

1939: The Rice Diet ñ Duke University

2000cals a day, 5% protein,3% fat, complex carbs and 150 mg salt as a last chance for hypertense patients with renal failure. 107 of 192 chronically ill patients improved, 25 died and 60 remained the same. The introduction of antihypertensive drugs eclipsed it, but it still exists in updated versions.

WW2

World War 2 saw food rationing introduced

If you wanted to buy meat, cheese, fats, canned fish, sugar, coffee, canned milk and other processed foods, you had to have government-issued coupons. Although many people bought restricted items on the black market, it was considered unpatriotic to eat more than your share of rationed foods, and wrong not to "finish all the food on your plate."

1942: The first Age and Weight Tables

Metropolitan Life created these tables that showed "ideal" weights for men and women based on their height.

1943: the U.S. federal government issues first guidelines for good nutrition.

Recommending seven food groups every day: vegetables, citrus and salad greens, potatoes and fruits, milk and dairy, meat and poultry, bread and cereals, and finally butter and margarine.

Sylvia of Hollywood, diet guru named catered to movie stars, offering them starvation diets plus "fat reduction" massages.

1946: "Diet the ice-cream way."

Cooking guru Marion White wrote this in 1946 promoting the idea that eating 1,000 calories per day, but you only could eat1000 cals a day in toto. Obviously, you would lose weight. Smoke and mirrors again. There was also a 2002 version of this book.

1948 Esther Manz creates TOPS, "Take Off Pounds Sensibly."
A support group which met once a week in Milwaukee, did not follow a diet plan but rather just discussed their mutual struggles and weighed themselves at every meeting. By 1958 TOPS had 30,000 members.

Mid-1940's "Plus-sized" clothing for women offered
Sears Roebuck and Montgomery Wards offer large sizes. The notation was a standard size with a plus-mark after it, such as Size 14+.

1949 National Obesity Society
Formed by American doctors to understand the causes, consequences, prevention and treatment of obesity.

1950: A British study
Had two groups of people overeat for a week. Thin people's metabolism raised when they overate to burn off the excess calories. Overweight peoples' did not rise, leading the researchers to conclude that, "Diet advice is heartless and out of date."

1950s newspapers serialize "The Fat Boy's Book" by Elmer Wheeler
How Elmer lost 40 pounds in 80 days." The work sold 112,000 copies as a hardbound.

The Mead Johnson company introduced "Metracal," a liquid shake advertised as "neither a drug nor food." You drank a can of Metracal instead of eating a regular meal. Similar meal replacement products quickly appeared: Bal-Cal by Sears Roebuck, Quota by Quaker Oats, and Sego by Pet Milk. By 1965 Sego and Metracal were a $450 million market.

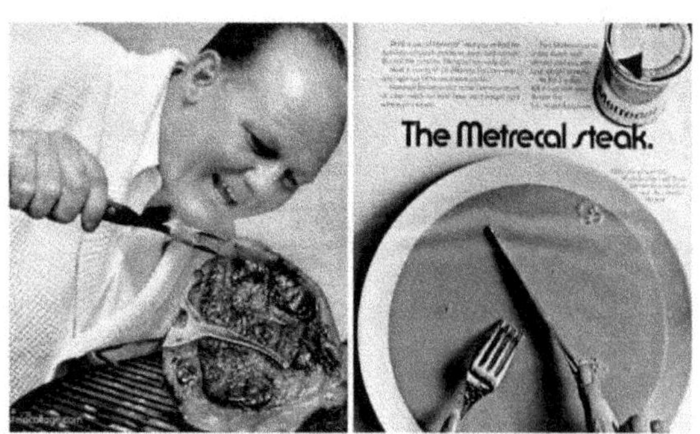

Some of the weight loss products sold through ads in women's magazines were "Doctor's Diet Reducing Tabs," the "Sauna Slim Suit" and the "VibaWay Tummer Trimmer."

Passive Exercise

One of the most expensive weight loss cures you could buy was the Staffer Home Reducing Plan that included a machine that looked like a backless padded couch. When you lay down on it, the "magic couch" would vibrate in such a way that your fat would disappear through "passive exercise." The appliance could also be used to rock a baby. Stauffer's ads were sometimes beamed to men, noting it was an item purchased by "understanding husbands."

1950: First Records of Obesity

In the early 1950s, the United States Center for Disease Control began keeping records of obesity for the first time, partly in an effort to combat obesity-related diseases. From 1950 to 1960 33% of adults were overweight, and an additional ten percent were clinically obese. By 1969, 35% of adults were overweight, while the obese percent had climbed to 15%.

Fat and Heart Disease

The general belief among the medical community in the 1950s was that a high fat diet causes heart disease. The market responded by manufacturing low-fat versions of cottage cheese, milk, sour cream, and other processed products.

1950s: The Cabbage Soup Diet

Re-emerges and promises you can lose 10ñ15 pounds in a week by eating a limited diet including cabbage soup every day. It was short, tough and ultra-boring which suits those dieters who like discipline and pain to avoid the gain. Its popularity has continued to the present day, even though, according to observations, ìit appears to be nothing more than a recipe for flatulence. The reason why it works is because cabbage is packed with insoluble fiber, so people end up spending a lot of time on the loo. Other soup diets have become popular in the decades since, such as the watercress soup.

1950s: Mediterranean Diet: At last! Some science!

The Mediterranean diet has been evolving for more than 5,000 years, with the superior health of the region's inhabitants first noted in a research paper published after World War II. As more research evolved, so did the diets popularity. It calls for eating little red meat, medium amounts fish and loads of plant -based foods.

Authors Note: This selection of foods has the most evidence for health and on what I base the recommend foods in Newtrition The Newtrition Micronutrient Revolution Diet.

1950s: The Sugar-based Diet

We need sugar for energy! And even 3 teaspoons of Domingo sugar contain fewer calories than your apple!

Does it have to be Domingo?

And as you will read, fruit is high in fiber, which drags its sugar through our gut, so less is absorbed. But further, fruits are full of micronutrients which donate many health benefits. Too much pure sugar has now been recognised as being deleterious for health.

1952 The Tuna Round the Clock Diet

Tuna for breakfast, morning tea, lunch, afternoon tea, dinner, supper and snacks. How could it possibly fail?

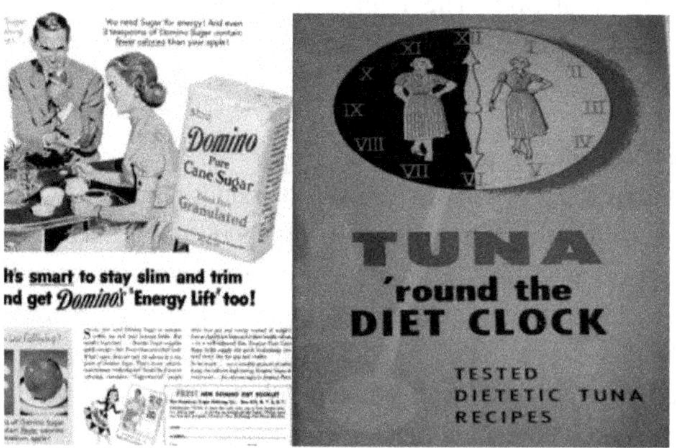

1954: The Tapeworm Diet (again)

Urban legend has it that opera singer Maria Callas dropped 65 pounds on the Tapeworm Diet, allegedly by swallowing a parasite-packed pill.

1956 Dr Hugh Sinclair writes a letter to *The Lancet*, entitled "Deficiency of essential fatty acids and atherosclerosis, etcetera"

1956: New government guidelines for a healthy diet
recommending four food groups: vegetables and fruits, milk/dairy, meat, and breads/cereal. Butter was no longer a food group.

1957: "Pray Your Weight Away." by Charles Shedd
A preacher who lost 100 pounds, wrote, "We fatties are the only people on earth who can weigh our sin."

Deborah Pierce "I Prayed Myself Slim."
She said, "if gluttony were a sin, then God would help me overcome it" and she lost enough weight to become a fashion model.

An ad for RyCrisp crackers featured the headline, "No one loves a fat girl." Hollywood diet guru Benjamin Hauser wrote in 1951, "There is no such thing as stylish stout."

1957: Pray Your Weight Away
A book by Revered Charlie Shed published in 1957 that was, depressingly enough, a bestseller. In it, Shedd writes, "If our bodies really are to be temples of the Holy Spirit, we had best get them down to the size God intended."

1958: Dr Jarvis The Alkaline Diet

Again - see 1920 The Hay Diet

The 1960s fashions called for a slim, boyish, androgynous body. The top model of the decade, a tiny Brit with cropped hair, was nicknamed Twiggy because she was as thin as a twig. At 89 pounds and five foot six, Twiggy was seriously underweight with a BMI of 14.

Magazines focus on the Baby Boomers with articles like "How to Look Like Your Favorite Model" and "The Prom Diet" in magazines like Seventeen, Glamour, and Cosmopolitan.

The main approach to dieting was to count calories, cut out sweets and high fat foods. This was based on the science of the times, particularly by studies done by Ancel Keys, a leading nutritionist. One of his earliest studies was about men on starvation diets during World War II. He found that they became anxious, depressed, unable to concentrate, and preoccupied with food and cooking. Some would sneak food into the study area, and one participant cut off the tip of his finger to get out of the experiment. These behaviours and problems are typical of any person on an extremely low-calorie regime.

Keys developed the idea that high fat foods cause high cholesterol, which in turn leads to heart disease. After studying diets all over the world, Keys concluded that the Mediterranean diet was the healthiest, and convinced government nutritionists to promote a similar low-fat diet in the United States. Today many believe that was a mistake, and that Keys dishonestly arranged the statistics he collected to link high cholesterol with heart disease.

Keys never said high fat foods elevated blood cholesterol and the accusation of falsifying his statistics was because he reduced his studies from 21 Nations to seven. He claims that this was because the other 14 Nations records were unreliable due to WW2.

There is no doubt that a high cholesterol causes heart attacks.

Keys had a big fight with the British Nutritionist Yudkin. Keys won. But Yudkin was also right as he though processed sugar was the problem.

Newtrition incorporates both their research.

Whatever: The Mediterranean Diet has been shown to be the healthiest, free of all these fads and absurd claims and easy to follow. Modern research endorses it. But, the absence of processed foods, added sugar and salt is mandatory.

Calorie counting, low fat foods, and "diet" foods stayed in style until the Atkins revolution in 1972. Dieters in the 1960s would typically buy a "calorie counter" that usually included an "ideal" weight chart based on gender, height and age.

Grocery stores began to offer "diet foods" like low-calorie bread, salad dressings, gelatin desserts, and hundreds of other "low-calorie" products that contained artificial sweeteners.

1960: The Zen Macrobiotic Diet

Launched by the Japanese philosopher, George Ohsawa, classing foods into Yin and Yang and claiming, without evidence, to treat cancer such that the AMA and American Cancer Society had to issue a warning that it poses a serious hazard to health and is not beneficial in the treatment of cancer. It was also known as 'The Brown Rice Diet'. Basically it was a vegetarian diet with some benefits but strict adherence led to vitamin deficiencies. Electric stoves, copper, aluminium and Teflon pots were to be avoided.

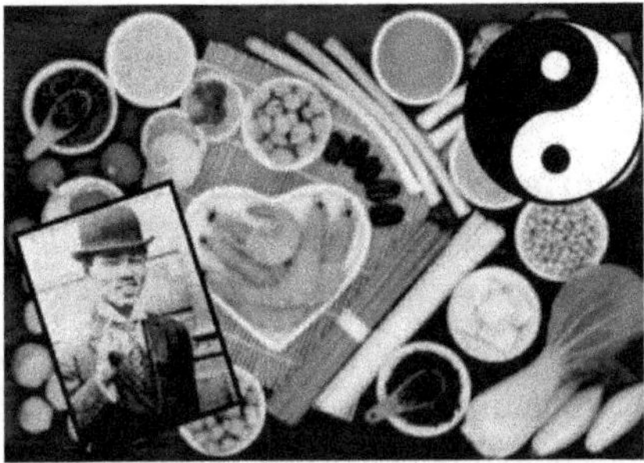

1960: the first Overeaters' Anonymous group was formed to use a 12-step system to fight food addiction based on the success of Alcoholics Anonymous.

1961: It's A Sin to Be Fat

Authors note: As I stated at the outset it is sad when Medical Men exploit the situation. This is double whammy fat shaming in the name of the Lord. Disgusting, sick and disturbed. I wonder if Dr Podolsky read Inge's book (1968).

1961: Dr Max Jacobson, "Dr. Feelgood," injected his patients with a combination of B vitamins, hormones and methamphetamine for energy and weight control.

He treated an incredible number of famous individuals. Tennessee Williams. Dubbed "Dr. Feelgood", Jacobson was known for his "miracle tissue regenerator" shots, which consisted of amphetamines, animal hormones, bone marrow, enzymes, human placenta, painkillers, steroids, and multivitamins.

John F. Kennedy first visited Jacobson in September 1960, shortly before the 1960 presidential election debates. Jacobson was part of the presidential entourage at the Vienna summit in 1961, where he administered injections to combat Kennedy's severe back pain. Some of the potential side effects included hyperactivity, impaired judgment, nervousness, and wild mood swings. Kennedy, however, was untroubled by FDA reports on the contents of Jacobson's injections, and proclaimed: "I don't care if it's horse piss. It works." Jacobson was used for the most severe bouts of back pain. By May 1962, Jacobson had visited the White House to treat the president 34 times, although such treatments were stopped by President Kennedy's White House physicians, who realized the inappropriate use of steroids and amphetamines administered by Jacobson. It was later observed that President Kennedy's leadership (e.g. the 1962 Cuban Missile Crisis, and other events during 1963) improved greatly once Jacobson's treatments were discontinued and replaced by a medically appropriate regimen.

1961: Formula 37, CorpuLean, Odrinex, Benzadrine, Prolamine Control were over-the-counter diet drugs which often contained an amphetamine compound called ephedra and/or the decongestant phenylpropanolamine. When people developed heart problems, strokes, addictions or even fatal reactions to these ingredients, the manufacturers replaced them with green tea extract, caffeine, and sometimes dehydroepiandrosterone (DHEA), a steroid.

1961: fewer than one in four American adults said they exercised regularly, according to Dr. Marc Stern, an expert on the history of fitness, but by 1987, 69% of adults said they did. Between those years, commercial fitness centers like L.A. Fitness and Gold's Gym were expanding their operations, and large companies began to offer on-site exercise facilities for their employees. In the early 1960s, however, all this was just beginning.

Calories Don't Count -The Vegetable Oil Diet:

This was a national bestseller. Obstetrician Dr Herman Taller's claimed eat as much as you want, and wash it down with vegetable oil, via his pill. The FDA later charged Taller with just peddling safflower oil and he was convicted of mail fraud.

Dr Irwin Stillman's "The Doctor's Quick Weight Loss Plan"

1963: Weight Watchers (now WW)

A self-described overweight housewife obsessed with cookies as a young wife in her 20s, Jean Nidetch decided to finally get control of her body, but even after losing 20 pounds in 10 weeks using a diet sponsored by the New York City Board of Health, she found she couldn't seem to stick to the plan in the long term. That was when she realized she needed the support of her friends. Nidetch began holding weekly meetings at her house, passing copies of the Board of Health Diet to anyone who came, with the hope that the more people were dieting together the better they all would do. While this predates the self-help movement and its attendant support-group networks it was, nevertheless, based on Alcoholics Anonymous. Nidetch and her friends were making this all up from scratch, and it turned out to be an addictive recipe. Within three months of her first meeting, more than 40 people were cramming into Nidetch's house on a weekly basis. Over the next year, she started several different groups around the New York metro area, finally incorporating her fledgling business in May of 1963. Now down to a trim 142 pounds, Nidetch hosted her first official Weight Watchers meeting, drawing more than 400 attendees.

Authors Note: She is to be congratulated for people who need support.

1963: Coca-Cola introduces Tab soda. You could also buy "Sweet-n-Low" in packets to use as a sugar replacement at the table.

1964: The Drinking Man's Diet
Was a page paperback by aerial photographer, Robert Cameron, and became a cultural phenomenon and, as a high-protein, low-carb diet paved the way for the Atkins and Dukan Diets. It was criticized by experts but sold 2.4 million copies and is still in print.

1968: The Sexy Pineapple Diet
According to a 1976 Chicago Tribune review "almost guarantees 24-hour dismay," and does not contain much more than illustrations of pineapples, women next to pineapples, and in "a surprise finish of five hamburger patties in a fry pan."

Another scam.

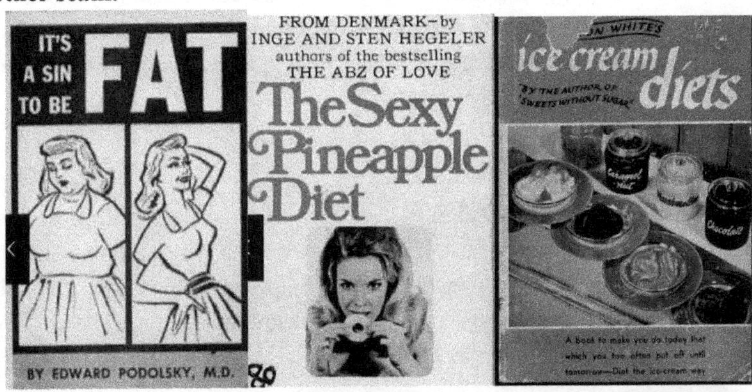

1969: Cyclamate banned. Coca-cola sweetened Tab with saccharin instead.

1970: Congress passed a law banning cigarette advertising on radio and TV. The last TV ad for cigarettes aired just before midnight on January 1, 1971, on the *The Johnny Carson Show.*

1970: 8% of all prescriptions were for amphetamines with many sold by "diet doctors" at "diet clinics." Amphetamines were not only chic, they were considered harmless and non-addictive. Neither was true.

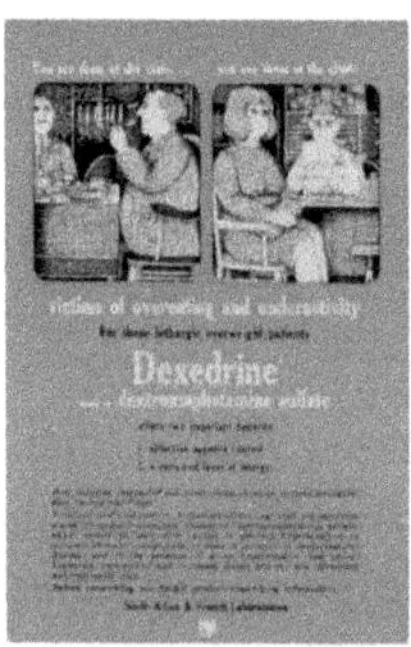

1970 – 1979: the percent of overweight adults remained about 35%, but the percent of obese adults climbed from 11% to 17%, meaning that for the first time the majority of Americans were too fat, despite all the diet books, weight loss products, pills, equipment and low-calorie foods now available.

1970s: New exercise equipment that you used at home, such as the "Twist and Tone," a wheel that spun when you wiggled your hips, stationary bicycles, and vibrating belts designed to jiggle the fat away. You could also buy a sauna suit that looked like something an astronaut would wear in order to sweat your fat away, or you could wear inflatable "air shorts" designed to eliminate water weight.

1970s: HCG Diet

This diet involves eating around 500 calories a day combined with injections of Human Chorionic Gonadotropin, a hormone taken from pregnant womens' urine. HCG is supposed to boost your metabolism to help you lose weight, although the massive calorie restriction is certainly a contributing factor. The diet made headlines in the 70s, and again in 2011.

Authors note: When I was specializing in London one of my colleagues supplemented his pittance by administering this in Harley Street. I thought it was a con then and it still is.

1970: The Sleeping Beauty Diet,

Involved risky sedation, is rumoured to have been tried by Elvis. If so, it didn't work. It was about taking sleeping pills and not eating for a few days while you were comatozed.

1970s: Ayds:

Were a popular appetite-suppressing candy called but taken off the market in 1980 after the AIDS crisis hit. They were phenylpropanolamine in chocolate, caramel, or butterscotch.

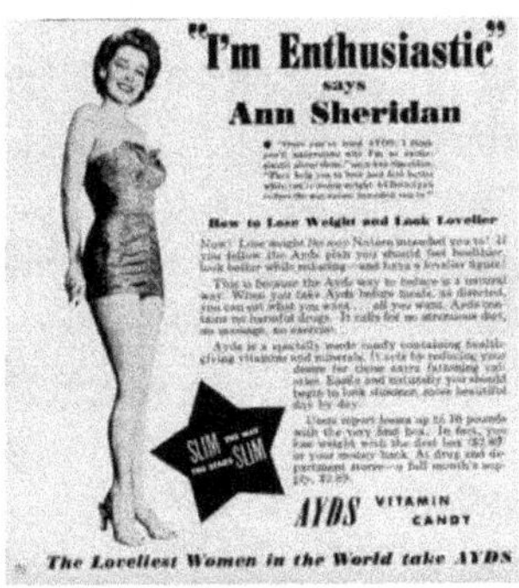

1972: Nutrisystem

Nutrisystem is a weight loss program that home delivers shelf-stable and freeze dried, portion controlled packaged meals. It has helped people achieve short-term weight loss goals but has received criticism from some customers not being able to sustain their weight loss.

1972: The Atkins Diet Lo-carbs again

The low-carb movement came into full swing with Dr Robert Atkins Diet Revolution book. The eating plan advised limiting carbohydrates to reduce weight as well as the risk of diabetes, high blood pressure and metabolic syndrome. The diet gained new popularity with Atkins 2002 follow-up, New Diet Revolutions.

Atkins made the controversial argument that the low-carbohydrate diet produces a metabolic advantage because 'burning fat takes more calories so you expend more calories[a]. He cited one study in which he estimated this advantage to be 950 Calories (4.0 MJ) per day. A review study published in Lancet, concluded that there was no such metabolic advantage and dieters were simply eating fewer calories.

In 1972 Dr. Roger Atkins published "Dr. Atkins' Diet Revolution." The title was no mistake -- his ideas actually caused a revolution in the diet industry. Atkins was telling people you could stay low-carb for the rest of your life. You did not have to count calories, and you did not have to restrict the amounts of food you were eating, but you did have to restrict what you ate. You had to cut out fruit, fleshy vegetables like potatoes, bread, cereal, pasta, desserts, sugary sodas, and everything but foods containing very few carbohydrates, such as meat, poultry, butter, fats, oils, nuts, and salad greens. People were having breakfasts of bowls of sour cream with fried eggs, lunches of five hamburgers without buns, and dinners of unlimited steaks with butter. Despite ingesting thousands of calories a day, Atkins fans claimed they were losing weight without feeling hungry.

The diet caused immediate controversy in the medical community, with most doctors assuming that it would increase heart disease by raising cholesterol levels. Some studies showed the immediate weight loss of between five and ten pounds the first week was mostly water loss, and if you stayed with Atkins, your results would be about the same as if you stayed on a healthier low-calorie diet.

Dr. Atkins went on to build a diet empire that manufactured all kinds of weight loss foods to use with the diet. At the height of its popularity, one in 11 Americans were on Atkins.

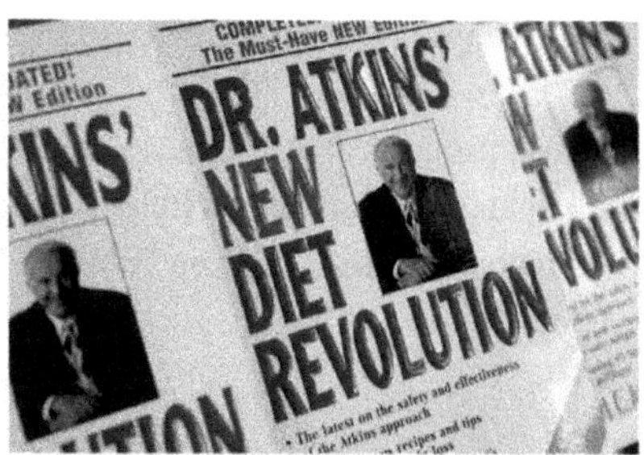

Atkins slipped on black ice in 2003 in New York and hit his head, never regained consciousness and died aged 72. His widow didn't allow an autopsy, but rumours were that he was overweight. His success stimulated a plethora of imitators and many companies released low-carb diets and low-carb foods but after his death, the popularity of Atkins' diet waned, with these other low-carb diets eroding its market share and questions being raised about its safety. In 2005, Atkins Nutritionals filed for bankruptcy.

1973 The Beautiful People's Diet Book by Luciana Avedon & Jeanne Molli

"For heightened perception without drugs plus rapid weight loss, nothing beats the oldest known treatment for obesity: total starvation."

1973: The Diet Clinic plan and Nutrisystem founded. Weight loss centers that sold prepackaged meals and had you report to a counsellor every week.

1974: The American Psychiatric Association recognized bulimia and anorexia as mental diseases of childhood and adolescence.

1975: The Cookie Diet

Florida Doctor Sanford Siegal baked up a specially designed diet cookie that's packed with a blend of amino acids. Eating six to nine of these cookies each day, along with sensible meals, was the diet's recipe for losing weight. Hollywood eats it up.

1975: The Stone Age Diet (East African, Inuit and Paleo Diets)

Gastroenterologist, Walter Voegtlin, proposed meats, animal fats and plants but eliminated dairy and grains.

In the 1980s Dr Stanley Eaton published his similar version of the East African diet while others explored the Inuit diet. These prehistoric diets took off in 2002 with the Paleo Diet (see below).

1975: Guzzle milk.

In 1975, the Dairy Farmers of Washington wrote, "Your response to our no-fad, no-gimmick, '7 Day Milk Diet for Women' has been overwhelming."

1976: The Prolin Diet or Last Chance Diet.

This plan involved foregoing food in favour of drinking a concoction called Prolin created by Robert Linn. It contained hooves, horns, bones and other slaughterhouse by products but no nutrients. At least 58 people had heart attacks while following this diet, although it was unclear if the attacks were due to fasting, drinking the Prolin or both.

1976: The Master Cleanser by Stanley Burroughs

Also called the lemonade diet or lemon detox diet is a modified "Juice fasting" juice fast that doesn't allow any food substituting lemonade made with maple syrup and cayenne pepper.

Burroughs, who initially marketed it in the 1940s and revived it his 1976 book. Proponents claim that the diet tones, reduces and cleanses the body, allowing the body to heal itself. There is no evidence that the diet removes any toxins (see below) or that it achieves anything beyond temporary weight loss, followed by rapidly regaining the lost weight. Though unlikely to be harmful over the short term, Master Cleanse and similar programs can be harmful over the long term. The diet lacks protein, fatty acids, and other essential nutrients and depends entirely on carbohydrates for calories.

1977: Slim Fast
Slim Fast started with a shake for breakfast, a shake for lunch and a sensible dinner. The weight loss product line has since grown to include snack bars, protein meal bars and a handful of shake flavors.

1977: Help Lord! The Devil Wants Me Fat by C.S. Lovett
The advice is as follows: 1. Be wary of the Devil at all times because he is trying to drop the "eat idea" into your mind. 2. Consume nothing but water for 10 days.

Authors note: **He should team up with Dr Podolsky (1961) and Dr Don Colbert (2002)**

1977: The FDA tried to take saccharin off the market as a carcinogen, but instead put warning labels on products containing it.

1978: The Scarsdale Diet
Dr Herman Tarnower's The Complete Scarsdale Medical Diet outlines a plan for eating carbohydrates, proteins and fats in precise proportions. A jilted girlfriend shot Tarnower two years after the book's publication.

1977: Dexatrim

A diet drug containing phenylpropanolamine (PPA), appears on drugstore shelves. Its formula changes after PPA is linked to an increased risk of stroke in 2000.

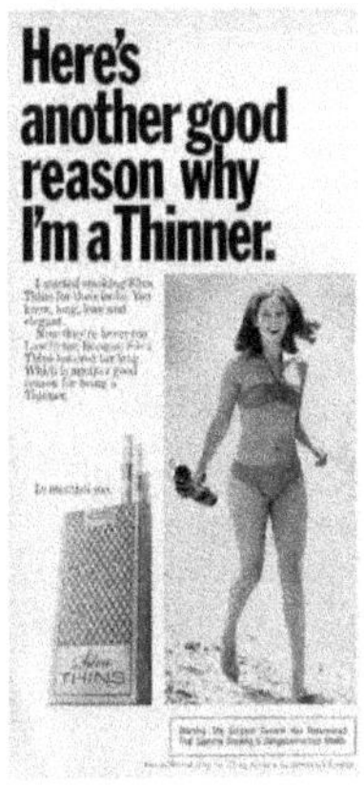

Just in case amphetamines weren't enough, Liggett Myers and Philip Morris companies introduced cigarettes marketed to women and with ads that synched with the women's movement. The slogan for "Virginia Slims" was "You've Come A Long Way, Baby -- You've got your own cigarette now." The Virginia Slims' message also implied if you smoked, you'd stay slim. The ads were not even that subtle, using language like "These cigarettes are longer and slimmer than the fat ones, men smoke." Eve cigarettes were deliberately packaged in a feminine way with flowers and an image of Eve in Eden. The Eve ads insisted that cigarette smoking was for ladies and used slogans like "Finally a cigarette as pretty as you" and "Every inch the lady."

It was still okay to be mean to fat people in the 1970s. As Washington Post columnist Ellen Goodman put it, "Eating has become the last bona-fide sin left in America." Dr. Thomas Szasz, a radical psychiatrist, wrote in 1973, "We used to go after Jews, homosexuals, the insane and drug addicts. Now it's fat people. We impose diets on them as part of the moral order. It's a national neurosis."

Although the percent of overweight Americans stayed steady around 35% between 1960 and 1990, the percent of obese adults began to skyrocket around 1980, climbing from 17% in 1980 to 35% by 1989. Scientists blamed the suburban lifestyle, too much reliance on cars, the increasing number of people eating out in restaurants, restaurants serving gigantic portions, sugary sodas, lack of breast-feeding, increased female participation in the work force, fewer people smoking, overly processed foods, fast foods, food advertising on television and radio, government advice on diets, and a too sedentary lifestyle. It was probably a combination of all of those things and more.

Some evidence implied that dieting itself could cause overweight because it may permanently lower the body's metabolic rate. Also, the vast majority of people gain back any weight they lose in diets, usually along with some extra pounds

1979: Dr Hugh Sinclair
Puts himself on an Inuit diet, consisting solely of seal, fish (including molluscs and crustaceans), and water for 100 days. His bleeding times rising from 3 min to over 50 min - a dramatic demonstration of the importance of long-chain fatty acids of fish oils in decreasing the aggregation of platelets and thus the incidence of thrombosis-heart attacks.

1979: Nathan Pritikin
No meat, no processed foods, low fat. Very popular.

Other low-fat reducing diets become popular in the 1980s featuring large amounts of fiber and whole grains but only 10% fat. Similar ones are the Ornish and Volumetrics.

1980s: The icon of the decade was England's Princess Diana, a tall slim woman who suffered from bulimia. As a result of the fitness craze, work-out clothes and jogging outfits came in style as street wear for the first time.

1980: 30 million people were using artificial sweeteners, a $2 billion market.

1981: The Breatharian Plan
Disciples eat air to liberate them from “the drudgery of food”. Several die from dehydration.

1981: The Beverly Hills Diet
The book, published in 1981, showed people how to follow a highly restrictive six-week food-combining regimen and turned its author, Judy Mazel, into a Hollywood diet guru but who had no science or nutritional training. Mazel, clearly inspired by William Hay, believed that the order in which we ate food was the main problem, confusing the enzymes in our bodies that digest the food and leading to weight gain. She advocated the eating of rather a lot of fat-burning

pineapple. For the first 10 days of the diet, only fruit was permitted; gradually other foods were introduced, but protein and carbohydrates were eaten separately.

It sold more than a million copies and attracted celebrity fans including Englebert Humperdinck Linda Gray and Liza Minnelli. Mazel died age aged 63.

1982: It was the decade when Americans, especially baby boomers nearing middle age, turned to physical fitness to help them control their weights. An estimated 25 million adults took up running, including President Jimmy Carter. Academy-award winning actress Jane Fonda released her book, "Jane Fonda's Work-Out," which became an immediate best-seller. She followed it up with the "Jane Fonda's Work Out" video in 1982 and produced 22 more exercise DVDs that sold over 17 million copies. Her advice was to work out until "you feel the burn."

1981: The Cambridge Diet

A fad diet in which 600 to 1500 cals are consumed per day, principally in liquids made from commercial products sold as part of the diet regime. These products are manufactured in the UK and include shakes, meal replacement bars, soups and smoothies. Banned.

1982: The F Plan

Is a high fiber diet created in the 1980s by British author Audrey Eyton, founder of Slimming Magazine and based on the work of Denis Burkitt (an Irish Missionary Physician who was correct in noting the reduced intake of fiber in the Western Diet compared with Africans and linking that to increased cancer of the colon in this Western Diet).

The F-Plan diet book was in the top ten best-selling books in America in April and May 1983. The diet works by restricting the daily intake of calories to less than 1,500 whilst consuming well-above the recommended level of dietary fiber. The fiber has a number of beneficial effects, such as making the dieter feel full for much longer than normal, reducing the urge to overeat, and promoting a healthy digestive system. The disadvantages include excessive flatulence in the first few weeks and having to eat food that is harder work to chew and swallow. Some people also express a dislike of the texture of such a high fiber diet. The dieter will need to consume more water than usual to prevent constipation.

Authors Note: I am a fan of Dr Dennis Burkitt and high fiber and include this in my Newtrition foods.

1982; The aerobics craze Jane Fonda
Launched her first exercise video, Workout: Starring Jane Fonda. Her catch phrase: No pain, no gain.

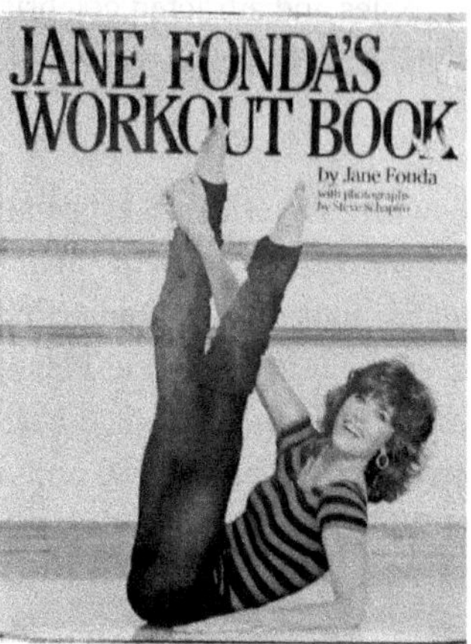

Authors Note: Exercise good but unfortunately it only accounts for 15% of weight loss.

1983: Jazzercise
Founded in 1969 by professional dancer Judi Sheppard Missett, hits all USA 50 states.

1983: Jenny Craig
Based on the motto Eat Well, Move More and Live Life, Jenny Craig was born in Louisiana and raised in New Orleans. In 1983, she and her husband created a nutrition, fitness, and weight loss program in Australia and began offering the program in the United States in 1985. The company became a part of Nestlé Nutrition in 2006. Each customized program combines frozen meals and other packaged foods, containing fruits, vegetables, lean meats, as well as meatless options. The couple sold the majority of their interest in the company in 2002. Nestlé purchased the company in 2006 for $600 million.

1983: Gloria Steinem, feminist icon, declared that eating disorders were a result of "gender prisons," and that 150,000 women died of them every year. The actual number recorded on death certificates in 1983 was 101. She also noted that the most powerful moment in her young adulthood was her recognition that she possessed an eating disorder, a realization that led to an interrogation of her own internalization of sexist values. An eating disorder, from this standpoint, becomes a rite of passage or admission into a community—an experience that signifies that you have suffered as your sisters have and can purify yourself through confession.

1984: FDA requires all Very Low Protein Diets carry a warning after 58 deaths.
Slim Fast escapes by recommending one sensible meal a day.

1984: The National Institutes of Health declared that fat is bad for people. Four years later, the United States Surgeon General said that ice cream is comparable to cigarettes when it comes to your health, and he linked a high-fat diet to heart disease, breast cancer, high blood pressure, and other health problems.

1985: Seattle Sutton's Healthy Eating
Illinois registered nurse Seattle Sutton eschewed dietary gimmicks and went for straightforward healthy eating with a plan that delivers well balanced, freshly prepared meals including fresh fruit and vegetables, right to people's doors.

Authors Note: These latter two would seem sensible.

1985: Fit for Life
Written by nutrition specialists, Harvey and Marilyn Diamond. Prohibits complex carbs and protein from being eaten during the same meal a throwback to the Hay diet. It lacks any scientific basis, no clinical trials, provokes vitamin, calcium and mineral deficiencies while potentially causing serious complications in diabetics. Nevertheless, it spent 40 weeks on the New York Times Best Seller list and sold over 12 million copies.

“Scams sell and science sucks” especially when it comes to diets.

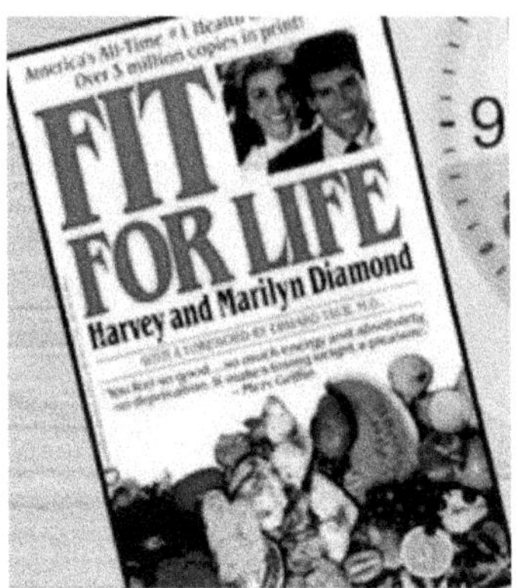

1985: The Caveman Diet aka Paleo

1986: The Rotation Diet
Launched by Martin Katahn, a professor of psychology at Vanderbilt University, involves diet, exercise and behaviour modification, it rotates different calorie restrictions over three weeks: 600, 900, 1200 for women and 1.200, 1,500 and 1,800 for men with a period of maintenance. It claims to prevent metabolic adaption as does the Zig-Zag diet.

1987: Elizabeth Takes Off
Actress Elizabeth Taylor lost over 50 pounds on a 1000-calorie diet, and then wrote about it. The first half of the book is a blunt description of how she gained the weight as bored wife of a senator in Washington, D.C. Her advise included to eat veggies and dip each day at 3 p.m.

1988: Oprah’s Liquid Diet
Wearing a pair of size 10 Calvin Klein jeans, Oprah walked onto the set of her show, pulling a wagon full of fat to represent the 67 pounds she lost. She had used the Optifast Liquid Protein Diet but she later said they did not fit by the following week once she started to eat real food again. After one year she was 17 pounds heavier and went on to regain most of her lost weight. Oprah’s “success” saw $200 million in profits for liquid diets that year.

As Ann La Berge wrote in the Journal of the History of Medicine, "the low-fat approach became an overarching ideology, promoted by physicians, the federal government, the food industry, and popular health media."

Hundreds of new low-fat versions of food products appeared alongside the low-calorie ones in grocery stores. However, many low-fat products contained starches and sugar to replace the fat originally in them, which meant they had fewer calories than the original products, but more carbohydrates. They were also less filling.

1990-2000: At the beginning of the 1990s, about 32% of American adults were overweight, 23% were obese, and 3% were extremely obese. Within ten years those figures were 34% overweight, 30% obese, and about 5% extremely obese, for a total of 67% of the entire population.

A 1990 Gallup Poll found that over 60% of women and 42% of men wanted to lose weight, but yet only 18% were on a reducing diet. Eighteen percent were dieting in 1950 when only 40% of American adults were overweight. These numbers indicate that many people were giving up.

1990: Chitosan

A non-prescription 'fat blocker' made from powdered crab shells. Didn't work.

1990s - The Low Fat Diet

The antithesis of the Atkins diet - and the rough eating plan still recommended today - is the low-fat diet. Prompted by government food pyramids, companies began marketing all of their food products as being low in fat, with many people believing that a diet high in saturated fat was conducive to heart disease and obesity.

1991: Optifast, Medifast and Ultrafast

Charged with Deceptive Advertising and agree to delete alleged deceptive claims as to long-term results and safety.

1991: Americans go low-fat

Eating foods like **McDonald's** McLean Deluxe burger.

1992: The United States government came up with a "food pyramid" to replace the old chart of essential food groups.

1994: Mode magazine clearly opened the door for some pretty niche publications.

When "Mode," a new magazine for "plus-sized" women appeared in 1994 featuring an actress who weighed 296 pounds, circulation climbed to 370,000 in the first month.

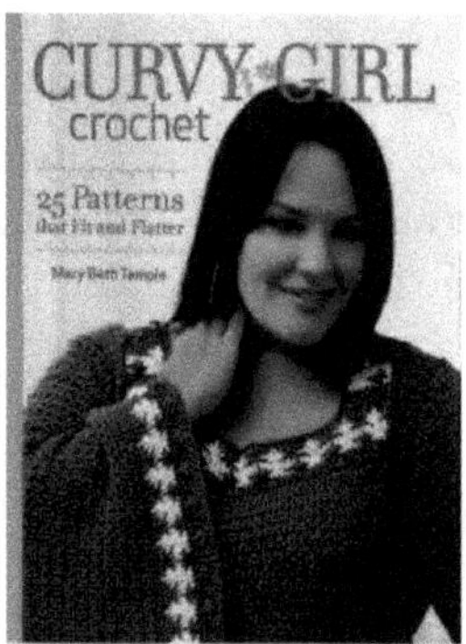

1994: the FDA required that all packaged foods must have a label that provides nutritional information.

1994: the American Psychiatric Association recognized anorexia, bulimia, and added "eating disorder not specified" to their list of mental disorders.

1993: The Carbohydrate Addict's Diet

1993: Eat More, Weigh Less

Dr Dean Ornish's diet emphasizes fiber and complex carbs, forbids nearly all animal products, and has only 10% fat. Dr Ornish served as President Bill Clinton's and Clint Eastwood's diet doctor.

1994: The Guide to Nutrition Labelling and Education Act (USA)

Requires food companies to include nutritional info on nearly all packaging.

1994: Fen-phen

A drug combining fenfluramine and phentermine. Withdrawn in 1997 after one third of users developed valvular heart problems.

1995: Cabbage Soup (again)

1995 Pills:

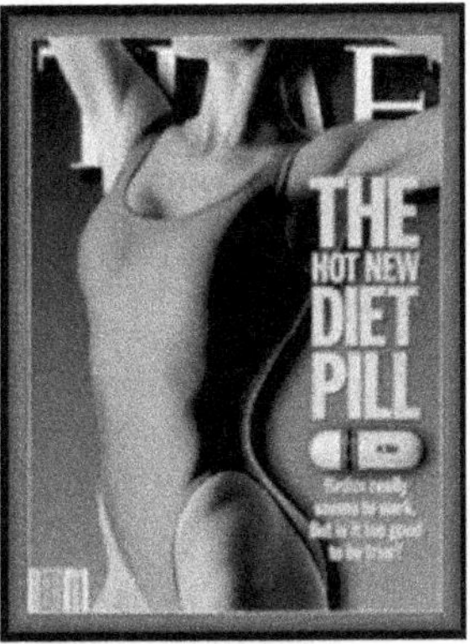

1995: The Zone Diet

Calls for a specific ratio of carbs, fat, and protein at each meal, begins to attract celeb fans.

1997: Eat Right for Your Type, Blood Type diet.

Peter D'Adamo, a naturopath, claimed that people should eat foods compatible with their blood type. He had no supporting evidence and subsequent studies found no evidence and findings do not support the Blood-Type diet hypothesis.

1997: Stacker 2

Originally developed for bodybuilders who engaged in the practice of stacking, or ingesting Ephedrine HCL, caffeine and aspirin for a lean look and extra energy.

1998: Sugar Busters! Protein Power

Fashion icons of the 1990s were extremely skinny supermodels like Linda Evangelista and Cindy Crawford, and very thin actresses like Michelle Pfeiffer, Meg Ryan.

The most recent government figures for obesity and overweight in United States are from 2012, showing that about 33% of the adult population is overweight and 36% obese. In the same year the government found that about half of all American children are either overweight or obese.

2000s:

Some of the popular diets in the early 21st century were the Breatharian, Blue Vision, South Beach, Paleo, Medifast, and Dukan.

The Blue Vision Diet requires you to wear blue tinted glasses in order to make food look blue and disgusting.

The Breatharian Lifestyle comes from the notion that a person who is truly spiritual and in harmony with the universe does not need to eat. Many try, some to the point of starving themselves to death.

Some of the more bizarre products for weight loss are high-tech leg wear that heats the skin and slims your legs by inches; fat-burning lip balm, aroma products designed to relax you and thereby suppress your food cravings, and ear staples that supposedly work like acupuncture to curb the appetite.

Authors note: I learned acupuncture from the London doctor, Felix Mann, who brought it out of China and used it with some success for migraines, sinusitis, arthritis and back pain in patients who didn't tolerate drugs. I even tried these ear staples but soon worked out it was the psychological support by seeing them regularly, that worked.

Yoga became very popular in the 2000s. Not only were health clubs and community centers offering classes, but many entrepreneurs were opening boutique gyms specializing in the ancient art that combines relaxation with stretching. Some other popular exercise regimes were Pilates, Zumba, spinning, ballet barre, and kick boxing.

Digital entered the fitness world around 2000 in the form of apps, websites and wearable electronic devices. Some are just hyped-up pedometers, but others are complex little machines that monitor calorie, carb and protein intake, sleep patterns, and calories burned during exercise. Some even give fitness advice.

Websites for dieters contain millions of listings for foods that include every bit of nutritional information about each one. You can even look up thousands of exact restaurant offerings.

Another Internet fad in the 2000s are cash rewards to those who lose weight. You pay to join and then by the month, and then you collect money if you lose weight.

2000: Gwyneth Paltrow lends publicity to the Macrobiotic Diet, a restrictive Japanese plan based on whole grains and veggies.

Authors note: The problem with Gwyneth is that she is so good looking she is believable but peddles rubbish. I think she could even sell poop on Goop.

2001: Torrid opened in 2001 as a store that sells plus-sized clothes for teenagers as well as women. Other mall favorites like Delia's, Gap and Old Navy began sizing up for "curvy teens." Big mainstream designers like Ralph Lauren and Tommy Hilfiger finally began making clothes in plus-sizes, after traditionally ending at Size 14. Carré Otis, who at five foot ten, 155 pounds and a size 12, became one of the first mainstream "plus-sized" models in 2001. Destination XL and other new stores for men began offering clothing in large sizes, finally giving this demographic a choice other than the "Big and Tall Shops."

The Dukan diet

A French GP, Pierre Dukan. Like the Atkins diet, it involves four stages of weight loss and stabilization, with the final stage being a diet for life. It is a throwback to both the Hay Diet and Atkins.

2002: The Paleo Diet

This high-protein diet by Loren Cordain PhD, includes lean meats, fish, fruit, vegetables and some animal fats, eggs and seeds while avoiding grains, legumes, processed foods, sugar, salt and potatoes. He claimed it was the diet of the Hunter-Gatherer and hence based on our genes. But Cordain was not a medical doctor and humans evolved salivary amylase to digest grains for essential vitamins and legumes have also been found to be nutritionally beneficial ñ so either Cordain didn't know this or he assumed our ancestors didn't eat grains or legumes ñ or potatoes ñ just don't tell the Peruvians or the Irish.

Our Paleo and Cavemen ancestors also had a varied diet and not just the one Cordain seemed to think and very similar to the Banting diet from 1863.

2002: Eat what Jesus ate by Don Colbert M.D.

There are no photos of Jesus, so we don't know if he was obese but as He walked everywhere, he was probably fit and slim. He ate fish, meat (but as He was a Jew probably not pork), fruit and vegetables and drank wine (just don't tell the Seven Day Adventists).

Authors note: Why it's the Mediterranean Diet! Funny that.

2003: The South Beach Diet

Miami Doctor Arthur Agatston, MD, adds fuel to the low-carb craze seen as a

2004 Gluten Free Diet

Gluten free diets have been around since WW2 when the Nazis took all the bread for themselves when occupying Holland. An astute Doctor then noticed some of his "Failure to Thrive" kids started to improve and grow normally. They had coeliac disease, and gluten, in wheat, rye and barley, is toxic to them. But gluten free diets started gaining widespread popularity with the Health Nutters around 2004 but have no place in weight control nor in imagined symptoms. Many people blame gluten for symptoms like excessive gas, bloating and joint pain, even though only one in 70 people are actually medically diagnosed with having Coeliac disease. There is, however, 'wheat sensitivity'.

2004: Ephedra Ban

The FDA bans the sale of diet drugs and supplements containing ephedra after it was linked to heart attacks.

2004: The Biggest Loser

TV debut, turning weight loss into a reality show. All regain weight and their fitness instructor has a heart attack.

2006: Master Cleanse (again)

Beyonce admits to using the Master Cleanse, a concoction of hot water, lemon juice, maple syrup, and cayenne pepper, to shed 20 pounds for Dreamgirls.

2006: F2

A revised version of the F-plan written in the light of subsequent medical discoveries, which claims to be faster and more effective and campaigns against low-carbohydrate diets, particularly the Atkins Diet.

2007: Alli

The non-prescription drug is taken with meals claiming to keep your body from absorbing some of the food you eat.

2007: Zantrex

Zantrex weight-loss products have been around since at least 2007, and they're apparently still going strong. Caffeine is one of the main components in their product line.

2009: Whole 30

Invented by a husband and wife. Nutritionists are generally critical about the Whole30 regimen. US News and World report consistently puts the plan near the bottom of its annual diet ranking.

It is not backed by science and a month isn't enough time to re-set your digestive system. Followers are encouraged to eat: Mostly home-cooked meals rich in veggies, meat, eggs, fish, and fruit.

It does not allow: Alcohol, bread (including gluten-free varieties), whole grains, beans, sugar, dairy (including butter), legumes like beans, peanuts, soy, MSG, processed snacks, or comfort foods like pancakes or desserts. There's also no weighing yourself allowed during the first month.

2009: The FDA approved Alli as effective for weight loss. The only FDA-approved drug sold over the counter, Alli comes with a "success plan" that includes a reducing diet. Its active ingredient, orlistat, interferes with how you digest fats. Many people cannot tolerate orlistat because it gives them diarrhea, or worse, causes discharges of oil.

2010:

New grocery store products became available for calorie-counters, grain eaters, and Atkins fans. You could buy Atkins low-carb entrees in the freezer section of the store, as well as Atkins packaged snacks. Boxes of popular snacks like potato chips and cookies appeared in packages of 100-calories each. Once obscure grain products like Bulgar wheat and quinoa became mainstream. Lean chicken was a diet fad in the 1990s. "Energy drinks," containing large amounts of caffeine, were beginning to equal the sales of traditional sodas.

Obesity is now double what it was in 1965, and the average American is about 24 pounds heavier than he or she was back then. Childhood obesity has tripled since 1980.

Even though overweight people are in the majority, discrimination against them at work, school and during social occasions continued in 2000s decade.

Joining the parade of endless fad diets, the 2010s saw the Baby Food Diet, the Clean Diet, Karl Lagerfeld, Pil-Sook, Five-Bite, Werewolf, Alkaline, Cotton ball, and KE.

The Baby Food Diet is what it sounds like. The Werewolf Diet, tried by Madonna and Demi Moore, makes you fast according to moon cycles. The Cotton Ball Diet, once used by 1950s models, has you eating them for filler. KE is one of the more insane diets, in that you don't eat food, you have it injected into your body through feeding tubes.

Juice cleanses became popular (again). You only drink fruit and/or green juices for 24 hours up to a week as a way to detox your system.

2010s - The Juice Cleanse

No! Not again!? Instagram bloggers and celebrities exploited the "organic" trendy fad and juice cleanses returned with companies offering a numbered package where people drink a certain juice at certain times in the day. People do lose weight, of course, because they're essentially consuming no calories at all and the medical profession persistently warned against trying them. See De-tox diets below.

2010: the "Air Diet"

The French magazine, Grazia, did an entire spread claiming the "Air Diet" as the new it weight loss method. You still make eating motions, and you can consume some hearty salt and water soup. This must be the best-seller follow-up to the 1973 Beautiful People starvation diet (see).

2010: Another major trend is to approach obesity as a societal problem. First Lady. Michelle Obama's project, the Let's Move! initiative begun in 2010, has the goal of "eliminating obesity in a generation" by focusing on a healthy start for babies and children. The Robert Wood Johnson Foundation spent $1 billion since 2007 on the same problem.

New laws made it mandatory for public schools and day care centers to serve more fruits and vegetables and less junk food.

2010: Expensive "craft beers" came in style and within a few years certain bars and restaurants were specializing in them.

2010: Gweneth Paltrow diagnosed at age 37 with osteopenia, a bone thinning disease common in older women. Extreme dieting can cause the condition.

2011: The U.S. government came up with "My Plate," a diagram of suggested nutrition for each meal. The plate was half veggies and fruits, and one fourth grain and protein with a glass of milk at the side.

2011: Three experts in nutrition and economics, writing in the Journal of the American Medical Association, have called for an across-the-board tax in the range of 10 to 30 percent on processed food, fast food and large chain restaurants.

2011: The HCG Diet (again)

Combines a fertility drug with a strict 500- to 800-calorie-a-day regimen, invites interest and criticism.

2012: Fasting Diets

Fasting Diets are as old as God's Dog but with increasing evidence as to their benefit. Recently popularized on the BBC as the 5:2 diet (eat normally for five days; restrict calories to 500 for women, and 600 for men, on two non-consecutive days), is the current diet trend as ñ though its supporters would describe it as advice for life rather than a fad diet.

2013: The Drunk Diet: How I Lost 40 Pounds...Wasted,

By Lady Gaga's ex-boyfriend Carl, he explains how he was able to get fit while being wasted and you can too! Being any sort of a drug addict also helps losing weight.

2012: Medifast a rival to Jenny Craig and Nutrisystem in that dieters buy prepackaged meals from clinics. In 2012 Medifast paid a $3.7 million civil claim for false advertising.

2013: New York City Council made it illegal to sell soft drinks over 16 ounces but the New York Appeals Court threw the law out before it went into force.

Some research indicates Americans may be giving up on dieting. In 1991, for example, 31% of adults were dieting, but in 2013 it was down to 20%. Only 23% of Americans said they believed that a certain weight would make you more attractive.

2013: The American Medical Association recognized obesity as a disease. This opened the door for some funds to pay for bariatric surgeries.

2013: The American Psychiatric Association changed its criteria for eating disorders by adding binge eating disorder, keeping anorexia and bulimia, and taking out "eating disorder unspecified." The National Institutes of Health estimates that anorexia affects 0.5% of women and 0.1% of men; bulimia is 1-3% of women and 0.1% of men; and binge eating is 3.3% of women and 0.8% of men. This means almost 8% or 2.5 million Americans have eating disorders. Some experts on eating disorders believe they only happen in places where there is a lot of food.

Grocery stores were still selling over-the-counter diet pills, but their ingredients were different than in other decades. Natural stimulants like acai berries and green tea were replacing laboratory formulas, mostly because the FDA had banned them.

2014: the FDA passed a rule that any chain operating 20 or more food establishments selling the same items has to provide nutritional information on all their menus. The FDA also changed labels on grocery store foods, making the calorie count bigger.

2015: some experts writing in various journals peg the obesity rate in the United States at 38%. The obesity epidemic is also spreading throughout the world: by 2014 almost two billion adults were overweight and more than 600 million were obese.

2015: Americans for the first time spent more money eating out in restaurants than they did in grocery stores. Restaurant patrons were demanding healthier foods, including options for people allergic to gluten and peanuts. The buzz words in the restaurant industry were organic, locally grown, pesticide-free, vegan, vegetarian, and non-genetically altered foods.

2015: A U.S. Advisory Panel suggested that Americans eat less red meat and sugar, and that "environmental factors should figure into a healthy diet." 2011 and 2015, Atkins fans immediately reacted to these government suggestions as ones that would make us even fatter.

2015: Artificial sweeteners were linked to causing obesity in that they may kill off bacteria gut helpful to digestion and elimination.

2015: it became possible to buy a DNA kit from online vendors who would in turn send you a personalized diet based on your heredity. The science behind this is by no means perfect and not expected to be accurate until 2020, according to an article in the journal Obesity.

2015: Amazon was selling over 23,000 weight loss books, 19,000 diet books, 31,500 fitness books, and 10,000 weight loss cookbooks. The Atkins diet category alone had 482 books.

2015: Americans New Year's Resolutions. At the top of the list was "to stay fit and healthy," mentioned by 37%, and next was "to lose weight," mentioned by 32%. The year before on January 1, 2014, 43% said they planned to lose weight, making it the perpetual No.1 New Year's resolution for all Americans.

2018: Optavia

Was named by Google as one of the top trending diets in 2018 in its year-end report It offers a few different structured weight loss programs ñ just order a box but it did not fare as well for long-term weight loss, nutrition, and heart healthfulness with a lack of fresh food, and highly processed products. It is also expensive.

The future of diets is probably in three trends: nutrigenomics, prescription drugs, and more governmental intervention in the food supply.

American drug companies are frantically searching for a medicine to cure obesity. Some promising research is being performed in the way hormones regulate appetite. One of the few prescription drugs available now for reducing is Contrave, approved in 2011. This drug is actually an anti-depressant combined with naltrexone, a drug that reverses the effects of narcotic drugs and is used in rehab programs. So far Contrave has been proven to be only mildly effective.

Nutrigenomics is the theory that your diet should be based on your DNA. People living in the Arctic, for example, eat a high fat diet full of whale blubber and remain slim, while people in the Tropics rely more on fruit and animal flesh. Where your ancestors came from, therefore, could determine whether whale blubber or fruit is the best diet for you. Nutrigenomics could explain why some people do well on low-carb/high protein diets like the Atkins, and others fare better on an opposite approach like the Ornish Diet.

Among the diets based on the theory of nutrigenomics are the Blood Type Diet, Body Type, Inuit Diet, the Noriska, Metabolic Type, and others.

The Weizmann Institute in Israel found vast differences in how some 800 people digested the same meal by monitoring their blood sugar levels and other factors. The researchers concluded that each person may need an individualized approach to dieting to succeed at it. This is the research direction that we seem to be taking now.

So far the childhood obesity rate in children ages six to 11 has leveled at 18% after years of increasing, and obesity in children two to five has fallen below 10% for the first time since the 1980s.

A few experts in the medical community are questioning whether you should put overweight patients on a diet when the long-term success rates are less than five percent. As Dr. Asheley Skinner of the University of North Carolina wrote, "Research assumes thin people are healthy but if someone loses weight, they will always need fewer calories and more exercise. Who knows what we are doing to their metabolisms."

And then there's Volumetrics, Flexitarian, Traditional Asian, Spark People, HMR, Flat Belly, Engine 2, South Beach, Abs, Eco-Atkins, Aitkins 40, Macrobiotic, Medifast, Supercharged Hormone, Body Reset, Whole 30, The Mono, Pizza (I kid you not), Wild, Disassociated, Military, The Taco (I kid you not again) and the Golo Diets (to name but a few).

As you can see from this history ALL weight loss diets depend on eating less (or getting a tapeworm to share your food). Of course, you have to eat less! We all know that! Losing weight is that simple, according to all these diets, yet it seems the hardest thing possible to achieve. Overweight and obesity, as per the History of Obesity chapter in my book Slim 4 Life, have always been a problem but obesity was only recognized as an epidemic in 1985 and coincides with the alteration to our foods.

These alterations of processed, ultra-processed, refined and additives, would seem implicated. Especially as they are delicious, cheap and readily available.

BUT IF YOU JUST WANT TO LOSE WEIGHT WITHOUT DIETING:

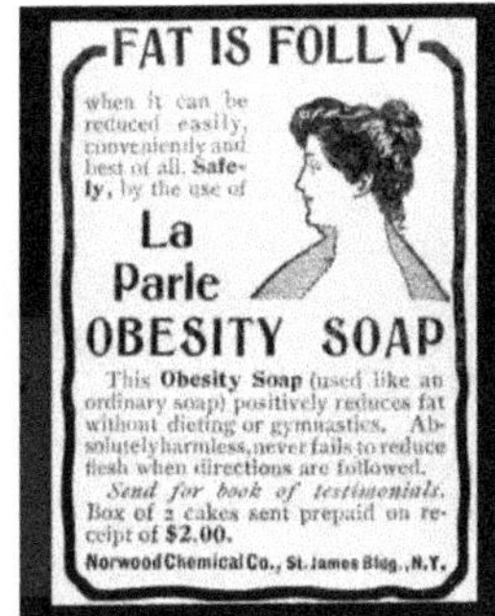

Rub a dub dub

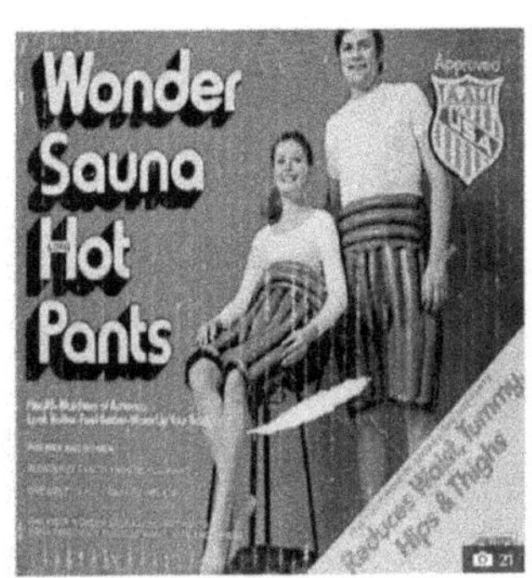

How can you go wrong! USA Approved!

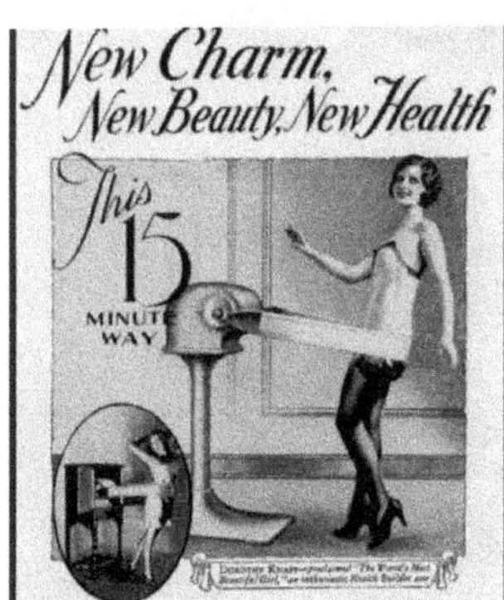

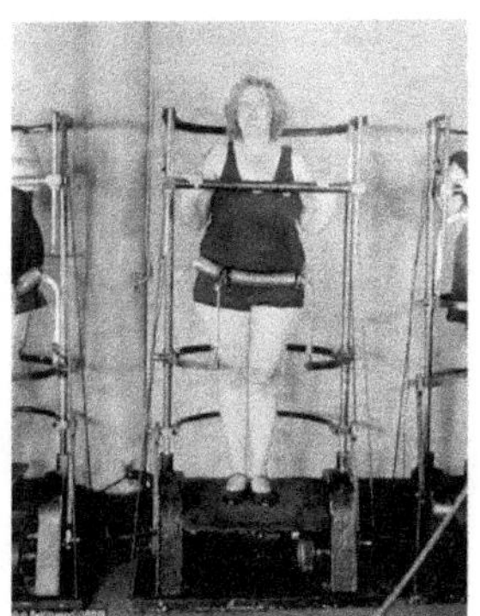

The Slendo Massager

Then there are the drugs all of which were found to have later severe side effects

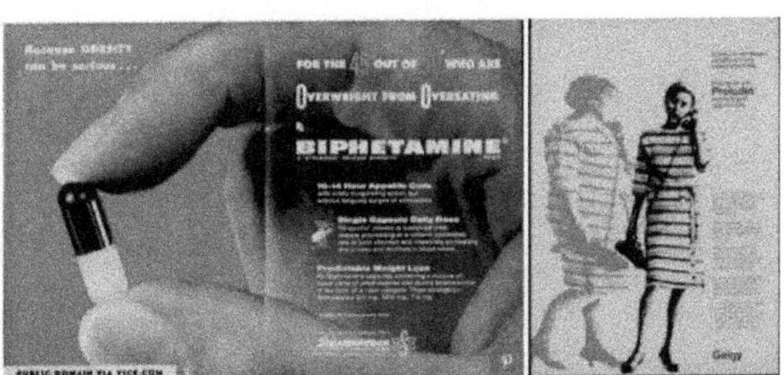

CHAPTER 33

DETOX DIETS - BEWARE

What are Detox Diets and Cleanses and Does Anyone Need Them?

Whether it's called a detox diet or a cleanse, it doesn't really matter. Neither has a clear-cut definition but both have similar goals -- to rid/cleanse the body of supposedly harmful substances (usually referred to as toxins).

Detox diets claim to rid the body of environmental toxins (pollution, chemicals in foods and household products, etc) or the by-products of metabolism through "clean eating" usually a strict diet of fruits, vegetables, whole grains, and raw nuts and seeds, plus lots of water, eliminating processed foods, and any personal sensitivities (dairy, gluten, eggs, and red meat). Cleanse diets go further, limiting intake of such fluids as smoothies for a period of several days.

By cutting out sugary and processed foods, patients may feel better in the short-term but there's no evidence detox and cleanse diets actually rid the body of "toxins", or that they're necessary.

According to MedlinePlus from the U.S. National Library of Medicine, Toxins are substances created by plants and animals that are poisonous to humans. Toxins also include some medicines that are helpful in small doses, but poisonous in large amounts. Toxins also include metals, such as lead, and certain chemicals in the environment.

However, in the context of commercial detox diets, the meaning of the term toxin is often vague or obscure.

In 2009, a group of early career scientists called The Voices of Young Science, created The Detox Dossier. They went to the manufacturers of 15 representative detox products and asked what toxin their product targeted and what evidence they had to support that claim. They came to the following conclusion:

No one we contacted was able to provide any evidence for their claims or give a comprehensive definition of what they meant by detox. We concluded that detox as used in product marketing is a myth. Many of the claims about how the body works were wrong and some were even dangerous.

Yes, folks, Detox and Cleanse Diets are yet just another scam.

Weight loss is often a secondary goal of detoxes or cleanses. All use a restrictive diet, often in conjunction with a variety of supplements (including herbs, vitamins, seasonings, and so on). For example, The Master Cleanse (see above), also called the Lemonade Diet, is a liquid-only diet consisting of water, lemon juice, maple syrup, and cayenne pepper taken for 10 days. It is essentially a starvation diet.

Unfortunately, most of the weight loss in a detox diet is water, and the weight returns just as quickly as it left as soon as a normal diet is resumed.

Detox diets falsely claim that they can help chronic conditions that occur when the body becomes victim to a build-up of toxins.

As Dr Junger claims in his book Clean which reached number 7 in Amazon sales rankings for alternative medicine books, "When our systems are overtaxed, they begin to break down in a multitude of ways. Allergies, headaches, depression, irritable bowel syndrome, fatigue, weight gain, and insomnia are just a few of the symptoms that can result. The majority of these common ailments are the direct result of toxin build-up in our systems that has accumulated during the course of our daily lives".

This is snake-oil garbage but 'Scams sell and science sucks'.

The science behind the detox theory is deeply flawed, says Peter Pressman, MD, an internal medicine specialist at Cedars-Sinai Medical Center in Los Angeles. The body already has multiple systems in place -- including the liver, kidneys, and gastrointestinal tract -- that do a perfectly good job of eliminating toxins from the body within hours of consumption.

Detox dieters often report a variety of benefits, but most of these improvements may be due to changes in the diet unrelated to any change in toxin levels. For instance, a decrease in headaches could be related to elimination of caffeine or alcohol in the diet. Decreased bloating just from eating less. Clearer skin may be related to better hydration.

Is there any scientific evidence to support the dubious claims of detox proponents?

Almost none. There is a 2015 study by Kim et al. Eighty-four premenopausal women were randomly divided into 3 groups: a control group without diet restriction (Normal-C), a pair-fed placebo diet group (Positive-C), and a lemon detox diet group (Lemon-D). The intervention period was 11 days total: 7 days with the lemon detox juice or the placebo juice, and then 4 days with transitioning food.

Women in the Lemon-D and Positive-C groups had significantly greater changes in body weight, BMI, and percentage of body fat than the control group. In addition, serum insulin levels, leptin, and adiponectin levels decreased in the Lemon-D and Positive-C groups. But there was no significant difference between the Lemon-D and Positive-C groups in any of these measurements- suggesting that the main contributing factor was caloric restriction.

A 2015 review by Klein and Kiat, in the Journal of Human Nutrition and Dietetics, pointed out a study on UltraClear (Metagenics Inc), the only commercial detox product to have been evaluated clinically. UltraClear is a medical food supplement that purports to detoxify the liver. A study, by MacIntosh and Ball, gave 25 naturopathy students UltraClear for 7 days. There was no placebo control group. They reported a statistically significant (47%) reduction in the Metabolic Screening Questionnaire [MSQ] scores. The MSQ is a series of questions used to gauge the severity of a variety of health conditions -- from acne, mood swings, and even dark circles under the eyes.

Klein reported that there were (at the time of his review) no current rigorous scientific studies that investigated the effectiveness of commercial detox diets for losing weight.

Are detox diets safe?

Possibly, for otherwise healthy people, if used for only a brief period of time. However, the diets can be stressful because of feelings of hunger and deprivation. But prolonged use of these diets can lead to electrolyte imbalances and protein and vitamin deficiencies. Occasionally, there have been reports of potential risks such as kidney damage from green smoothies (Makkapati, 2018) or liver failure from detox teas (Kesavarapu, 2017).

Despite the lack of evidence that detox diets have any real health benefits, they remain incredibly popular due to celebrity endorsements and intensive marketing of the diets and related products.

CHAPTER 34

PERSONALIZED DIETS

Not everybody responds to the same foods in the same way. The Human Genome Project, completed in 2003, laid the groundwork for scientific research on the environment's influence on gene expression. This led to the increased popularity of nutrigenomics, the field of discovery about how environmental factors, such as food intake and lifestyle impact on us.

It studies the effects of foods and food constituents on gene expression focusing on identifying and understanding molecular-level interaction between nutrients and other dietary bioactives. Peoplesí genes can be tested. Gene variants help determine the choice of foods and identifies deficiencies.

Testing can determine for example how quickly you metabolize caffeine, the efficiency with which your body can absorb different vitamins and minerals and even how motivated you are to exercise. But One study showed a nutrigenomic based diet did not increase weight loss compared to a standard balanced diet. A 2016 meta-analysis found no significant effects of communicating DNA-based risk estimates on diet or physical activity. Another study showed that knowledge of the MTHFR genotype, implicated in the absorption of folate from food, did not significantly improve dietary folate intake. And, although evidence is strong for some gene-diet associations, others remain unclear.

At the present state of knowledge, it is not regarded as good practice to counsel patients to change their diets or lifestyles based on genetics without considering individual clinical biomarkers, dietary and lifestyle preferences and ability to make changes. It may never be possible to prescribe a specific diet based on genetics alone. Using a nutrigenomic approach has not achieved better results than current nutrition counseling methods.

However, a modified approach is to measure your own blood glucose levels say one then, two hours after a meal: Some people get significant spikes while others do not, to the same food(s)!?

It is thought our gut bacteria, the microbiome, causes this. Good bacteria no spike, bad bacteria spikes. You can then either eat the foods that don't cause a spike or alter your microbiome.

As to the latter there is enormous research going into this with many laboratories offering to analyze your microbiome, but I am not sure if any have detailed successful transition methods from bad to good gut bacteria, as yet. So, I would be more inclined to do my own glucose levels and find out what foods, in essence, I don't metabolize well. You can buy a Glucometer at the Pharmacy and testing requires a finger prick and a drop of blood.

But all this seems so difficult and complicated.

My fundamental approach is that, as anyone can observe, people who starve lose weight. The corollary, which no one wants to hear, acknowledge or admit to (the Elephant in the room) is that, it is eating more than we need that puts on weight. However, I maintain, as you will see later, it is the eating more of the wrong foods.

But weight loss is not the main object of the NEWTRITION DIET. The main aim is to provide you with the healthiest diet known which minimises illnesses, especially our greatest cause of our premature demise ñ heart attacks ñ promotes longevity and in doing so also controls our weight.

CHAPTER 35

THE MICROBIOME

GUT FEELINGS

Until just a few decades ago, our bodies were accustomed to whole foods derived from natural sources, rather than the artificial, highly processed foods of today. Research provides shows how balance in the intestinal microbiota and gut-brain communication, which was well adjusted over millennia, might be disturbed by the introduction of modified foods high in fat and sugar. Disrupting that balance leads to the confused brain and inappropriate satiety feedback that can result in obesity; the brain no longer senses signals for fullness, which can cause overeating. In other words, a high-fat diet changes gut microbe populations and the brains ability to recognize fullness which is why eating one good-tasting French fry may lead you to eat the whole batch and leave you wanting more.[628]

It's increasingly clear that our gut bacteria, or microbiota, can communicate with the human brain. Both a high fat and a high-sugar diet, compared to a normal diet, cause changes in gut bacteria that appear related to a significant loss of "cognitive flexibility," or the power to adapt and adjust to changing situations. Mice have proven to be a particularly good model for studies relevant to humans on such topics as aging, spatial memory, obesity and other issues. After just four weeks on a high fat or a high-sugar diet, the performance of mice on various tests of mental and physical function began to drop, compared to animals on a normal diet. One of the most pronounced changes was in cognitive flexibility. A person with high levels of cognitive flexibility would immediately adapt to change and remember.[629]

The gut goes from the mouth, esophagus, stomach, duodenum, small then large intestine and rectum but the small intestine (SI) is one of the most important interfaces between the environment and our body. It has two major functions: it is responsible for absorbing nutrients from the food we eat and functions as a barrier to restrict the entry of harmful substances. The SI is a highly adaptive and

---

[628] Society for the Study of Ingestive Behavior. "High fat diet changes gut microbe populations and brain's ability to recognize fullness." ScienceDaily. ScienceDaily, 7 July 2015. <www.sciencedaily.com/releases/2015/07/150707212451.htm>.

[629] Relationships between diet-related changes in the gut microbiome and cognitive flexibility. Neuroscience, 2015; 300: 128 DOI: 10.1016/j.neuroscience.2015.05.016

dynamic organ, as it adapts to changes in nutrient intake or diet. The intestinal epithelium undergoes a process of continuous renewal, every 3-5 days.

Effects of aging and diet on the small intestine have been investigated. It is known that aging leads to reduced absorption of nutrients by the epithelium thus contributing to malnutrition in elderly people. In addition, anatomical differences between different regions of the SI are known.

Processed Food

The microbiome is the latest darling of the medical researchers but, as yet, there are no or few practical results. My take on it is that it is obviously complex, and one alteration may well result in an unforeseen result elsewhere.

Above all, as per Newtrition, we humans are omnivores who by necessity have evolved to be opportunistic and flexible. But this depends on eating fresh foods and not eating processed foods which, obviously, our microbiomes have not evolved to metabolize and which then have the potential to alter our microbiome.

THE GUT MICROBIOME

The gut microbiota are our normal microbes / bacteria that inhabit our digestive tract (gut). It has been said that the number of bacteria in our gut number more than the stars in the galaxy. They assist with digestion, make some vitamins, break down toxins, and tune our immune system. Over the past decade, scientists have uncovered compelling connections between different types of gut microbes and the development of obesity and diabetes — two factors closely tied to a higher risk of heart disease. Recently, several studies have explored how our gut microbes interact with the food we eat to spur artery-damaging inflammation and narrowing. These findings are still preliminary, but experts hope they'll one day lead to personalized diet recommendations or other therapies to lower the risk of heart disease.

Although the science of probiotic therapies is relatively young, the understanding of how microbiota contribute to our mental and medical well-being is rapidly advancing. It's clear that these commensal organisms co-evolved with us and are adapted to our diet. Our microbiomes contain well over 1 million genes, compared with our 23,000 genes. Furthermore, the commensal microbiome accounts for 90% of the cells in our bodies. Among other functions, these gastrointestinal symbiotes help form and maintain our immune system and aid in digestion, so their health is critical to our health. One of the most powerful interventions to alter our microbiome is diet. Research shows that stressed mice experienced changes in the gastrointestinal microbiota, reflecting the gut-brain relationship.[630] There are 260 million neurons connecting the gut and the brain; furthermore, many commensal gut bacteria make neurotransmitters and communicate with the brain via the vagus nerve. Diet is the principal regulator of the GI microbiome, the ecosystem of the human GI tract which contains trillions of bacteria (microbiota) which use the remnants from digestion to create new signaling molecules that allow the microbiota to communicate with a person's metabolic and GI regulatory system.

The microbiome needs a diverse diet to function optimally. However, current agricultural practices have contributed to a loss of that diversity, with about 75% of the world's population consuming only five animal species and 12 plant species. Of those 12, rice, corn (maize) and wheat contribute 60% of all the calories. Like any ecosystem, the one that is most diverse in species is the one that is going to be the healthiest.

In almost every disease state that has been studied so far, the microbiome has lost diversity. There are just a few species that seem to dominate. People with prediabetes and Type 2 diabetes had a different microbiome makeup than people without those health conditions. A made-up formulation of inulin, beta glucan and antioxidants saw a shift in the makeup of the microbiome and, consequently, health benefits that included improved glucose control, increased satiety and relief from constipation. "Heirloom" foods that once were popular are now rarely eaten. A made-up meal derived from whole soybean pods resulted in positive health benefits on obese mice, including protection from colon inflammation and decreased weight gain.

Think, how can we get more diversity into our diets and less about fad diets where you eliminate a certain component to your diet. Diversifying your diet may make your gut healthier.[631]

---

[630] Alterations in the vaginal microbiome by maternal stress are associated with metabolic reprogramming of the offspring gut and brain. Endocrinology, 2015 Jun 16:en.20151177. [Epub ahead of print]

[631] Institute of Food Technologists (IFT). "Diversifying your diet may make your gut healthier." ScienceDaily. ScienceDaily, 14 July 2015. <www.sciencedaily.com/releases/2015/07/150714142231.htm>.

Gut Microbiota Regulates Antioxidant Metabolism:[632]

The effect of bacteria has been identified by studying the metabolic differences between the many gut, liver and fat tissues obtained from normal and bacteria-free mice. Studies show that gut microbiota regulates the glutathione and amino acid metabolism. Glutathione is a key antioxidant, found in every cell in our body and is our body's most powerful antioxidant and the main detoxifying agent. It plays a vital role in enabling the immune system, nutrient metabolism and regulation of other important cellular events. It is a very small protein, produced inside the cells from three amino acids ultimately obtained from food. Deficiency of glutathione contributes to oxidative stress, which plays a major role in lifestyle diseases such as obesity, type 2 diabetes, atherosclerosis, non-alcoholic fatty liver disease as well as the opposite end of the spectrum, for example malnutrition, which have been associated with imbalance in human gut microbiota. Hence, the interactions between the gut microbiota of the gastrointestinal tract and other peripheral tissues as well as diet are known to be highly relevant for the health of the host. Some bacteria in our gut consume glycine, which is required for the synthesis of the glutathione and imbalances in the composition of bacteria may lead to the progression of the chronic diseases. The plasma levels of glycine are decreased in all subjects with the above-mentioned diseases compared to the healthy subjects.

Artery damage

The initial discovery connecting the gut microbiota to cardiovascular disease came from researchers at the Cleveland Clinic. They discovered that when gut microbes feed on a chemical called choline (found in eggs, red meat, and dairy products), they produce a compound called TMA. In the liver, TMA is converted to TMAO, which causes hardening of the arteries (atherosclerosis) in mice and is linked to a higher risk of heart disease in humans. "For the first time, they showed how the relationship between a dietary component, bacterial metabolism, and human metabolism can have adverse consequences for blood vessels".

Avoiding blockages

The investigators then tested a molecule that blocks the production of TMA, which they gave to mice prone to atherosclerosis, thanks to their genes and a high-fat diet. The molecule, called DMB, occurs naturally in olive oil and red wine.

[632] The gut microbiota modulates host amino acid and glutathione metabolism in mice. *Molecular Systems Biology*, 2015; 11 (10): 834 DOI: 10.15252/msb.20156487

The mice that got DMB in their water had healthier, clearer arteries than those that didn't.

Gut check?

These findings suggest that altering the gut microbiota in different ways might minimize blood vessel damage. There's also some evidence that the gut microbiota may influence the levels of cholesterol and other fats in the bloodstream, as well as blood pressure.

A more diverse mix of bacteria seems to be healthier than a limited one. People who eat a traditional, plant-based Mediterranean or Asian diet tend to have a greater diversity of intestinal bacteria than Americans and Europeans, whose diets are heavier in red meat, sugars, and other refined carbohydrates, and lighter in fruits and vegetables.

Changing our Gut Microbiome[633]

Research suggests it is possible to improve our gut microbiome.

Scientists harvested the gut bacteria from people who followed sharply different diets. One group ate a fairly typical American diet, consuming about 3,000 calories a day, high in animal proteins with few fruits and vegetables. Some of their favorite foods were processed cheese, pepperoni and lunch meats.

The other group consisted of people who were devotees of calorie restriction. They ate less than 1,800 calories a day and had meticulously tracked what they ate for at least two years, sticking to a mostly plant-based diet and consuming far less animal protein than the other group, a third fewer carbohydrates and only half the fat.

This calorie-restricted group, the researchers found, had a far richer and more diverse microbial community in the gut than those eating a typical American diet. They also carried several strains of "good" bacteria, known to promote health, that are unique to their plant-based diet.

It is thought that the best way to cultivate a healthier microbiome is to eat more fiber by consuming more fruit, vegetables, whole grains, legumes, and nuts or seeds and aim for 40 to 50 grams of fiber daily.

633Prior Dietary Practices and Connections to a Human Gut Microbial Metacommunity Alter Responses to Diet Interventions DOI: http://dx.doi.org/10.1016/j.chom.2016.12.006

Gut Health: Probiotics

The gut health diet focuses on probiotics—foods that boost the population of gut bacteria thought to impede the proliferation of disease-causing microorganisms.

They might also reduce gastrointestinal symptoms, such as gas and bloating, and reduce inflammation throughout the body.

Probiotic foods include cultured yogurt, kefir, kimchi, sauerkraut, miso, and tempeh and kombucha tea.

There is little evidence that they improve the gut microbiome except for one small study that found Kefir and kombucha tea did seem to provide a good bacteria boost.

There have been reports of side effects ranging from nausea to allergic reactions but in the main side effects are mild and all people can do is try them and see if you feel better. If you pay enough you will have to feel better.

CHAPTER 36

THE COMPLETE:

BIAS, MISINFORMATION, FAKE NEWS, RELIGIOUS ZEALOTS and VEGANMANIA

Please read the introductory Chapter 8 first.

"There is no greater indignation than that of threatened vested interests".

There is a great deal of increasing nutritional bias, misinformation and manipulation as to nutritional advice and not just from the unqualified wellness industry but from formerly respected University or Nutrition Organizations some of whom seem to have been infiltrated by the Vegan Lobby.

Revealing their inroads and methods may hopefully alert you to the bias, misinformation, fake news and veganmania being perpetrated by a religious cult affecting legitimate but biased research and who have adopted such user friendly welcoming euphuisms as "Wellness", "Lifestyle", "Responsible", "True", "Animal Rights" which offer a health halo of legitimacy and authority while peddling veganism.

Again, I am not opposed to a vegan diet, nor am I pro-meat but these people are vehemently anti-meat, seldom if ever, reveal their religious compulsion, and I think any such disguised bias and secrecy should be declared or otherwise exposed.

Cognitive bias in clinical medicine is increasingly recognized as an important source of medical error,[634] but it is not so easily recognized when applied to nutrition.

[634] J R Coll Physicians Edinb 2018; 48: 225-232

Lessons from the Covid-19 Pandemic

As reported in the BMJ (2nd May 2020): *"Inevitably perhaps, people are using aspects of the covid-19 pandemic to argue in support of something they already believed in. Vegetarians point to the origin of the virus to show the harms of eating meat. Libertarians fear that the pandemic is herding us towards a police state. Religious leaders see it as a timely reminder of eternal truths. Sometimes the evidence points both ways (https://www.spectator.co.uk/article/we-re-all-guilty-of-recruiting-this-virus-to-our-cause). Supporters of the NHS think the pandemic shows the value of socialised medicine. Detractors, on the other hand, say that it reveals a monolithic organization unable to react fast enough to avoid a population lock down".*

We all have our own views based mostly on our family upbringing and we then are attracted to and tend to mix with like-minded people. This 'herd association' while socially normal can, as will be seen, influence whole University and Hospital Departments wherein all Researchers are 'persuaded' to the one cause or belief. But this then does not allow any contrary view, checks or balances. Invariably it's the Head of the Departments' "Way, or the Highway".

I am old enough to have seen many vogues in medicine, most well-meant, but nevertheless vogues which, after the evidence evolves, are seen to have been just that and not the best medical practices.

The current vogue is "Plant Based Diets" which is often a soft sell, deceitful euphuism to recruit people to a total Vegetarian-Vegan Diet, where meat is portrayed as toxic based on spurious "evidence". This vogue or fad is, however, being aggressively promoted by fundamentalist religious zealots who believe in creation, not evolution, and whose dietary advice was handed by the Lord Himself to an uneducated woman in 1863 in one of her 2,000 such "visions".

This is curious because Jesus, Himself, ate meat and drank wine (also a no-no to these zealots).

To correct the "advice" I find questionable or, at least, provide another point of view, I may have to step on a few corns. I have been 'counselled' not to alienate the Bloggers, Influencers, the Loonies and the Religious Zealots for, as you will read, these people can be extremely devious, vicious and persistent – nearly ruining one surgeon's career when he had the temerity to advise his patients to lose weight (which is world's best practice).

In my introduction, I pointed out how I now have concerns about nutrition articles in prestigious medical journals and Epidemiologists who have to "publish or perish".

There is also this rapidly expanding religious cult who have infiltrated, funded and corrupted arguably every nutrition organization or university department. They never declare their religion but gradually embed and institute their "veganmania".

Epidemiologists, Fake News and Bhakts

Epidemiologists are not clinicians. They are historians and data gatherers. Of course, they can and do provide valuable information, but their limitations should be understood.

The Covid-19 pandemic exposed their limitations. In Australia the senior epidemiologist conceded that national guidelines were not followed prescriptively enough in the New South Wales Health Department's dealings with ships carrying Covid-19 infected passengers and let them disembark, thus causing the only mistake and fatally spreading the virus, in the Nation's otherwise remarkable containment of less than 1% mortality.

Epidemiologists are not trained to diagnose a clinical disease or equipped to react quickly. The incredible delays in containing the covid virus in Italy, Spain, the UK and the USA are further testimony to this slow interpretation of a clinical scenario. And this calls into question how correct are their conclusions, let alone their recommendations, in other health matters. In many cases, in nutrition, they are dubious and questionable.

Epidemiologists use mathematical models but according to Rebecca Morrison, an assistant professor of computer science at the University of Colorado Boulder, *"There are very few situations where a model perfectly corresponds with reality. By definition, models are simplified from reality,"* Morrison said. *"In some way or another, all models are wrong"* and she has combined with Brazilian mathematician Americo Cunha using the 2016 outbreak of the Zika virus as a test case to develop an "embedded discrepancy operator" might be able to help scientists fix models that fall short of their goals -- effectively aligning model results with real-world data.[635]

---

635 Chaos: An Interdisciplinary Journal of Nonlinear Science, 2020; 30 (5): 051103
DOI: 10.1063/5.0005204

While we need data on the prevalence of a health entity like heart attacks, any conclusions as to how to diagnose and reduce these is mostly a clinical matter and not that of an epidemiologist but more and more, they are seeking the limelight and making theoretical recommendations.

The other identified problem with researchers and epidemiologists is that they often mine data that agrees with their preconceived beliefs and often just trawl through other studies that support their bias, claiming their 'meta-data' as original work but which may draw the wrong conclusions. Or they follow the 'Party Line' that the Head of Department 'suggests'. The more controversial the better as they will attract funding.

In one article alleging a high cholesterol was beneficial in old people, at least five of the study authors had previously written books questioning the links between cholesterol and heart disease, while another of the authors is a prominent campaigner against statins. The consensus of informed experts is that they are wrong and biased.

Now there is an epidemic of papers by the vegans, who have been, they claim, instructed by the Lord, to say all meat, milk, dairy, fish and wine are bad.

But, in addition, they publish articles which are flagrantly, boosting their business interests and, while ostensibly promoting health, they manufacture ultra-processed, sugar laden breakfast cereals which, to my research, cause more health problems than meat ever has. Just try Kellogg's Frosty Loops.

I am annoyed with myself for not waking up sooner as I recommended walnuts above all other nuts as there were so many articles recommending them. But these are all from Seventh Day Adventist (SDA) sources such as Loma Linda University and, guess what? Yep, the SDA own walnut groves. These articles are pure marketing exercises.

The truth is that all nuts are beneficial, including pea or groundnuts.

And if such papers are queried then there would now seem and organized army to immediately object. The intrusion of Medical Journalists is also very much resented with those challenged Doctors claiming the health moral high ground when, in truth, these journalists, at least the best of them, have the time and diligence to investigate further. I don't always agree with some, but I do enjoy and respect their "lancing of the boil".

We need them because, unfortunately, clinicians like myself, are too busy consulting or operating to question articles in prestigious journals as they are ostensibly peer reviewed. But what is the peers have been infiltrated?

This sounds like a conspiracy theory but over the last decade I also noticed how, not only did they ever so strongly recommend plant-based diets, carefully avoiding the words vegetarian or vegan, but how they also increasingly went out of their way to make meat sound as deadly as they could.

John Ionaddis, MD, Professor of Medicine and Professor of Epidemiology and Population Health at Stanford, has, reassuringly, been particularly vocal and insightful about the limitations of nutrition studies, writing: "A large majority of human nutrition research uses nonrandomized observational designs, but this has led to little reliable progress. This is mostly due to many epistemologic problems (how do we discern what is true), the most important of which are as follows:

- difficulty detecting small (or even tiny) effect sizes reliably for nutritional risk factors and nutrition-related interventions;
- difficulty properly accounting for massive confounding among many nutrients, clinical outcomes, and other variables;
- difficulty measuring diet accurately; and suboptimal research reporting.
- Tiny effect sizes and massive confounding are largely unfixable problems that narrowly confine the scenarios in which nonrandomized observational research is useful.

Medical proof depends on Koch's postulates which basically say something has to be found that causes the illness, and by removing it the illness is cured but reoccurs when that 'something' is reintroduced.

The best studies and evidence is by Random Controlled Trials (RCT) where for example an identical drug and a placebo are administered by people who don't know which is which, to a statistically valid number of volunteers and the results assessed by yet more independent researchers – they are thus "double blind" studies.

Nutrition studies are, by necessity, observational and RCTs, the 'Gold Standard', are not just unlikely, but practically impossible, owing to the enormous cost of recruiting >100,000 participants and maintaining them on their monitored respective diets (and not just self-reported recall) for several years.

Unfortunately, even the best nutrition studies most often depend on participants recall as to what they ate. And this, as we all know, is most unreliable.

However, meta-analyses at least provide a degree of evidence and certainty.

Newtrition has used only the best of these meta-analyses and studies.

Confounders

A confounder is a variable, often not considered, that could be affecting the results of a trial or study.

Such as, vegetarians can claim their diet is the healthiest as they-live longer. But to then extrapolate that meat is bad is spurious. Vegetarians are 'food obsessed' and invariably lead a healthier lifestyle of no smoking, no booze and keeping trim. But if you add some grass-fed meat to this, as in twin studies, there is no real difference.

The opposite confounders are the Good Ol' Boys who char their steaks while smoking, drinking, eating sausages and junk food and who are invariably overweight, sedentary and have reduced lifespans. They could spuriously claim, to use the vegan argument, that it the accompanying vegetables and cornbread that shorten the Good Ol' Boys' lives.

Looks like I'm not alone and not paranoid as to my concerns: In an article in the BMJ (British Medical Journal) as to the latest US Dietary Guidelines, *Nina Teicholz* wrote:

"Much has been written about how industries try to influence nutrition policy, so it is surprising that unlike authors in most major medical journals, guideline committee members are not required to list their potential conflicts of interest. A cursory investigation shows several such possible conflicts: one member has received research funding from the California Walnut Commission and the Tree Nut Council, as well as vegetable oil giants Bunge and Unilever. Another has received more than $10,000 (£6400; €8800) from Lluminari, which produces health related multimedia content for General Mills, PepsiCo, Stonyfield Farm, Newman's Own, and "other companies." And for the first time, the committee chair comes not from a university but from industry: Barbara Millen is president of Millennium Prevention, a company based in Westwood, MA, that sells web-based platforms and mobile applications for self-health monitoring. While there is no evidence that these potential conflicts of interest influenced the committee members, the report recommends a high consumption of vegetable oils and nuts as well as use of self-monitoring technologies in programs for weight management".

I'd like to add that, to my dismay and concern, authors in most major medical journals, while listing potential conflicts of interests do not reveal full disclosure as to their funding, kickbacks or religious bias. I would recommend you check out the site at the end of this chapter to see just how much funding one such University Department gets and the handsome 'retainers' to their staff – all from vested interests who are not donating their funds unless they get payment in kind viz: articles promoting these businesses via their products. These are increasingly vegetarian-vegan.

According to Ian Leslie who wrote an article 'The Sugar Conspiracy' in the Guardian 7th April 2016, the response of the nutrition establishment to Teicholz's article, *"was ferocious: 173 scientists – some of whom were on the advisory panel, and many of whose work had been critiqued in Teicholz's book, signed a letter to the BMJ, demanding it retract the piece"*.

It reminds me of the observation; *"There is no greater indignation than that of threatened vested interests"*. This, as you will read later, was the trigger to cause the grain producers, the people whose products make breakfast corn and wheat flakes, who, with falling sales, complained about a surgeon who advised his obese patients to cut out such breakfast sugar laden cereals, and nearly ruined his career.

Onward Christian Soldiers Going as to War

In their aggressive business tactics, again under the pretence of "health", they take no prisoners as they promote breakfast cereals, soy, walnuts, olive oil and who knows what-else as they are a very secretive cult. With, as they claim, God on their side, it would seem they feel it is OK to destroy anyone who is not a vegetarian or better yet, a vegan.

As such they have conducted terror campaigns against farmers under the guise of "Animal Liberation" and have destroyed many farmers lives and livelihoods – all in the name of Jesus – so they claim. But, then again, as a Jewish Rabbi didn't Jesus partake in ritual animal sacrifices?

(The priests (rabbi) slaughtered animals, they took the animal carcasses on the altar, roasted the animals, dispensed the meat. When people brought their sacrifice to the Temple because say, a wife had a baby, say a child recovered from illness, or say at a pilgrimage festival celebrating. The priest takes it away and brings back roast beef or roast lamb in a little while where you and your family sit and eat.[636])

Author's Note: As a break from my medical textbook writings I relaxed investigating, on a whim, homosexuality and then misogyny in the Christian Church and wrote **"Holy Moly"** (Amazon-Kindle), which is how I know a little about this.

Publishing a rejoinder to this BMJ article by Nina Teicholz is one thing; requesting its erasure is another, conventionally reserved for cases involving fraudulent data. As a letter of response pointed out: *"Scientific discussion helps to advance science. Calls for retraction, particularly from those in eminent positions, are unscientific and frankly disturbing."*

Does Science Advance One Funeral at a Time or "Do It My Way".

Scientists, like the rest of society, attract or conform like-minded people. It is part of what the Polish philosopher of science Ludwik Fleck called a "thought collective": a group of people exchanging ideas in a mutually comprehensible idiom. The group, suggested Fleck, inevitably develops a mind of its own, as the individuals in it converge on a way of communicating, thinking and feeling.

This makes scientific inquiry, as Ian Leslie points out, 'prone to the eternal rules of human social life: Deference to the charismatic, herding towards majority opinion, punishment for deviance, and intense discomfort with admitting to error'. But such tendencies are precisely, as Leslie points out, what the scientific method was invented to correct.

National Bureau of Economic Research sought an empirical basis for physicist Max Planck observation: "A new scientific truth does not triumph by convincing its opponents and making them see the light, but rather because its opponents eventually die, and a new generation grows up that is familiar with it."

They found that the disciples, or junior researchers, of dead elites, now published less, but that the newcomers' articles increased and became more influential.

This, of course, accounts for the vogues and fads in all spheres of human activities but in nutrition the old meat eaters are out and the new veggies are in.

---

[636] Temple Culture **Shaye I.D. Cohen:** Samuel Ungerleider Professor of Judaic Studies and Professor of Religious Studies Brown University

Veggies Vs Meat Eaters[637]

A study published in October 2019, in the prestigious *Annals of Internal Medicine,* further raises concerns.

It was a thorough meta-analysis by an international review panel of 14 members from seven countries, including three lay members, who voted on the recommendations. The work was led by NutriRECS, which describes itself as an independent group "unencumbered by institutional constraints and conflicts of interest, aiming to produce trustworthy nutritional guideline recommendations based on the values, attitudes and preferences of patients and community members." The Polish and Spanish Cochrane centres are partners. Another author was Gordon Guyatt, a Canadian epidemiologist who first coined the term "evidence-based medicine."

They reached a conclusion directly contrary to the public health advice in that they suggested that adults should continue their current consumption of both red and processed meat.

This resulted in an incredible barrage by the articles detractors who targeted the Annals Editor with 2,000 near identical complaints in half and hour while there was still an embargo on the article. The Annals Editor, Christine Laine, blamed David Katz, director of the Yale-Griffin Prevention Research Center in Connecticut and she received a letter four days before the article was published, urging her to temporarily retract it for closer review.

Two signatories from Harvard, Walter Willett and Frank Hu, are on the board of the True Health Initiative, and David Katz is its president. Laine alleged that the True Health Initiative created the bot that flooded her inbox. This allegation is strongly denied by Willett and Hu.

But the chancellor of Texas A&M University, which employs two of the red meat article's authors, has written to Harvard's president demanding that Willett and Hu be investigated for having "mischaracterised scientific research and falsely accused Texas A&M scientists of selling out to industry interests." Willett, he wrote, had branded Texas A&M and one of its professors as representatives of "Big Beef" in a slide at a cardiology conference.

Laine, the *Annals*' editor, notes that some of the study's critics have written books promoting plant-based diets. The California Walnut Commission has funded

[637] BMJ 2020;368:m397

Harvard's TH Chan School of Public Health, where Willett and Hu work. The school put out a statement criticising the *Annals* guidance. The True Health Initiative has "for-profit partners" such as the pasta maker Barilla and a *JAMA* article listed grants that Katz had received totalling more than US$1.7m (£1.3m; €1.5m) from several food industries, including Hershey Foods, the Egg Nutrition Center, and ISOThrive, described as a "microfood" that tackles bacterial imbalances in the gut that are "at the root of chronic health conditions." (The Microbiome is another current medical vogue).

Willett also chaired the discredited EAT Commission (see later) which tried to turn the world vegetarian.

What Does All This Mean

Simply it is that, even in University or Hospital Departments that were once independent and excellent, the researchers inevitably have to bend to the Head of the Department's views and bias - "My way or the Highway". If (s)he is a vegan, then there will be a spate of articles endorsing veganism. And if they depend on vegetarian funding, well "he who pays the Piper calls the tune" and that would seem to now be the case.

All this is of concern. It would seem many nutritional organizations have been herded toward a unified opinion - "plant good, meat bad" and, I suspect, they are handsomely funded, one way or another, by vested interests such as The Walnut Lobby of California, Kellogg's and other SDA businesses whose advocates proclaim it is their religious obligation to promote vegetarianism. However, they seem to be doing so, more and more aggressively, while at the same time, surreptitiously infiltrating nutrition organizations while not declaring their bias.

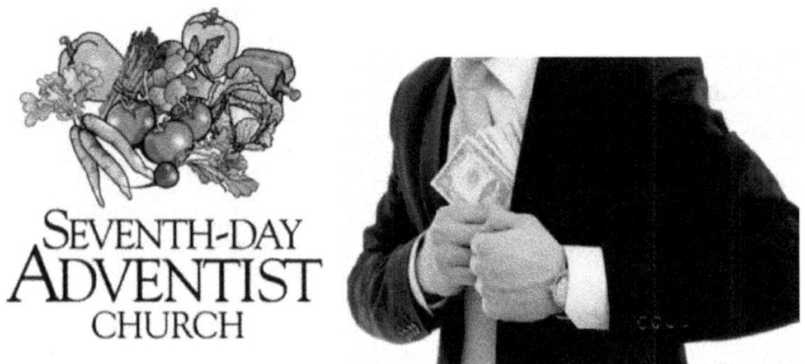

In the meantime, with breathtaking hypocrisy, while claiming the moral health high ground they promote their ultra-processed, sugar and salt laced breakfast cereals and don't acknowledge that the healthiest coronary arteries in this world, are in meat eaters, or how, as Joanna Blythman observes, *"Vegan products are often just high-protein flours with gums, glues, water and a range of additives. A lot contain a rogues' gallery of additives and dodgy ingredients that I wouldn't touch with a bargepole"*[638].

That's OK, the meat, dairy, sugar and Fast Food industries fund biased studies too. But my concern is that all funding, Committee and Board Appointments, all paid consultancies, lectures, travel, endorsements and whatever, should be declared, including any religious nutritional taboos. I would now like to know which of these critics are, in fact, Seventh Day Adventists. If they, or any of them are, then I must treat their publications with suspicion as they are biased. If they are not, then they gain greater credibility. What have they got to lose?

These deluges or tsunamis of complaints to the Annals and BMJ articles, would infer a well organised anti-meat, pro-veg lobby. That is not to say they may not have a point but 2,000 similar emails in 30 minutes some requesting a retraction to an article in the Annals of Internal Medicine, and 173 signatures demanding an article be retracted from the BMJ, would suggest these are very organised groups, intent on shutting down what they perceive are views contrary to theirs which would seem increasingly vegetarian.

However, despite their best (or worst) efforts, a meta-analysis, published online February 3, 2020, in *JAMA Internal Medicine,* supports, to my way of thinking, the pro-meat recommendation more than the vegetarian lobby.

It found that greater consumption of processed meat, unprocessed red meat, and, unexpectedly, poultry, but not fish, is significantly associated with a *small* increased risk for incident cardiovascular disease (CVD), which included cardiovascular deaths.

The large 6-cohort study found that a higher intake of processed meat and unprocessed red meat, but not poultry or fish, significantly correlates with a *small* increase in the risk for all-cause mortality and increased relative risks for these associations, ranging from approximately 3% to 7% and increased absolute risks for less than 2% during a follow-up period that lasted up to 30 years.

This is the longest study so far (30 years and ~30,000 participants) and based on a larger and more diverse sample and longer follow-up than most published studies.

---

[638] "Swallow This: Serving Up the Food Industry's Darkest Secrets" by Joanna Blythman.

An absolute risk of just 2% over 30 years with it not being clear if this included processed meat, but eating meat four times a week, I would regard as 'acceptable', and certainly modifiable by reducing all meat and cutting out processed meats, as Newtrition recommends. And it certainly does not warrant further hysterical outbursts of the Veggie Loonies, as above.

It is interesting to me that this article did not come out of Harvard which seems, now, to be the focus of veganmania. The other interesting but odd finding was that that poultry intake was positively associated with CVD. It was suggested that eating fried skin may be the culprit.

I wonder if this poor author got 2,000 emails and demands he recant and retract.

Science Fiction: The EAT-Lancet Commission

In 2019 a group, the EAT-Lancet Commission, held a conference in Norway.

It was co-chaired by Prof. Walter Willett from the Harvard T.H. Chan School of Public Health and Prof. Johan Rockstr.m, PhD from the Potsdam Institute for Climate Impact Research & Stockholm Resilience Centre and brought together 19 Commissioners and 18 co-authors from 16 countries in various fields including human health, agriculture, political science and environmental sustainability.

It produced an amazingly beautiful report in several languages which purported to deliver the diet that would make the world sustainable with its "planetary health diet".

This diet was essentially vegetarian.

When analysed, however, critics found not only was it methodologically flawed with false conclusions but that it was too expensive for the diets it wanted to replace and was deficient in some essential nutrients resulting in low intakes of iron, retinol, and vitamins B12 and D3, according to at least one dietitian's analysis.

The study's authors say that the diet—which calls for major increases in consumption of whole grains, legumes, fruits and vegetables, and conversely, decreases in anything that comes from animals—would go a long way in reducing weight-related disease and mortality.

Strange that they did not include reducing the ultra-processed breakfast cereals. But then again…

Further, as it advocated the culling of cows as they claimed their methane was causing global warming (that would also get rid of the 'evil' dairy and meat) it was pointed out that the then deforestation of land needed to grow the vegetarian crops, was more likely to cause global warming.

It even resulted in Italy's ambassador to the United Nations, questioning the diet's impact on public health concluding "A standard diet for the whole planet, regardless of the age, sex, metabolism, general state of health and eating habits of each person, has no scientific justification at all." "Moreover, it would mean the destruction of millenary healthy traditional diets which are a full part of the cultural heritage and social harmony in many countries."

And as Ioannidis pointed out, "There are few exceptions, but the status of epidemiological literature is not at a level to allow us to make these types of very detailed, specific recommendations," and for that reason, the health claims in the EAT-Lancet diet are "science fiction. I can't call it anything else."

The Italian Ambassador and others, publicly criticising them, caused a confusing retreat by the WHO. The British Medical Journal, in fact, reported that the World Health Organization (WHO), the arm of the United Nations charged with monitoring global health, had dropped its sponsorship of the EAT-Lancet Commission's planetary health diet.

Over Population

It would seem, rather than save the planet, EAT was just yet another vegetarian inspired proposal. But, judging from their brochure, a very expensive one.

When I first read it, I shook my head in disbelief as it was so ludicrously theoretical. I could not imagine, for example, a pale Norwegian dietician telling a cow-blood, milk drinking Masai how he now needed to stop his traditional diet, plant beans, stop growing taller than Norwegians and to stop jumping…and on and on.

As an aside, the Maasai diet traditionally consisted of raw meat, raw milk, and raw blood from cattle and in 1935 it was reported that most tribes were disease-free. Many had not a single tooth attacked by dental caries nor a single malformed dental arch. Later electrocardiogram tests applied to 400 young adult male Maasai found no evidence whatsoever of heart disease, abnormalities or malfunction. Further study with carbon-14 tracers showed that the average cholesterol level was about 50 percent of that of an average American.[639]

The other fact which calls into question EAT's whole deluded pretence of saving the planet by exterminating cattle and forcing us all to be vegetarians, is that the cause of Global Warming, denudation of fish stocks and malnutrition, is over-population.

But this is obviously too difficult a subject for them to address. Besides which, the more people the more they will contribute to their business model of walnut, soya and olive products and why, they might even get the Masai to eat Frosty Loops and Coca Cola for breakfast.

The SEVENTH DAY ADVENTIST CHURCH and ATMOSPHERIC POLLUTION

The SDA, who want to get rid of all cattle as they feel they are a major cause of atmospheric pollution, may look at these photos of major, cattle-free cities, Los Angeles and Sydney, when cars were taken off the streets and planes grounded.

And while the vegans may argue that animals use more primary resources, 80% (+) of the world's almonds are grown in California and is their number one agricultural export. But California is a very dry state and almonds require 1.1 gallons or 4.15 litres of water to grow one almond and to grow a pound or 454 grams takes 1,900 gal/ lb or 7,192 litres i.e. approximately 2000 litres of water to grow half a kilo of almonds.

[639] *The Last of the Maasai.* Mohamed Amin, Duncan Willetts, John Eames. 1987. Page 87. Camerapix Publishers International. ISBN 1-874041-32-6

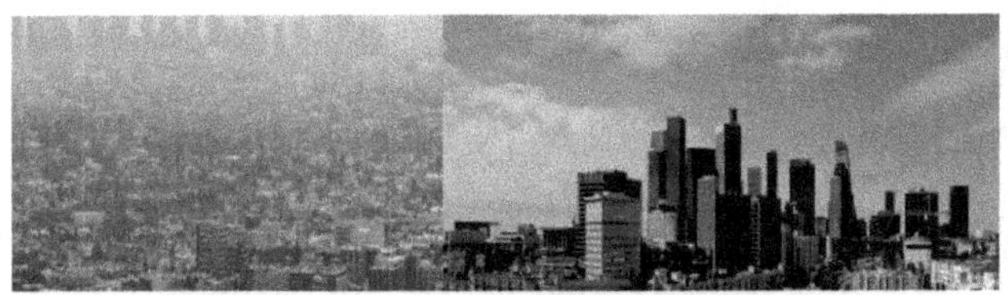

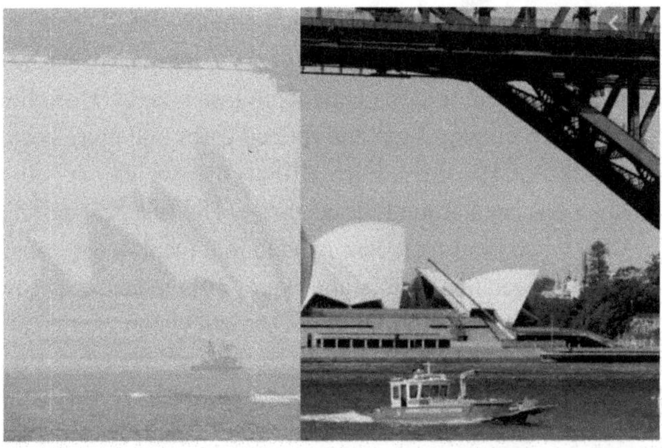

The SDA claim the Lord told them not to eat meat but they now pursue this incredibly aggressive agenda of trying to exterminate cattle. But the problem is over-population and human pollution.

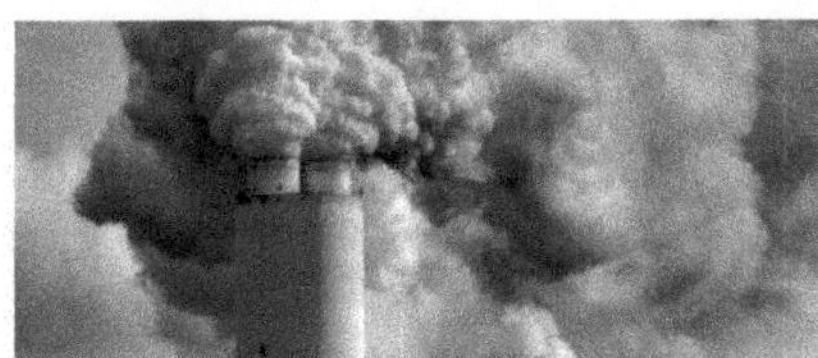

e producing methane?
:ould it even be a factory
lucing breakfast cereals?

I had, I thought, finished this chapter until I remembered the following case:

The Plot Thickens

"The phenomenon of "*medical evangelism*" the activities of medical doctors and dietitians belonging to the Seventh-day Adventist Church".

Dr Gary Fettke is a Tasmanian Orthopedic surgeon who after a serious medical illness which saw him gain weight and "balloon", finally tried a Low carb diet which worked for him. Many of his patients were overweight and, as any good orthopod will advise, he told his patients to lose weight. Unfortunately, for him, he recommended reducing sugar and refined carbs and more healthy fats and red meat. This is the LCHF (Low Carb Hi Fat) diet which, as you can read in the history chapter has been around for centuries. The first best-selling diet book was LCHF in 1863 when Banting recommended four meals a day consisting of simple food like meat, vegetables, fruits and wine. This is somewhat poignant as that same year was when the Lord told the SDA, in a vision, that meat was bad.

I recommend the Mediterranean Diet and, while I have written a book "Slim 4 Life", for weight loss, it often comes down to 'whatever works for you' and, as I point out, people like being disciplined and if LCHF works for you, then do it. And, in actual fact, the latest and very complete review of 14 of the most popular diets,[640] (BMJ, April 2020) has Low-Carb as the fastest way to lose weight short-term. So, it would seem to me Dr Fettke's pre-op advice was the best available and calls into question the poor nutritional knowledge of these dieticians as well as their and AHPRA's contemptable lack of ethics.

What happened next is long, circuitous and disgusting revelation as to the aggression and snide tactics of the SDA and I recommend you follow it all on Google on "isupportgary.com" for the details but, in summary:

The SDA laid anonymous complaints against Dr Fettke via two dietitians who reported him to the Australian Health Practitioners Regulatory Agency (AHPRA). AHPRA held a behind-closed-doors investigation, then told Fettke to stop what he was doing. Bizarrely, AHPRA said that even if LCHF became mainstream in future, he still could not speak about nutrition. (?!)

It would seem there was a small cabal of cereal industry CEOs who had become concerned about the fall in cereal consumption among consumers. The SDA

---

[640] BMJ 2020;369:m696. Published 1 April 2020.

produce the ultra-processed breakfast cereals, falsely advertised as "whole-grain" and very aggressively push the eating of processed grains. These industry executives meet annually to plot ways to increase consumption of their products, according to former Senator Cori Bernardi, and identified a list of individuals to target and Fettke was the target doctor on these cereal makers' "hit-list". They appear to have then "enlisted the Dieticians Association of Australia (DAA) to do their dirty work. The processed food industry appears to have spent 20 years funding the DAA to "push an anti-dairy, anti-meat message".

Medical Evangelism

In preparing evidence in his defence against the dietitians' complaints, Fettke and his wife also uncovered the phenomenon of "medical evangelism" as a contributing factor. And in particular, the activities of medical doctors and dietitians belonging to the Seventh-day Adventist Church.

- They align clearly with the WHO and its "meat causes cancer stance"
- Another partner is the Physicians Committee for Responsible Medicine (PCRM). By snide inference, doctors not belonging to it are practising "irresponsible" medicine? Neat trick guys – see the "True" Health Initiative below.
- PCRM founder, Dr Neal Barnard, has links PETA
- PETA (People for Ethical Treatment of Animals).
- Adventists' recent strategic alliance is with kindred spirits in fringe medical groups under the guise of "lifestyle medicine". These operate under similar names in most continents. Lifestyle medicine is a *"potential front for serious medical evangelism pushing Adventist vegetarian ideology"*.
- Lifestyle Medicine Global Alliance (LMGA). It's a new venture outside the US that reaches to many countries. It includes the American College of Lifestyle Medicine and the Australasian Society of Lifestyle Medicine. In the US, the Joslin Diabetes Centre has a lifestyle-medicine arm. So too does Harvard Medical School.
- LMGA strategic partners include the True Health Initiative (THI). THI founder is Dr David Katz who openly advocates for vegetarian diets as "greener". Katz has taken to using "plant-based" rather than vegetarian. He has also co-published with Barnard.
- Big Food is high on the list, of course. The sugar industry, the grain and cereal industries as well as the processed food industries don't like the LCHF message of fresh, "real" food. Nor did they much like Fettke saying that grain and cereals products are products of the food industry, not nature.

Fettke's research pointed to a second group attempting to silence him: those with a belief that animal fat is bad for health in body and mind. Chief among those are vegetarians, vegans and animal rights activists.

He then also found an intriguing connection between AHPRA's star witness against him and a similar vendetta being carried out in South Africa against Professor Peter Noakes in that AHPRAs star witness was Monash University emeritus professor Mark Wahlqvist and in South Africa it was retired North-West University professor Hester "Este" Vorster. Wahlqvist and Vorster have known each other for years. Both were involved in the International Union of Nutritional Sciences. Both have links to the International Life Sciences Institute (ILSI), a Coca-Cola and Kellogg's front and both seldom, if ever, reveal these potential conflicts of interest. They all also push the lifestyle medicine mantra: "Exercise is medicine," a theme Coca-Cola and others continue to push the idea that people can outrun a bad diet whereas exercise only accounts for some 15% of weight loss. Despite that, ADSA, DAA, Harvard Medical School, all support this flawed advice. Wahlqvist is also associated with the Sanitarium Health and Wellbeing company that the Adventist Church wholly owns. Wahlqvist apparently doesn't admit that he or his wife are Adventists.

How he "appeared" at AHPRA's Kangaroo Court is an unexplained mystery but AHPRA had to finally apologise to Fettke.

It only took two and a half years.

One can only wonder if AHPRA has also been infiltrated by SDA.

The Seventh Day Adventists (SDA)

I don't want to waste my time on this, but the SDA is making incredible inroads into health advice and their advice is biased and dubious and needs to be corrected.

It's no longer "vegetarian" but "plant-based" – sounds less threatening and more friendly eh? (Like "Wellness, True, Lifestyle, Responsible" and other mealy mouth euphuisms they employ).

No one can dispute advocating fresh fruit and vegetables but to extrapolate this to then say meat is bad because the Lord created us and told us, and us alone, that meat is a no-no, is, in my opinion, Loony Land. But that's OK. That's their business except they have embarked on an incredibly aggressive mission to veganise the world and have infiltrated every nook and cranny of nutrition organizations while expanding their breakfast cereal, walnut, soya and olive oil businesses. That's OK too but to do so by undermining any opposition, let alone trying to ruin the career of a surgeon, is more than sinister. It would seem they believe God has sent them on this mission and nothing should stand in their way.

The Seventh-day Adventist Church is the largest of several Adventist groups which arose from the Millerite movement of the 1840s. William Miller predicted that Jesus Christ would return (The 'Advent') to Earth between the spring of 1843 and the spring of 1844. When Jesus failed to appear Miller chose another, then another date. Miller's failed predictions became known as the "Great Disappointment".

After which the followers fractionated, and the Prophetess Ellen White emerged claiming to have received a vision from the Lord on the subject in 1863 "when the great subject of health Reform was opened before me in vision. ... The Lord presented a general plan before me. I was shown that God would give to His commandment-keeping people a reform diet..."

The Lord apparently advised Ellen not to eat meat, not to smoke, not to drink, (which is odd because Jesus drank and ate meat) and to go to Australia where she started Sanitarium to make breakfast cereals in the tradition of other SDAs, the Kellogg brothers.

Ellen did seem to have some hang-ups as, according to her, meat in your diet will do the following to you: Clouds the brain, Benumbs the intellect, Enfeebles and deadens the moral nature, Weakens the higher powers, Lessens spirituality, Renders mind incapable of understanding truth, Causes insubordination, Stimulates lustful propensities, Strengthens the lower passions, Animalizes you, strengthens the animal appetites, Interferes with the religious life, Causes you to miss out on companionship with heavenly angels, May cause God to decide not to heal your sickness, Causes sickness and disease, endangers physical, mental, and spiritual health.

Little wonder the SDAs don't like meat as they accept these as gospel truths.

Ellen was knocked out for three weeks with no retrograde memory when aged 9 years. She had no formal education but over 2,000 visions of angels and the Lord and despite her 'healthy diet' seemed to be sick all the time.

(If you are wondering about religious visions I have written about their psychiatric implications and explanations in my book ***"Holy Moly".)***

The SDA

- don't believe in evolution, so I wonder how they explain our canine teeth
- they don't ordain women despite Ellen White's major contribution
- are still waiting for Jesus (when, I assume, they will have to hide the booze, get Him on the wagon and hide the fish and the lamb)
- some SDA believe the Pope is the Anti-Christ
- all naughty people will be exterminated
- they did not recognise psychiatric illnesses
- they do not approve of same-sex marriages but don't seem to query if Jesus was homosexual as many think[641]

While they are a minor cult, they are aggressively expanding rapidly and sneakily, infiltrating and assuming low profiles. They have a Medical School at Loma Linda California but it is listed as "unranked" by U.S. News & World Report Best Colleges Ranking and listed as the 994th best university in the world and the 213th best university in the United States by the Center for World University Rankings.

As part of their infiltration they sponsor medical and health meetings and, in Australia, they even somehow managed to get their 'Fact Sheets' hard-wired into the back end of software packages run in 50% of medical practices around Australia, encouraging vegetarianism and turning the unsuspecting doctors into de facto missionaries for their vegetarian message.

In Australia, as well as Sanitarium processed food products, they own extensive farms such as Cobram Estate Olive Oil, many Soya plantations around the world and I assume Walnut groves in California. They pay no tax as a religious organization claiming their profits go into health care and such.

Again, one is left to wonder just who are SDAs in the Nutrition world, as they have obviously targeted, infiltrated and influenced it. But they believe in creation, not evolution, and as such, do not believe in most science but blindly follow the edicts of Ellen White with a ruthless missionary, blinded, focused zeal. While I don't know how many SDAs contributed to the ludicrous EAT Report, those that aren't have been corrupted and seduced. And one wonders now about the Harvard T.H. Chan School of Public Health funded by the Walnut industry.

I advocate the Mediterranean Diet (obviously!) but to spend now every seeming article urging the extinction of all cattle while promoting their walnuts, soy and olive oils is, well, here goes, "nuts".

---

[641] "Holy Moly" by Mileham Hayes, Amazon-Kindle 2020.

My personal conclusions are that, while I initially had respect for their "research" I now regard their papers as incredibly biased and flawed.

This Fettke vendetta was a disgusting, vicious and reprehensible saga. It seems the BMJ contributing author, Nina Teicholz, and the Annals of Internal Medicine Editor, Christine Laine, were also given the SDA treatment.

Who's next? I'd better keep looking over my shoulder while I await AHPRA's midnight door knock.

Conclusion

The bottom line is that we now need full disclosure, *including any religious affiliations or funding,* who have nutrition taboos, obligations or bias for any papers published in Journals.

As a Specialist Physician the truth is the truth, and the evidence is the evidence, even if it goes against their (and my) beliefs.

And so, to the best of my unfunded, non-kickback ability, Newtrition is the truth based on the best evidence and studies with no vested interests or trying to convert you to a cult. Neither has God spoken to me personally to advise me as to what to eat.

I am sorry for those whom the truth offends: This book is not for you.

Animal Liberation

I don't know how many so-called animal liberationists are SDA but I suspect, if they are not, then they are duped by the SDA into their terrorist tactics against farmers. One might have had some sympathy for their cause until the horrific drought then bushfires in Australia saw hundreds of thousands of both domestic and wild-life dying under dreadful conditions. But these people were now nowhere to be seen or to help, and it was left to the farmers, they had previously tried to destroy, to attend to these animals.

Breakfast Cereals

As detailed elsewhere these are highly processed foods denuded and stripped of nutrients.

- How they claim these as "whole grain" when they are highly processed is beyond me.
- How they infer they are "healthy" is beyond me.
- How the SDA who manufacture, peddle and promote these, which are much more likely to cause CVD and dental caries than meat, which they condemn, is beyond me.

1. Kellogg's Frosties Breakfast Cereal (41.3% sugar!)
2. Kellogg's Fruit Loops (38% sugar)
3. Kellogg's Coco Pops Chex (37.4% sugar)
4. Kellogg's Coco Pops (36.5% sugar)
5. Kellogg's Hersheys Chocolatey Bites Cereal (32.5% sugar)
6. Kellogg's Crunchy Nut Cornflakes (31.7% sugar)
7. Nestle Nesquik (29.9% sugar)
8. Kellogg's Crunchy Nut Clusters (28.9g)
9. Kellogg's Just Right Apricot & Sultana Cereal (28.7% sugar)
10. Kellogg's Sultana Bran High Fiber Breakfast Cereal (28.2% sugar)
11. Nestle Milo Cereal (26.9% sugar)
12. Weet-Bix blends cranberry and coconut: Here's the result

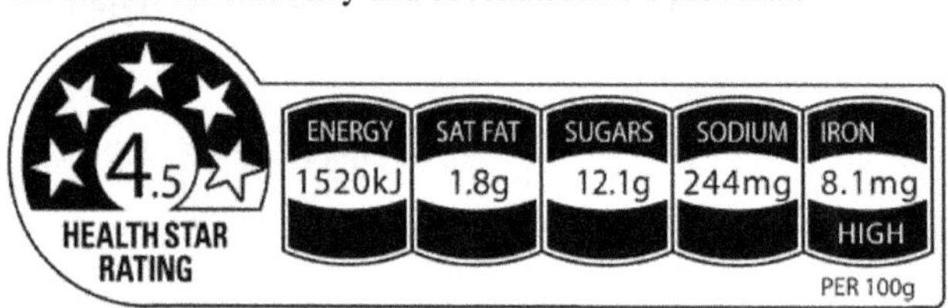

The recommended content for sugar is < 4g per 100g.

- How this achieves a 4.5 "Health" Star Rating is beyond me

Finally

The donations and funding of the Harvard T.S. Chan School of Public Health would seem mostly from firms or organizations that would most profit promoting articles on vegetarianism. The school received between $455,000 and $1,500,000 from companies or groups interested in promoting vegetarian products or the vegetarian diet generally.

While writing articles favouring those who fund you is commercially understandable, to then close a blind eye to potentially damaging nutrition as in sugar laden ultra-processed breakfast cereals and not address or even comment on these, is biased censorship.

For those interested in the full revelation of this financial-vegan intrigue google

Dr. Walter Willett – isupportgary.

I hasten to add that in no way is this meant to criticize Dr Willett, who has for many years authored articles I have devoured and admired. But, as per my Position Statement, I feel all funding and influences by all authors should be declared and, as stated, especially after the EAT-Lancet debacle, the T.S.Chan School of Harvard, like Loma Linda University, seems to only publish not just ‘Plant good’ articles, but ‘Meat bad’ ones, with no balance as with the Tsmaine Studies. Nor have they investigated, to my knowledge, the benefits or otherwise of small amounts of grass fed, organic beef.

CHAPTER 37

AND NOW A WORD FROM OUR SPONSORS

And it's not just the SDA that have infiltrated and corrupted the Dietician Organizations. I would recommend reading the complete reports for those interested but they are a sad inditement especially if you read the Dr Gary Fettke case in the last chapter.

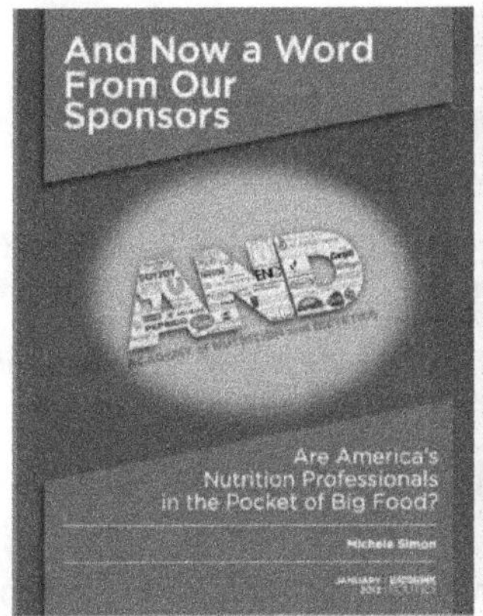

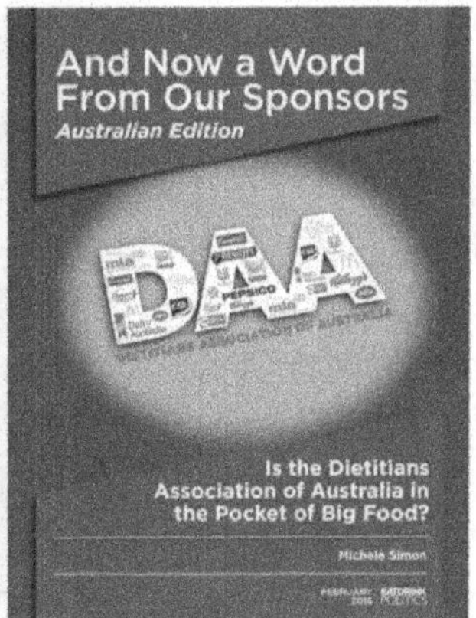

Michele Simon is a public health lawyer who has been researching and writing about food policy since 1996. Her work has been featured on CNBC, CBS News, *The New York Times*, *San Francisco Chronicle*, *Chicago Tribune*, Reuters, and Forbes. She has written extensively on the politics of food, and her book, *Appetite for Profit: How the Food Industry Undermines Our Health and How to Fight Back*, was published by Nation Books in 2006. Simon has also written extensively about alcohol policy.

In 2013 she wrote "And Now a Word from Our Sponsors" as to sponsorships for the (American) Academy of Nutrition and Dietetics in which she states in summary:

"By any measure, the nation is currently suffering from an epidemic of diet-related health problems. According to the U.S. Centers for Disease Control and Prevention, chronic diseases – such as heart disease, stroke, cancer, and diabetes – "are among the most common, costly, and preventable of all health problems."

Against this backdrop, we must ask: what is the role of the Academy of Nutrition and Dietetics (AND)—the nation's largest association of nutrition professionals—in preventing or at least stemming the tide of diet-related health problems? What responsibility does this influential group of registered dietitians bear to be a leading advocate for policy changes to make eating healthfully more accessible? Does forming partnerships with the food industry compromise such a group's credibility? And what does the food industry gain from such partnerships?

Why does it matter? As this report will show, the food industry's deep infiltration of the nation's top nutrition organization raises serious questions not only about that profession's credibility, but also about its policy positions. The nation is currently embroiled in a series of policy debates about how to fix our broken food system. A 74,000-member health organization has great potential to shape that national discourse – for better and for worse.

Findings:

- Beginning in 2001, AND listed 10 food industry sponsors; the 2011 annual report lists 38, a more than three-fold increase.
- The most loyal AND sponsor is the National Cattleman's Beef Association, for 12 years running (2001-2012).
- Processed food giants ConAgra and General Mills have been AND sponsors for 10 of the last 12 years.
- Kellogg and the National Dairy Council have been AND sponsors for 9 of the last 12 years.
- Companies on AND's list of approved continuing education providers include Coca-Cola, Kraft Foods, Nestlé, and PepsiCo.
- Among the messages taught in Coca-Cola- sponsored continuing education courses are: sugar is not harmful to children; aspartame is completely safe, including for children over one year; and the Institute of Medicine is too restrictive in its school nutrition standards.
- At AND's 2012 annual meeting, 18 organizations – less than five percent of all exhibitors – captured 25 percent of the total exhibitor space. Only two out of the 18 represented whole, non-processed foods.
- Based on square footage, only about 12 percent of the expo floor was taken up by fruit and vegetable vendors, using AND's own generous classification.
- The AND Foundation sells "nutrition symposia" sponsorships for $50,000 at the annual meeting. In 2012, Nestlé presented a session on "Optimal Hydration."
- The Corn Refiners Association (lobbyists for high fructose corn syrup) sponsored three "expo impact" sessions at the AND 2012 annual meeting.

- Roughly 23 percent of annual meeting speakers had industry ties, although most of these conflicts were not disclosed in the program session description.
- In an independent survey, 80 percent of registered dietitians said sponsorship implies Academy endorsement of that company and its products.
- Almost all RDs surveyed (97 percent) thought the Academy should verify that a sponsor's corporate mission is consistent with that of the Academy prior to accepting them.
- A majority of RDs surveyed found three current AND sponsors "unacceptable." (Coca-Cola, Mars, and PepsiCo.)
- The AND lobbying agenda reveals mostly safe issues benefiting registered dietitians. To date, AND has not supported controversial nutrition policies that might upset corporate sponsors, such as limits on soft drink sizes, soda taxes, or GMO labels.
- AND's sponsors and their activities appear to violate AND's own sponsorship guidelines.
- In 2011, AND generated $1.85 million in sponsorship revenue, which represents about 5% the total revenue. This is down from 9% in both 2010 and 2009.
- For the AND Foundation, corporate contributions were the single largest source of revenue in 2011: $1.3 million out of a total of $3.4 million or 38 percent.
- In 2011, the AND Foundation reported more than $17 million in net assets, more than six times its expenses for that year.

Academy Sponsors 2001-2012
BEEF USA National Cattlemen's Beef Association
12 years
ConAgra Foods
10 years
GENERAL MILLS
10 years
Kellogg's
9 years
NATIONAL DAIRY COUNCIL
9 years
Academy Partners 2008-2012
ARAMARK
The Coca-Cola Company
NATIONAL DAIRY COUNCIL
Partners or Premier Sponsors 2008-2012
Abbott Nutrition
GENERAL MILLS
Kellogg's
MARS
PEPSICO

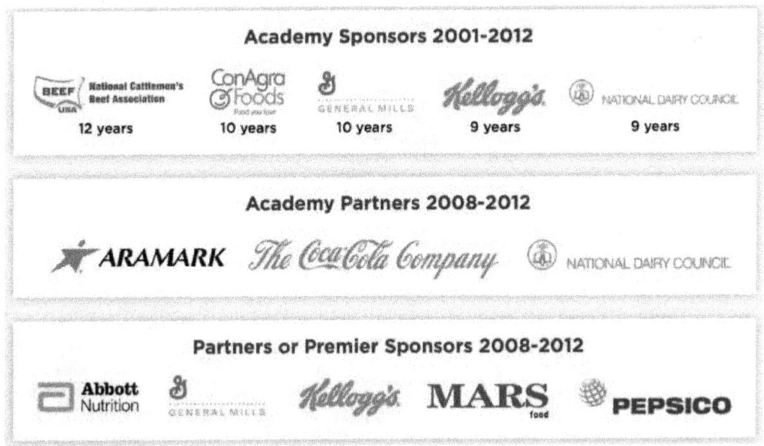

In 2015 Michelle Simon followed up examining the Dietitians Association of Australia (DAA) and found the DAA:

- Is sponsored by Meat and Livestock Australia, Nestlé, Unilever, Dairy Australia, and the Egg Nutrition Council
- Is a partner in the "Nestlé Choose Wellness Roadshow"
- Has important members who work for Kellogg and PepsiCo
- Has a spokesperson who is paid by Coca-Cola to present his research denying a connection between sugars and obesity
- Displays recipes from corporate sponsors with branded products despite policies against such things
- Is believed to have stripped a dietitian of her earned credential for speaking out against such conflicts of interest [*but see additional comments below].

The DAA offers its corporate sponsors the following benefits:

- Credible, independent, expert partner for nutrition communications
- Unparalleled opportunity to inform the Australian public through members and the DAA profile
- Access to members and interest groups for advice
- Information and expert advice on all nutrition and health issues
- Opportunities to sponsor DAA programs

DEFINITIONS

Health

"A state of complete physical, mental and social wellbeing and not merely the absence of disease or infirmity." —World Health Organization, 1946

Quality of Life (QOL)

A relatively new concept with over a hundred definitions. As society becomes more complex, so the criteria increase. It is important to consider the broader concerns of the individual. This is a changing concept that takes into account the general well-being of individuals and societies, outlining negative and positive features of life, and observing life satisfaction, including physical health, family, education, employment, wealth, religious beliefs, finance and the environment.

Live Longest

Optimization of present health and fitness: to minimize illnesses and disabilities; to stay mentally alert, active, healthy, independent and socially integrated, with the capacity to cope with change; for the whole predicted lifespan with respect to personal, social, spiritual, emotional and economic goals and restrictions.

Cost-Effectiveness

"Health improvement gained dollar for dollar."

Cost Beneficial

Major illnesses involve an immeasurable amount of disruption, both emotionally and financially, to the patient, family and employer. It may well thus be more beneficial, but not as cost-effective, to the patient to pay more to minimize these downstream effects.

Compression of Morbidity

Postponement of disabling conditions without necessarily extending life itself.

Focus

The most cost-effective optimization of present and future health. In effect this means concentrating on those illnesses that can be prevented or cured.

Preventive Medicine

The cost-effective prevention or early diagnosis of illness by evidence-based criteria to maximize health, longevity, independence and minimize disabilities.

Ideal food is low-density, nutrient-rich.

High-/Low-Density Food = High or low calorie content
Nutrient-Rich/-Poor = Good and beneficial food or poor-quality junk and pap.

ABBREVIATIONS

BMJ – British Medical Journal
JAMA – Journal of the American Medical Association
NEJM – New England Journal of Medicine
BG – Blood Glucose
BMD - bone-mineral density
BMI - Body Mass Index
BP – Blood Pressure
CA, Ca - Cancer
CAC – Cancer of the Colon
CAD – Coronary Artery Disease
CDC – Centers for Disease Control and Prevention
cf - compared to / with
CHD - Coronary Heart Disease
CVD- Cardiovascular Disease
COPD – Chronic Obstructive Pulmonary Disease
DHA Docosahexaenoic acid
EAR-Estiamted Average Requirement
EPA - Eicosapentaenoic acid
EPIC-European Prospective Investigation into Cancer and Nutrition
EVOO -Extra Virgin Olive Oil
ECG/EKG - Electrocardiogram
FDA – Federal Drug Administration
FV - Fruit and Vegetables
GI(T) - Gastro Intestinal (Tract)
HEI - Healthy Eating Index
HFCS - High Fructose Corn Syrup
H/L DL – High- or Low-Density Cholesterol
HT – Hypertension – raised BP
IHD – Ischemic Heart Disease – essentially the same as CAD
IARC - International Agency for Research on Cancer
MD - Mediterranean Diet
MIND - Mediterranean-DASH Intervention for Neurodegenerative Delay.
MUFA - Monounsaturated Fatty Acid
MVA/RTA – Motor Vehicle/Road Traffic Accidents
n–3 LCPUFAs (Long Chain Polyunsaturated fatty Acids)—mainly eicosapentaenoic acid (EPA) and docosahexaenoic acid (DHA)
NHANES - National Health and Nutrition Examination Survey
NHS National Health Scheme - the UK Government Health system
OO - Olive Oil
PAH Polycyclic aromatic hydrocarbons
PCB Polychlorinated biphenyls
PFA Perfluoroalkylated substances
POPs Persistent organic pollutants
PUFA - Polyunsaturated Fatty Acid
QOL - Quality of Life
RDA Recommended daily Allowance
RCT -Random Controlled Trial/Test
SCS Seven Countries Study
SFA - Saturated Fatty Acids
SSB - sugar-sweetened beverages
TF(A) - Trans fats (Acid)
TMD - Traditional Mediterranean Diet
WHO - World Health Organisation

AUTHOR PROFILE

Mileham Hayes graduated in Medicine from the University of Queensland and was subsequently appointed to positions in Teaching Hospitals in Brisbane, Sydney, Edinburgh and London passing his Specialist Physician exams in 1974 and later being elevated as a Fellow of the Royal College of Physicians of both Edinburgh and London. He was appointed to the world's first Coronary Care Unit that revolutionized the treatment of heart attacks, as well as early pioneering Sports and Obesity Clinics. In Edinburgh he was exposed to the same methods of observation that Conan Doyle, who had also been a doctor there, had used to create Sherlock Holmes. These experiences stimulated his interest in Preventive Medicine. In addition his father, also a clinician, had witnessed the introduction of vitamins, antibiotics and had seen both the miracles they brought but also the unforeseen downstream damage of processed foods with the current epidemic of the Diseases of Affluence and his shrewd observations alerted Mileham to the benefits of good nutrition and a holistic approach and his intensive training, international experience and 50 years of clinical practice, uniquely equips him to write the definitive series on Living Longest.

He was commissioned by the world's largest medical publisher to write a surgical textbook, which then became two but now they are finished and successful he has returned to his passion to rewrite a series of Preventive Medicine seminars he first presented at the University of Queensland.

On a personal note he played sports at a high level even getting the occasional game from a Wimbledon and US Champion and driving so fast BP offered him sponsorship. He volunteered for Viet Nam but ended at the Hospital treating the soldiers just twelve hours after they were wounded and had many adventures flying with the CIA and RAF. He put himself through medicine farming and playing jazz and ended touring the world and appearing with many of the world's greats and sharing the Tourism Award for his Jazz and Blues Festival with the Indie 500. He loves music, wine, food, cooking, literature, art and gardening. He writes bad poems but great limericks. He was awarded the Order of Australia in 1996. He is married with five children.

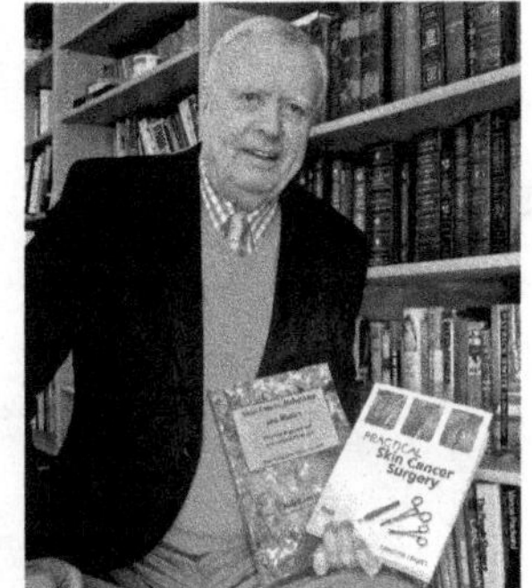

www.ingramcontent.com/pod-product-compliance
Lightning Source LLC
Chambersburg PA
CBHW070604030426
42337CB00020B/3691
* 9 7 8 0 9 9 5 3 9 9 6 8 6 *